Terri Hamlin, BScPharm, ACPR
Clinical Informatics Pharmacist
Alberta Health Services
Calgary AB

Robyn Harrison, MD FRCPC
Infectious Disease Specialist
Grey Nuns Hospital
Edmonton AB

Jill Henderson-Grainger, RN, BScN
Nurse Consultant, Communicable Disease
Surveillance and Assessment Branch,
Family and Population Health Division,
Alberta Health
Edmonton AB

Holly Hoang, MD FRCPC
Infectious Diseases Specialist
Covenant Health
Edmonton AB

Stan Houston, MD DTM&H FRCPC
Professor of Medicine (Infectious Disease &
General Internal Medicine) & Public Health
Director, Northern Alberta HIV Program
University of Alberta
Edmonton AB

Jim Hutchinson, MD, FRCP(C)
Medical Director - Antimicrobial Stewardship
Program
Vancouver Island Health Authority
Victoria BC

Ari Joffe, MD, FRCPC
Pediatric Critical Care and Infectious
Diseases
Stollery Children's Hospital
Edmonton AB

A. Mark Joffe, MD, FRCP(C)
Infectious Diseases Specialist
University of Alberta
Edmonton AB

Jennifer Jupp, BscPharm, BCOP
Clinical Practice Leader - Hematology,
Oncology, Transplant Program
Alberta Health Services
Calgary AB

Kevin Katz, MD
Medical Director of IP&C
North York General Hospital
Toronto ON

Bonita Lee, MD, FRCP(C)
Pediatric Infectious Diseases Specialist
University of Alberta
Edmonton AB

... MD SM FRCPC
Toronto ON

Susan Nolt, RN, BScN
Nurse Consultant, Communicable Disease
Surveillance and Assessment
Branch, Family and Population Health
Division, Alberta Health
Edmonton AB

Neesh Pannu, MD SM FRCP
Associate Professor
Divisions of Nephrology and Critical Care
University of Alberta
Edmonton AB

David Patrick, MD, FRCPC, MHSc
Director and Professor
UBC School of Population and Public Health
and Medical Epidemiology Lead,
Antimicrobial Resistance, BC CDC
Vancouver BC

Rita Pon, BSP, ACPR
Drug Information Pharmacist
Alberta Health Services
Edmonton AB

Joan L. Robinson, MD, FRCP (C)
Pediatric Infectious Diseases Specialist
Stollery Children's Hospital
Edmonton AB

Marcel Romanick, BSc Pharm
Pharmacist
UAH/Stollery Children's Hospital
Edmonton AB

Stuart J. Rosser, MD FRCPC MPH
Clinical Assistant Professor, Division of
Infectious Diseases
University of Alberta
Edmonton AB

Lynora Saxinger, MD, FRCPC, CTropMed
Chair, Antimicrobial Stewardship and
Resistance Committee, AMMI Canada
Associate Professor, Infectious Diseases,
University of Alberta
Edmonton AB

S. Nan Schuurmans, MD, FRCSC
Zone Clinical Department Head, Women's
Health Program
Alberta Health Services, Edmonton Zone
Edmonton AB

Ameeta Singh, BMBS(UK), MSc, FRCP(C)
Clinical Professor, Division of Infectious
Diseases
University of Alberta
Edmonton AB

Wendy Sligl, MD, MSc, FRCP(C)
Critical Care/Infectious Diseases Specialist
University of Alberta
Edmonton AB

Stephanie W. Smith, MD, MSc., FRCPC
Infectious Diseases Specialist
University of Alberta
Edmonton AB

Daniel J.G. Thirion, B.Pharm., M.Sc.,
Pharm.D., FCSHP
Pharmacist, McGill University Health Centre
Clinical Associate Professor, Faculté de
pharmacie, Université de Montréal
Montreal QC

Bharti Thomas, BScPharm, ACPR
NICU Clinical Pharmacist
Alberta Health Services
Edmonton AB

Wendy Vaudry, MDCM, FRCPC
Director of Pediatric Infectious Diseases
Stollery Children's Hospital
Edmonton AB

Gary Victor, MD, FRCP(C)
Internal Medicine/Infectious Diseases
Kelowna General Hospital
Kelowna BC

Denise Werry, BScPharm, ACPR, PharmD
Clinical Pharmacy Specialist - Infectious
Diseases
Kelowna General Hospital
Kelowna BC

Cover Design: Doug Driediger, Metrographics

Funding provided by: Alberta Health Services
                       Alberta Health
                       BC Ministry of Health, Pharmaceutical Services Division

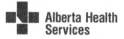

ISBN: 978-0-9916769-0-3

PREFACE

The information presented in this book is solely for educational purposes. It is not our intention to supersede any institution's current policies or guidelines but only to provide general recommendations for appropriate antibiotic use and care of patients with infectious diseases.

Recommendations made in this book are based on our experience in infectious diseases, microbiology, and pharmacotherapy; an extensive review of the literature, and consultation with multiple specialists. We are extremely indebted to all of our colleagues for their valuable contributions.

Antimicrobial resistance has become a major threat to the successful treatment of many infectious diseases. This book represents an antimicrobial stewardship tool to limit the development of resistance through the judicious use of antibiotics.

The Bugs & Drugs® book is supported by Alberta Health Services, Alberta Health, the BC Ministry of Health, and the Do Bugs Need Drugs?® program. The Do Bugs Need Drugs?® program is another longstanding antimicrobial stewardship initiative that addresses antimicrobial resistance by promoting three key messages to the public and healthcare professionals:

1. Handwashing is the most important way to stop the spread of infections.
2. Bacteria and viruses are different and antibiotics do not work against viruses.
3. Antibiotic resistance is a problem therefore antibiotics must be used wisely.

As before, this book is dedicated to our children. Future generations will be the beneficiaries of good antimicrobial stewardship.

Edith Blondel-Hill
Susan Fryters

TABLE OF CONTENTS

TABLE OF CONTENTS

ANTIMICROBIAL SPECTRUM OF ACTIVITY[†]

[†]**Legend**

Predictable Activity:

Most strains are susceptible and empiric therapy is reasonable until susceptibility results available.

Unpredictable Activity:

Empiric therapy not advised due to potential for resistance but antibiotic may be used if susceptibility confirmed.

No/Insufficient Activity:

Organism demonstrates intrinsic resistance, widespread acquired resistance, or antibiotic has unfavourable pharmacodynamics, documented clinical failures, or has not been sufficiently studied in the treatment of infections due to this organism.

ANTIMICROBIAL SPECTRUM OF ACTIVITY[†]

ORGANISM GROUPS

Staphylococci spp	Viridans group Streptococci	Streptococcus pneumoniae

Methicillin susceptible S. aureus - MSSA
Methicillin resistant S. aureus - MRSA
Vancomycin intermediate S. aureus - VISA
Vancomycin resistant S. aureus - VRSA
Coagulase negative staphylococci - CoNS
	Streptococcus anginosus group
	Streptococcus mitis group
	Streptococcus mutans group
	Streptococcus salivarius group
	Streptococcus sanguis group
	Streptococcus bovis/equinus group*
	
	* includes S. gallolyticus, S. infantarius
		Penicillin susceptible (Pen-S)
		MIC:
		    ≤ 2µg/mL (parenteral-nonmeningitis)
		    ≤ 0.06µg/mL (parenteral-meningitis)
		    ≤ 0.06µg/mL - oral penicillin
		Penicillin intermediate - (Pen-I)
		MIC:
		    4µg/mL - parenteral-nonmeningitis
		    0.12-1µg/mL - oral penicillin
		Penicillin resistant - (Pen-R)
		MIC:
		    ≥ 8µg/mL - parenteral-nonmeningitis
		    ≥ 0.12µg/mL - parenteral-meningitis
		    ≥ 2µg/mL - oral penicillin

Enterococci spp	**Coryneform bacteria**	
Vancomycin resistant enterococci - VRE	Arthrobacter spp Brevibacterium spp Cellulomonas spp Dermabacter spp Microbacterium spp Turicella spp Oerskovia spp Curtobacterium spp Exiguobacterium spp	

ORGANISM GROUPS

Enterobacteriaceae	Enterobacteriaceae that produce inducible cephalosporinase	
Cedecea spp Citrobacter spp Cronobacter spp Edwardsiella spp Enterobacter spp Escherichia spp Hafnia spp Klebsiella spp Morganella spp Proteus spp Providencia spp Salmonella spp Serratia spp Shigella spp Yersinia spp	Enterobacter spp Citrobacter freundii complex Serratia spp Morganella spp Providencia spp Proteus vulgaris Proteus penneri Hafnia spp	

ANTIMICROBIALS

ANTIMICROBIAL SPECTRUM OF ACTIVITY†

AMIKACIN

Predictable Activity	Unpredictable Activity	No/Insufficient Activity
Actinomyces spp (aerobic) Campylobacter spp Enterobacteriaceae Haemophilus influenzae/H. parainfluenzae Mycobacterium spp (selected species) Nocardia spp (most) Pasteurella spp Pseudomnonas spp	Acinetobacter spp Staphylococcus spp	Actinomyces spp (anaerobic) Alcaligenes spp Anaerobes Burkholderia spp Chlamydia/Chlamydophila spp Enterococcus spp Legionella spp Mycoplasma spp Stenotrophomonas maltophilia Streptococcus spp

ANTIMICROBIAL SPECTRUM OF ACTIVITY†

AMOXICILLIN-CLAVULANATE

Predictable Activity	Unpredictable Activity	No/Insufficient Activity
Actinomyces spp (aerobic/anaerobic)	Acinetobacter spp	Bartonella spp
Anaerobes (most)	Aeromonas spp	Burkholderia cepacia
β-haemolytic Streptococci (Group A,B,C,G)	Campylobacter spp	Chlamydia/Chlamydophila spp
Capnocytophaga spp	Corynebacterium spp	Enterobacteriaceae producing:
Eikenella spp	Escherichia coli	• inducible β-lactamases
Enterococcus faecalis	Haemophilus ducreyii	• extended spectrum β-lactamases (ESBL)
Haemophilus influenzae/H. parainfluenzae	Neisseria gonorrhoeae	Enterococcus faecium
Klebsiella spp	Viridans group Streptococci	Legionella spp
Moraxella catarrhalis	Yersinia spp	Mycobacterium spp
Neisseria spp		Mycoplasma spp
Pasteurella spp		Pseudomnonas spp
Proteus mirabilis		Staphylococcus aureus (MRSA)
Staphylococcus aureus (MSSA)		Stenotrophomonas maltophilia
Staphylococcus lugdunensis		Streptococcus pneumoniae (Pen-R)
Staphylococcus saprophyticus		
Streptococcus pneumoniae (Pen-S, Pen-I)		

ANTIMICROBIAL SPECTRUM OF ACTIVITY[†]

AZITHROMYCIN IV/PO

Predictable Activity	Unpredictable Activity	No/Insufficient Activity
Actinomyces spp	Anaerobic Gram positive cocci/bacilli	Anaerobic Gram negative bacilli
Bordetella pertussis	β-haemolytic Streptococci (Group A,B,C,G)	Burkholderia spp
Chlamydia/Chlamydophila spp	Bacillus spp	Coxiella burnetii
Enteropathogenic E. coli	Borrelia spp	Ehrlichia spp
Legionella spp	Brucella spp	Enterobacteriaceae
Leptospira spp	Campylobacter spp	Enterococcus spp
Moraxella catarrhalis	Coagulase negative Staphylococci (CoNS)	Listeria monocytogenes
Mycoplasma spp	Corynebacterium spp	Pseudomnonas spp
Plesiomonas shigelloides	Haemophilus influenzae	Staphylococcus aureus (MRSA)
Salmonella spp (including S. typhi/paratyphi)	Helicobacter pylori	
Treponema pallidum	Lactobacillus spp	
Ureaplasma urealyticum	Mycobacterium spp (other than M. avium complex)	
Vibrio spp (including V. cholerae)	Neisseria gonorrhoeae	
Yersinia enterolitica	Neisseria spp	
	Shigella spp	
	Staphylococcus aureus (MSSA)	
	Staphylococcus lugdunensis	
	Streptococcus pneumoniae	
	Viridans group Streptococci	

ANTIMICROBIAL SPECTRUM OF ACTIVITY†

CEFACLOR		
Predictable Activity	**Unpredictable Activity**	**No/Insufficient Activity**

β-haemolytic Streptococci (Group A,B,C,G)
Streptococcus pneumoniae (Pen-S)
	Escherichia coli
	Haemophilus influenzae*
	Klebsiella spp
	Moraxella catarrhalis
	Proteus mirabilis
	Staphylococcus aureus (MSSA)
	Viridans group Streptococci
		Acinetobacter spp
		Actinomyces spp
		Anaerobic Gram negative bacilli
		Bacillus spp
		Bordetella spp
		Capnocytophaga spp
		Chlamydia/Chlamydophila spp
		Corynebacterium spp
		Eikenella spp
		Enterobacteriaceae producing:
		  • inducible β-lactamases
		  • extended spectrum β-lactamases (ESBL)
		Enterococcus spp
		Listeria monocytogenes
		Mycoplasma spp
		Nocardia spp
		Pseudomonas spp
		Staphylococcus aureus (MRSA)
		Stenotrophomonas maltophilia
		Streptococcus pneumoniae (Pen-I, Pen-R)

* Cefaclor is less stable against β-lactamase producing H. influenzae than cefuroxime axetil, cefixime, or amoxicillin-clavulanate. β-lactamase negative ampicillin resistant (BLNAR) strains are resistant to cefaclor.

ANTIMICROBIAL SPECTRUM OF ACTIVITY†

CEFAZOLIN

Predictable Activity	Unpredictable Activity	No/Insufficient Activity
β-haemolytic Streptococci (Groups A,B,C,G)	Actinomyces spp	Anaerobic Gram negative bacilli
Klebsiella pneumoniae	Clostridium spp	Bacillus spp
Staphylococcus aureus (MSSA)	Escherichia coli	Bordetella spp
Staphylococcus lugdunensis	Klebsiella oxytoca	Chlamydia/Chlamydophila spp
Streptococcus pneumoniae (Pen-S)	Moraxella catarrhalis	Corynebacterium spp
	Proteus mirabilis	Eikenella spp
	Streptococcus pneumoniae (Pen-I)	Enterobacteriaceae producing:
	Viridans group Streptococci	• inducible β-lactamases
		• extended spectrum β-lactamases (ESBL)
		Enterococcus spp
		Haemophilus influenzae/H. parainfluenzae
		Legionella spp
		Listeria monocytogenes
		Mycoplasma spp
		Nocardia spp
		Pasteurella spp
		Pseudomonas aeruginosa
		Rickettsia spp
		Salmonella spp
		Staphylococcus aureus (MRSA)
		Streptococcus pneumoniae (Pen-R)

ANTIMICROBIAL SPECTRUM OF ACTIVITY[†]

CEFEPIME

Predictable Activity	Unpredictable Activity	No/Insufficient Activity
Aeromonas spp	Alcaligenes spp	Acinetobacter spp
β-haemolytic Streptococci (Group A,B,C,G)	Comamonas spp	Actinomyces spp
Haemophilus influenzae/H. parainfluenzae	Enterobacteriaceae producing:*	Anaerobic Gram negative bacilli
Enterobacteriaceae*	• inducible β-lactamases	Bacillus spp
Moraxella catarrhalis	Pseudomonas spp (other than P. aeruginosa)	Bordetella spp
Neisseria spp	Ralstonia spp	Burkholderia cepacia
Pasteurella spp	Shingomonas spp	Chlamydia/Chlamydophila spp
Pseudomonas aeruginosa	Staphylococcus lugdunensis	Clostridium spp
Staphylococcus aureus (MSSA)	Streptococcus pneumoniae (Pen-R)	Corynebacterium spp
Streptococcus pneumoniae (Pen-S, Pen-I)	Viridans group Streptococci	Enterobacteriaceae producing:*
		• extended spectrum β-lactamases (ESBL)
		Enterococcus spp
		Listeria monocytogenes
		Mycoplasma spp
		Rickettsia spp
		Staphylococcus aureus (MRSA)
		Stenotrophomonas maltophilia

* May retain activity against Enterobacteriaceae producing inducible (Amp C) β-lactamase, but not reliable against those producing ESBLs.

ANTIMICROBIAL SPECTRUM OF ACTIVITY[†]

CEFIXIME

Predictable Activity	Unpredictable Activity	No/Insufficient Activity
β-haemolytic Streptococci (Group A,B,C,G)	Moraxella catarrhalis	Acinetobacter spp
Escherichia coli	Neisseria gonorrhoeae	Actinomyces spp
Haemophilus influenzae/H. parainfluenzae	Shigella spp	Anaerobes (Gram positive and Gram negative)
Klebsiella spp	Staphylococcus saprophyticus	Bacillus spp
Pasteurella spp	Streptococcus pneumoniae (Pen-S)	Burkholderia spp
Proteus mirabilis	Yersinia enterolitica	Bordetella spp
Salmonella spp		Campylobacter spp
		Chlamydia/Chlamydophila spp
		Corynebacterium spp
		Enterobacteriaceae producing:
		• inducible β-lactamases
		• extended spectrum β-lactamases (ESBL)
		Enterococcus spp
		Legionella spp
		Listeria monocytogenes
		Mycoplasma spp
		Pseudomonas spp
		Staphylococcus aureus (MSSA, MRSA)
		Stenotrophomonas maltophilia
		Streptococcus pneumoniae (Pen-I, Pen-R)

ANTIMICROBIAL SPECTRUM OF ACTIVITY†

CEFOTAXIME

Predictable Activity	Unpredictable Activity	No/Insufficient Activity
Aeromonas spp	Abiotrophia spp	Achromobacter spp
Aggregatibacter spp	Actinomyces spp	Acinetobacter spp
β-haemolytic Streptococci (Group A,B,C,G)	Campylobacter spp	Alcaligenes spp
Bartonella spp	Clostridium spp	Anaerobic Gram negative bacilli
Capnocytophaga spp	Fusobacterium spp	Bacillus spp
Escherichia coli	Granulicatella spp	Burkholderia spp
Haemophilus influenzae*/ H. parainfluenzae	Leuconostoc spp	Chlamydia/Chlamydophila spp
Kingella kingae	Nocardia spp	Chryseobacterium spp
Klebsiella spp	Pediococcus spp	Corynebacterium spp
Moraxella catarrhalis	Porphyromonas spp	Enterobacteriaceae producing:
Neisseria spp	Prevotella spp	• inducible β-lactamases
Pasteurella spp	Staphylococcus aureus (MSSA)	• extended spectrum β-lactamases (ESBL)
Propionibacterium spp	Staphylococcus lugdunensis	Enterococcus spp
Proteus mirabilis	Streptococcus pneumoniae (Pen-R)	Legionella spp
Streptococcus pneumoniae (Pen-S, Pen-I)		Listeria monocytogenes
Vibrio spp		Mycoplasma spp
Viridans group Streptococci		Pseudomonas spp
		Staphylococcus aureus (MRSA)
		Stenotrophomonas maltophilia

* Some β-lactamase negative, ampicillin resistant (BLNAR) H. influenzae may rarely exhibit resistance to cefotaxime.

ANTIMICROBIAL SPECTRUM OF ACTIVITY†

CEFOXITIN

Predictable Activity	Unpredictable Activity	No/Insufficient Activity
Actinomyces spp	Anaerobic Gram negative bacilli	Acinetobacter spp
Anaerobic Gram positive cocci	Clostridium spp	Campylobacter spp
β-haemolytic Streptococci (Group A,B,C,G)	Escherichia coli	Chlamydia/Chlamydophila spp
Klebsiella pneumoniae	Klebsiella oxytoca	Corynebacterium spp
Mycobacterium abscessus	Mycobacterium fortuitum	Enterobacteriaceae producing:
Pasteurella spp	Neisseria gonorrhoeae	• inducible β-lactamases
Propionibacterium spp	Neisseria meningitidis	Enterococcus spp
Salmonella spp	Proteus mirabilis	Haemophilus influenzae/H. parainfluenzae
Shigella spp	Staphylococcus aureus (MSSA)	Lactobacillus spp
Streptococcus pneumoniae (Pen-S)	Streptococcus pneumoniae (Pen-I)	Legionella spp
	Viridans group Streptococci	Listeria monocytogenes
		Mycobacterium chelonae
		Mycoplasma spp
		Nocardia spp
		Pseudomonas aeruginosa
		Staphylococcus aureus (MRSA)
		Stenotrophomonas maltophilia
		Streptococcus pneumoniae (Pen-R)

ANTIMICROBIAL SPECTRUM OF ACTIVITY[†]

CEFPROZIL

Predictable Activity	Unpredictable Activity	No/Insufficient Activity
β-haemolytic Streptococci (Group A,B,C,G)	Escherichia coli	Acinetobacter spp
Moraxella catarrhalis	Haemophilus influenzae*/H. parainfluenzae	Actinomyces spp
Pasteurella spp	Klebsiella spp	Anaerobic Gram negative bacilli
Streptococcus pneumoniae (Pen-S)	Proteus mirabilis	Bacillus spp
	Staphylococcus aureus (MSSA)	Bordetella spp
	Streptococcus pneumoniae (Pen-I)	Capnocytophaga spp
		Chlamydia/Chlamydophila spp
		Corynebacterium spp
		Eikenella spp
		Enterobacteriaceae producing:
		• inducible β-lactamases
		• extended spectrum β-lactamases (ESBL)
		Enterococcus spp
		Legionella spp
		Listeria monocytogenes
		Mycoplasma spp
		Pseudomonas spp
		Staphylococcus aureus (MRSA)
		Stenotrophomonas maltophilia
		Streptococcus pneumoniae (Pen-R)

* Haemophilus coverage not as good as cefuroxime. β-lactamase negative, ampicillin resistant (BLNAR) strains are resistant to cefprozil.

ANTIMICROBIAL SPECTRUM OF ACTIVITY[†]

CEFTAZIDIME

Predictable Activity	Unpredictable Activity	No/Insufficient Activity
Bordetella bronchoseptica	Acinetobacter spp	Anaerobes (Gram positive and Gram negative)
Comamonas spp	Alcaligenes spp	Chlamydia/Chlamydophila spp
Escherichia coli*	β-haemolytic Streptococci (Group A,B,C,G)	Chryseobacterium spp
Haemophilus influenzae/H. parainfluenzae	Burkholderia spp	Enterobacteriaceae* producing:
Klebsiella spp*	Leuconostoc spp	• inducible β-lactamases
Proteus mirabilis*	Moraxella catarrhalis	• extended spectrum β-lactamases (ESBL)
Pseudomonas aeruginosa	Pediococcus spp	Enterococcus spp
	Pseudomonas aeruginosa	Listeria monocytogenes
	Shingomonas spp	Mycoplasma spp
	Streptococcus pneumoniae (Pen-S)	Ochrobactrum spp
		Ralstonia spp
		Rickettsia spp
		Staphylococcus aureus (MSSA, MRSA)
		Stenotrophomonas maltophilia
		Streptococcus pneumoniae (Pen-I, Pen-R)
		Viridans group Streptococci

* Cefotaxime and ceftriaxone have better activity than ceftazidime against Enterobacteriaceae.
NB: Ceftazidime will induce β-lactamases much more rapidly than other third-generation cephalosporins.

ANTIMICROBIAL SPECTRUM OF ACTIVITY[†]

CEFTRIAXONE		
Predictable Activity	**Unpredictable Activity**	**No/Insufficient Activity**
Aeromonas spp	Abiotrophia spp	Achromobacter spp
Aggregatibacter spp	Actinomyces spp	Acinetobacter spp
β-haemolytic Streptococci (Group A,B,C,G)	Campylobacter spp	Alcaligenes spp
Bartonella spp	Clostridium spp	Anaerobic Gram negative bacilli
Borrelia burgdorferi	Fusobacterium spp	Bacillus spp
Brucella spp	Granulicatella spp	Burkholderia spp
Capnocytophaga spp	Leuconostoc spp	Chlamydia/Chlamydophila spp
Haemophilus influenzae*/H. parainfluenzae	Nocardia spp	Chryseobacterium spp
Escherichia coli	Pediococcus spp	Corynebacterium spp
Kingella kingae	Porphyromonas spp	Enterobacteriaceae producing:
Klebsiella spp	Prevotella spp	• inducible β-lactamases
Moraxella catarrhalis	Staphylococcus aureus (MSSA)	• extended spectrum β-lactamases (ESBL)
Neisseria spp	Staphylococcus lugdunensis	Enterococcus spp
Pasteurella spp	Streptococcus pneumoniae (Pen-R)	Legionella spp
Propionibacterium acnes		Listeria monocytogenes
Proteus mirabilis		Mycoplasma spp
Salmonella spp**		Pseudomonas spp
Shigella spp**		Staphylococcus aureus (MRSA)
Streptococcus pneumoniae (Pen-S, Pen-I)		Stenotrophomonas maltophilia
Vibrio spp		
Viridans group Streptococci		
Yersinia spp**		

* Some β-lactamase negative ampicillin resistant (BLNAR) strains may exhibit resistance to ceftriaxone.
**Ceftriaxone preferred over cefotaxime for serious infections as it achieves higher intraluminal concentrations in the gastrointestinal tract.

ANTIMICROBIAL SPECTRUM OF ACTIVITY[†]

CEFUROXIME AXETIL PO

Predictable Activity	Unpredictable Activity	No/Insufficient Activity
β-haemolytic Streptococci (Group A,B,C,G)	Clostridium spp	Acinetobacter spp
Haemophilus influenzae*/H. parainfluenzae	Escherichia coli	Actinomyces spp
Neisseria spp	Klebsiella spp	Anaerobic Gram negative bacilli
Pasteurella spp	Moraxella catarrhalis	Bacillus spp
Staphylococcus aureus (MSSA)	Propionibacterium acnes	Bordetella spp
Streptococcus pneumoniae (Pen-S)	Proteus mirabilis	Capnocytophaga spp
	Shigella spp	Chlamydia/Chlamydophila spp
	Streptococcus pneumoniae (Pen-I)	Corynebacterium spp
	Viridans group Streptococci	Eikenella spp
	Yersinia spp	Enterobacteriaceae producing:
		• inducible β-lactamases
		• extended spectrum β-lactamases (ESBL)
		Enterococcus spp
		Listeria monocytogenes
		Mycoplasma spp
		Nocardia spp
		Pseudomonas spp
		Staphylococcus aureus (MRSA)
		Stenotrophomonas maltophilia
		Streptococcus. pneumoniae (Pen-R)

* β-lactamase negative ampicillin resistant (BLNAR) strains are resistant to cefuroxime.

ANTIMICROBIAL SPECTRUM OF ACTIVITY[†]

CEFUROXIME IV		
Predictable Activity	Unpredictable Activity	No/Insufficient Activity
β-haemolytic Streptococci (Group A,B,C,G)	Klebsiella oxytoca	Acinetobacter spp
Escherichia coli	Streptococcus pneumoniae (Pen-I)	Actinomyces spp
Haemophilus influenzae*/H. parainfluenzae		Anaerobic Gram negative bacilli
Klebsiella pneumoniae		Bacillus spp
Moraxella catarrhalis		Bordetella spp
Pasteurella spp		Capnocytophaga spp
Proteus mirabilis		Chlamydia/Chlamydophila spp
Staphylococcus. aureus (MSSA)		Corynebacterium spp
Streptococcus pneumoniae (Pen-S)		Eikenella spp
		Enterobacteriaceae producing:
		• inducible β-lactamases
		• extended spectrum β-lactamases (ESBL)
		Enterococcus spp
		Listeria monocytogenes
		Mycoplasma spp
		Nocardia spp
		Pseudomonas spp
		Staphylococcus aureus (MRSA)
		Stenotrophomonas maltophilia
		Streptococcus. pneumoniae (Pen-R)

* β-lactamase negative ampicillin resistant (BLNAR) strains are resistant to cefuroxime.

ANTIMICROBIAL SPECTRUM OF ACTIVITY†

CEPHALEXIN

Predictable Activity	Unpredictable Activity	No/Insufficient Activity

β-haemolytic Streptococci (Groups A,B,C,G)
Staphylococcus aureus (MSSA)
	Proteus mirabilis (urine only)
	Streptococcus pneumoniae (Pen-S)
	Viridans group Streptococci
		Actinomyces spp
		Anaerobic Gram negative bacilli
		Bacillus spp
		Bordetella spp
		Capnocytophaga spp
		Chlamydia/Chlamydophila spp
		Corynebacterium spp
		Eikenella spp
		Enterobacteriaceae producing:
		  • inducible β-lactamases
		  • extended spectrum β-lactamases (ESBL)
		Enterococcus spp
		Escherichia coli
		Haemophilus influenzae/H. parainfluenzae
		Klebsiella spp
		Legionella spp
		Listeria monocytogenes
		Moraxella catarrhalis
		Mycoplasma spp
		Nocardia spp
		Pasteurella spp
		Pseudomonas aeruginosa
		Salmonella spp
		Staphylococcus aureus (MRSA)
		Streptococcus pneumoniae (Pen-I, Pen-R)
		Yersinia spp

ANTIMICROBIAL SPECTRUM OF ACTIVITY[†]

CIPROFLOXACIN IV/PO		
Predictable Activity	Unpredictable Activity	No/Insufficient Activity
Aeromonas spp	Acinetobacter spp	Achromobacter spp
Aggregatibacter spp	Alcaligenes spp	Actinomyces spp
Bacillus spp	Bartonella spp	Anaerobes
Brucella spp	Capnocytophaga spp	β-haemolytic Streptococci (Group A,B,C,G)
Campylobacter spp	Coagulase negative Staphylococci (CoNS)	Borrelia spp
Eikenella spp	Corynebacterium spp	Burkholderia cepacia
Enterobacteriaceae (other than E. coli and	Escherichia coli	Chlamydia/Chlamydophila spp
Serratia spp)	Mycobacterium spp	Enterococcus spp
Francisella tularensis	Neisseria gonorrhoeae*	Listeria monocytogenes
Haemophilus influenzae/H. parainfluenzae	Neisseria meningitidis	Mycoplasma spp
Legionella spp	Nocardia spp	Rhodococcus spp
Leptospira spp	Pseudomonas spp (other than P. aeruginosa)	Staphylococcus aureus (MSSA, MRSA)
Moraxella catarrhalis	Serratia spp	Stenotrophomonas maltophilia
Pasteurella spp		Streptococcus pneumoniae
Pseudomonas aeruginosa		Viridans group Streptococci
Staphylococcus saprophyticus		
Vibrio spp		
Yersinia spp		

* Quinolones are no longer recommended for empiric therapy of N. gonorrhoeae due to increasing resistance.

ANTIMICROBIAL SPECTRUM OF ACTIVITY[†]

CLARITHROMYCIN

Predictable Activity	Unpredictable Activity	No/Insufficient Activity
Bordetella pertussis	Anaerobic Gram positive cocci/bacilli	Acinetobacter spp
Borrelia burgdorferi	β-haemolytic Streptococci (Group A,B,C,G)	Anaerobic Gram negative bacilli
Chlamydia/Chlamydophila spp	Bacillus spp	Burkholderia spp
Coxiella burnetii	Campylobacter spp	Enterobacteriaceae
Haemophilus ducreyi	Coagulase negative Staphylococci (CoNS)	Enterococcus spp
Legionella spp	Corynebacterium spp	Listeria monocytogenes
Leptospira spp	Haemophilus influenzae/H. parainfluenzae	Pseudomonas spp
Moraxella catarrhalis	Helicobacter pylori	Staphylococcus aureus (MRSA)
Mycobacterium avium intracellulare (MAI) complex	Lactobacillus spp	Stenotrophomonas maltophilia
Mycoplasma spp	Mycobacterium spp (other than MAI complex)	
Rickettsia rickettsii	Neisseria spp	
	Staphylococcus aureus (MSSA)	
	Streptococcus pneumoniae	
	Viridans group Streptococci	

- 20 -

ANTIMICROBIAL SPECTRUM OF ACTIVITY[t]

CLINDAMYCIN IV/PO

Predictable Activity	Unpredictable Activity	No/Insufficient Activity
Actinomyces spp	Anaerobic Gram negative bacilli	Acinetobacter spp
Capnocytophaga spp	β-haemolytic Streptococci (Group A,B,C,G)	Aeromonas spp
Chlamydia trachomatis	Bacillus spp	Aggregatibacter spp
Coxiella burnetii	Campylobacter spp	Cardiobacterium spp
Gardnerella vaginalis	Chlamydophila spp	Eikenella corrodens
Nocardia spp	Clostridium spp	Enterobacteriaceae
Streptococcus pneumoniae	Coagulase negative Staphylococci (CoNS)	Enterococcus spp
Viridans group Streptococci	Corynebacterium spp	Haemophilus influenzae/H. parainfluenzae
	Haemophilus ducreyi	Kingella spp
	Lactobacillus spp	Legionella spp
	Peptostreptococcus spp	Listeria monocytogenes
	Propionibacterium spp	Moraxella catarrhalis
	Staphylococcus aureus (MSSA/MRSA)	Mycoplasma spp
	Staphylococcus lugdunensis	Neisseria spp
		Pasteurella spp
		Pseudomonas spp
		Ureaplasma spp

ANTIMICROBIAL SPECTRUM OF ACTIVITY[†]

COLISTIN

Predictable Activity	Unpredictable Activity	No/Insufficient Activity
Acinetobacter spp	Stenotrophomonas maltophilia	Anaerobes
Citrobacter spp		Bacillus spp
Enterobacter spp		Burkholderia spp
Escherichia coli		Chlamydia/Chlamydophila spp
Klebsiella spp		Corynebacterium spp
Pseudomonas aeruginosa		Enterococcus spp
		Gram positive organisms
		Lactobacillus spp
		Legionella spp
		Listeria monocytogenes
		Morganella spp
		Mycoplasma spp
		Neisseria spp
		Proteus spp
		Providencia spp
		Salmonella spp
		Serratia spp
		Shigella spp
		Staphylococcus spp
		Streptococcus spp

ANTIMICROBIAL SPECTRUM OF ACTIVITY[†]

DAPTOMYCIN - Note: do not use for pulmonary infections as drug inactivated by pulmonary surfactant.		
Predictable Activity	Unpredictable Activity	No/Insufficient Activity
β-haemolytic Streptococci (Group A,B,C,G)	Anaerobes (Gram positive)	Actinomyces spp
Bacillus spp	Clostridium spp	Aerobic Gram negative bacilli - nonfermenters
Coagulase negative Staphylococci (CoNS)	Lactobacillus spp	Aeromonas spp
Corynebacterium spp	Listeria monocytogenes	Anaerobic Gram negative bacilli/cocci
Enterococcus spp		Burkholderia spp
Leuconostoc spp		Enterobacteriaceae
Pediococcus spp		Haemophilus influenzae/H. parainfluenzae
Staphylococcus aureus (MSSA, MRSA, VISA, VRSA)		Moraxella catarrhalis
		Mycobacterium spp
Streptococcus pneumoniae		Neisseria spp
Viridans group Streptococci		Nocardia spp
		Pasteurella spp
		Plesiomonas spp
		Pseudomonas spp
		Rhodococcus spp
		Stenotrophomonas maltophilia
		Vibrio spp

ANTIMICROBIAL SPECTRUM OF ACTIVITY[†]

DORIPENEM

Predictable Activity	Unpredictable Activity	No/Insufficient Activity
Actinomyces spp	Acinetobacter spp	Burkholderia cepacia
Anaerobes	Aeromonas spp	Chlamydia/Chlamydophila spp
Alcaligenes spp	Bacillus spp	Chryseobacterium spp
β-haemolytic Streptococci (Group A,B,C,G)	Corynebacterium spp	Enterococcus faecium
Haemophilus influenzae/H. parainfluenzae	Enterococcus faecalis	Legionella spp
Enterobacteriaceae	Listeria monocytogenes	Mycoplasma spp
Leuconostoc spp	Mycobacterium spp	Staphylococcus aureus (MRSA)
Moraxella catarrhalis	Nocardia spp	Stenotrophomonas maltophilia
Neisseria spp	Streptococcus pneumoniae (Pen-R)	
Pasteurella spp		
Pediococcus spp		
Pseudomonas aeruginosa		
Staphylococcus aureus (MSSA)		
Streptococcus pneumoniae (Pen-S, Pen-I)		
Viridans group Streptococci		

ANTIMICROBIAL SPECTRUM OF ACTIVITY†

DOXYCYCLINE		
Predictable Activity	Unpredictable Activity	No/Insufficient Activity
Aeromonas spp	Acinetobacter spp	Listeria monocytogenes
Bartonella spp	Actinomyces spp	Pseudomonas spp
Borrelia burgdorferi	Anaerobes (Gram positive and Gram negative)	
Campylobacter spp	Bacillus spp	
Chlamydia/Chlamydophila spp	β-haemolytic Streptococci (Groups A,B,C,G)	
Coxiella burnetii	Brucella spp	
Francisella tularensis	Burkholderia spp	
Haemophilus influenzae/H. parainfluenzae	Chryseobacterium spp	
Legionella spp	Coagulase negative Staphylococci (CoNS)	
Leptospira spp	Enterobacteriaceae	
Moraxella catarrhalis	Enterococcus spp	
Mycobacterium abscessus	Helicobacter pylori	
Mycobacterium chelonae	Mycoplasma genitalium	
Mycobacterium fortuitum	Neisseria spp	
Mycoplasma pneumoniae	Nocardia spp	
Pasteurella spp	Propionibacterium spp	
Rickettsia spp	Stenotrophomonas maltophilia	
Staphylococcus aureus (MSSA, MRSA)	Streptococcus pneumoniae	
Treponema pallidum	Ureaplasma urealyticum	
Tropheryma whippleii	Vibrio spp	
Yersinia spp		

ANTIMICROBIAL SPECTRUM OF ACTIVITY[†]

ERTAPENEM

Predictable Activity	Unpredictable Activity	No/Insufficient Activity
Actinomyces spp	Aeromonas spp	Acinetobacter spp
Anaerobes	Alcaligenes spp	Chlamydia/Chlamydophila spp
β-haemolytic Streptococci (Group A,B,C,G)	Bacillus spp	Chryseobacterium spp
Bergeyella zoohelcum	Bilophila wadsworthia	Enterococcus spp
Haemophilus influenzae/H. parainfluenzae	Burkholderia cepacia	Lactobacillus spp
Eikenella spp	Corynebacterium spp	Legionella spp
Enterobacteriaceae	Streptococcus pneumoniae (Pen-R)	Listeria monocytogenes
Moraxella catarrhalis		Mycoplasma spp
Neisseria spp		Pseudomonas aeruginosa
Pasteurella spp		Staphylococcus aureus (MRSA)
Staphylococcus aureus (MSSA)		Stenotrophomonas maltophilia
Streptococcus pneumoniae (Pen-S, Pen-I)		
Viridans group Streptococci		

ANTIMICROBIAL SPECTRUM OF ACTIVITY[†]

FOSFOMYCIN - for urinary tract infections only

Predictable Activity	Unpredictable Activity	No/Insufficient Activity
Citrobacter spp	B-haemolytic Streptococci (Group A,B,C,G)	Acinetobacter spp
Escherichia coli	Enterobacter spp	Anaerobes
Enterococcus faecalis	Enterococcus faecium	Corynebacterium spp
Proteus mirabilis	Klebsiella spp	Haemophilus influenzae/H. parainfluenzae
	Proteus vulgaris/penneri	Moraxella catarrhalis
	Providencia spp	Morganella morganii
	Serratia spp	Neisseria spp
		Pseudomonas aeruginosa
		Staphylococcus aureus (MSSA, MRSA)
		Staphylococcus saprophyticus
		Streptococcus pneumoniae
		Viridans group Streptococci

ANTIMICROBIAL SPECTRUM OF ACTIVITY†

IMIPENEM		
Predictable Activity	**Unpredictable Activity**	**No/Insufficient Activity**
Actinomyces spp	Acinetobacter spp	Burkholderia cepacia
Alcaligenes spp	Aeromonas spp	Chlamydia/Chlamydophila spp
Anaerobes	Corynebacterium spp	Chryseobacterium spp
β-haemolytic Streptococci (Group A,B,C,G)	Enterococcus faecalis	Elizabethkingia meningosepticum
Bacillus spp	Morganella morganii	Enterococcus faecium
Burkholderia spp (other than B. cepacia)	Mycobacterium spp	Legionella spp
Cardiobacterium hominis	Nocardia spp	Listeria monocytogenes
Citrobacter spp	Plesiomonas spp	Mycoplasma spp
Eikenella corrodens	Proteus spp	Staphylococcus aureus (MRSA)
Enterobacter spp	Providencia spp	Stenotrophomonas maltophilia
Escherichia coli	Pseudomonas spp (not P. aeruginosa)	
Haemophilus influenzae/H. parainfluenzae	Streptococcus pneumoniae (Pen-R)	
Kingella kingae		
Klebsiella spp		
Leuconostoc spp		
Moraxella catarrhalis		
Neisseria spp		
Pasteurella spp		
Pediococcus spp		
Pseudomonas aeruginosa		
Salmonella spp		
Serratia spp		
Shigella spp		
Staphylococcus aureus (MSSA)		
Streptococcus pneumoniae (Pen-S, Pen-I)		
Viridans group Streptococci		

ANTIMICROBIAL SPECTRUM OF ACTIVITY[†]

LEVOFLOXACIN IV/PO		
Predictable Activity	Unpredictable Activity	No/Insufficient Activity
Chlamydia/Chlamydophila spp	β-haemolytic Streptococci (Group A,B,C,G)	Actinomyces spp
Enterobacteriaceae (other than E. coli)	Coagulase negative Staphylococci (CoNS)	Anaerobes
Haemophilus influenzae/H. parainfluenzae	Escherichia coli	Burkholderia cepacia
Legionella spp	Mycobacterium spp	Enterococcus spp
Moraxella catarrhalis	Neisseria gonorrhoeae*	Listeria monocytogenes
Mycoplasma spp	Nocardia spp	Stenotrophomonas maltophilia
Neisseria meningitidis	Pseudomonas aeruginosa	
Streptococcus pneumoniae	Staphylococcus aureus (MSSA, MRSA)**	
	Ureaplasma spp	
	Viridans group Streptococci	

* Quinolones no longer recommended for empiric therapy of N. gonorrhoeae due to increasing resistance.
**Despite in vitro susceptibility, resistance may develop. Monotherapy not recommended.

ANTIMICROBIAL SPECTRUM OF ACTIVITY[†]

LINEZOLID IV/PO		
Predictable Activity	Unpredictable Activity	No/Insufficient Activity
β-haemolytic Streptococci (Group A,B,C,G)	Actinomyces spp	Acinetobacter spp
Bacillus spp	Aerococcus spp	Bacteroides fragilis group
Coagulase negative Staphylococci (CoNS)	Anaerobic Gram negative bacilli	Chlamydia/Chlamydophila spp
Corynebacterium spp	Anaerobic Gram positive cocci	Enterobacteriaceae
Coryneform bacteria	Chryseobacterium meningosepticum	Haemophilus influenzae/H. parainfluenzae
Enterococcus spp	Clostridium spp	Helicobacter pylori
Lactobacillus spp	Listeria monocytogenes	Legionella spp
Lactococcus spp	Mycobacterium spp	Moraxella catarrhalis
Micrococcus spp	Pasteurella spp	Mycoplasma spp
Nocardia spp	Viridans group Streptococci	Neisseria spp
Pediococcus spp		Pseudomonas spp
Rhodococcus equi		Stenotrophomonas maltophilia
Staphylococcus aureus (MSSA, MRSA, VISA, VRSA)		Ureaplasma spp
Streptococcus pneumoniae		

Although linezolid shows good activity against some anaerobes (Clostridium, Peptostreptococcus, Bacteroides, Fusobacterium), there are not enough data to prove that it has reliable, broad-spectrum antianaerobic activity.

ANTIMICROBIAL SPECTRUM OF ACTIVITY[†]

MEROPENEM		
Predictable Activity	Unpredictable Activity	No/Insufficient Activity
Actinomyces spp	Acinetobacter spp	Chlamydia/Chlamydophila spp
Alcaligenes spp	Aeromonas spp	Chryseobacterium spp
Anaerobes	Bacillus spp	Enterococcus spp
β-haemolytic Streptococci (Group A,B,C,G)	Burkholderia cepacia	Legionella spp
Haemophilus influenzae/H. parainfluenzae	Corynebacterium spp	Mycoplasma spp
Enterobacteriaceae	Lactobacillus spp	Staphylococcus aureus (MRSA)
Erysipelothrix rhusiopathiae	Listeria monocytogenes	Stenotrophomonas maltophilia
Moraxella catarrhalis	Mycobacterium spp	
Neisseria spp	Nocardia spp	
Propionibacterium acnes	Streptococcus pneumoniae (Pen-R)	
Pseudomonas spp		
Staphylococcus aureus (MSSA)		
Streptococcus pneumoniae (Pen-S, Pen-I)		
Viridans group Streptococci		

ANTIMICROBIAL SPECTRUM OF ACTIVITY[†]

MINOCYCLINE

Predictable Activity	Unpredictable Activity	No/Insufficient Activity
Burkholderia pseudomallei	Acinetobacter spp	Enterobacteriaceae
Chlamydia/Chlamydophila spp	Actinomyces spp	Enterococcus spp
Haemophilus influenzae/H. parainfluenzae	Aeromonas spp	Listeria monocytogenes
Legionella spp	Anaerobes (Gram positive and Gram negative)	Pseudomonas spp
Moraxella catarrhalis	β-haemolytic Streptococci (Group A,B,C,G)	
Mycobacterium marinum	Bacillus spp	
Mycoplasma spp	Brucella spp	
Pasteurella spp	Coagulase negative Stephylococci (CoNS)	
Staphylococcus aureus (MSSA, MRSA)	Helicobacter pylori	
Ureaplasma urealyticum	Neisseria spp	
	Nocardia spp	
	Stenotrophomonas maltophilia	
	Streptococcus pneumoniae	
	Vibrio spp	

ANTIMICROBIAL SPECTRUM OF ACTIVITY[†]

MOXIFLOXACIN IV/PO - not recommended for urinary tract infections

Predictable Activity	Unpredictable Activity	No/Insufficient Activity
Bordetella spp	Acinetobacter spp	Actinomyces spp
Chlamydia/Chlamydophila spp	Anaerobes	Burkholderia cepacia
Enterobacteriaceae (other than E. coli)	β-haemolytic Streptococci (Group A,B,C,G)	Enterococcus spp
Haemophilus influenzae/H. parainfluenzae	Coagulase negative Staphylococci (CoNS)	Listeria monocytogenes
Legionella spp	Corynebacterium spp	Pseudomonas aeruginosa
Moraxella catarrhalis	Escherichia coli	Staphylococcus saprophyticus
Mycoplasma spp	Mycobacterium spp	
Neisseria meningitidis	Neisseria gonorrhoeae*	
Pasteurella spp	Nocardia spp	
Streptococcus pneumoniae	Pseudomonas spp (not P. aeruginosa)	
	Staphylococcus aureus (MSSA, MRSA)**	
	Staphylococcus lugdunensis	
	Stenotrophomonas maltophilia	
	Ureaplasma spp	
	Viridans group Streptococci	

* Quinolones are no longer recommended for empiric therapy of N. gonorrhoeae due to increasing resistance.
**Despite in vitro susceptibility, resistance may develop. Monotherapy not recommended.

ANTIMICROBIAL SPECTRUM OF ACTIVITY[†]

NITROFURANTOIN - for urinary tract infections only		
Predictable Activity	**Unpredictable Activity**	**No/Insufficient Activity**
Coagulase negative Staphylococci (CoNS)	Anaerobes	Acinetobacter spp
Escherichia coli	Citrobacter spp	Corynebacterium spp
Enterococcus spp	Enterobacter sp	Listeria monocytogenes
Staphylococcus aureus	Klebsiella spp	Morganella spp
Staphylococcus saprophyticus	Neisseria spp	Pseudomonas aeruginosa
Streptococcus agalactiae (Group B Strep)	Proteus spp	Rhodococcus equii
Streptococcus pyogenes (Group A Strep)	Providencia spp	Serratia spp
	Salmonella spp	
	Shigella spp	

ANTIMICROBIAL SPECTRUM OF ACTIVITY†

PIPERACILLIN-TAZOBACTAM

Predictable Activity	Unpredictable Activity	No/Insufficient Activity
Actinomyces spp	Acinetobacter spp	Burkholderia spp
β-haemolytic Streptococci (Group A,B,C,G)	Aeromonas spp	Chlamydia/Chlamydophila spp
Bacillus spp	Corynebacterium spp	Enterobacteriaceae producing:
Bordetella bronchoseptica	Lactobacillus spp	• inducible β-lactamases
Capnocytophaga spp	Mycobacterium spp	• extended spectrum β-lactamases (ESBL)
Enterococcus faecalis	Pseudomonas spp (not P. aeruginosa)	Enterococcus faecium
Escherichia coli	Streptococcus pneumoniae (Pen-I)	Legionella spp
Haemophilus influenzae/H. parainfluenzae	Viridans group Streptococci	Listeria monocytogenes
Klebsiella spp		Mycoplasma spp
Moraxella catarrhalis		Nocardia spp
Neisseria spp		Staphylococcus aureus (MRSA)
Pasteurella spp		Stenotrophomonas maltophilia
Proteus mirabilis		Streptococcus pneumoniae (Pen-R)
Pseudomonas aeruginosa		
Salmonella spp		
Staphylococcus aureus (MSSA)		
Streptococcus pneumoniae (Pen-S)		

ANTIMICROBIAL SPECTRUM OF ACTIVITY†

TICARCILLIN-CLAVULANIC ACID		
Predictable Activity	Unpredictable Activity	No/Insufficient Activity
Anaerobes	Aeromonas spp	Acinetobacter spp
Actinomyces spp	β-haemolytic Streptococci (Group A,B,C,G)	Burkholderia spp
Bordetella bronchoseptica	Escherichia coli	Chlamydia/Chlamydophila spp
Capnocytophaga spp	Klebsiella spp	Enterobacteriaceae producing:
Haemophilus influenzae/H. parainfluenzae	Pseudomonas aeruginosa	• inducible β-lactamases
Moraxella catarrhalis	Streptococcus pneumoniae (Pen-S)	• extended spectrum β-lactamases (ESBL)
Neisseria spp	Viridans group Streptococci	Enterococcus spp
Pasteurella spp		Legionella spp
Proteus mirabilis		Listeria monocytogenes
Salmonella spp		Mycobacterium spp
Staphylococcus aureus (MSSA)		Mycoplasma spp
		Nocardia spp
		Staphylococcus aureus (MRSA)
		Stenotrophomonas maltophilia*
		Streptococcus pneumoniae (Pen-I, Pen-R)
* May be used in combination if susceptible.		

ANTIMICROBIAL SPECTRUM OF ACTIVITY[†]

TIGECYCLINE - NOT recommended for bacteremia or urinary tract infections		
Predictable Activity	Unpredictable Activity	No/Insufficient Activity
Aeromonas spp	Acinetobacter spp	Listeria monocytogenes
Anaerobes (most)	Enterobacteriaceae producing inducible β-lactamases	Pseudomonas aeruginosa
β-haemolytic Streptococci (Group A,B,C,G)	Proteus spp	
Chlamydia/Chlamydophila spp	Stenotrophomonas maltophilia	
Coagulase negative Staphylococci (CoNS)		
Eikenella spp		
Enterococcus spp (includes VRE)		
Escherichia coli		
Haemophilus influenzae		
Klebsiella spp		
Moraxella catarrhalis		
Mycobacterium spp		
Mycoplasma spp		
Neisseria gonorrhoeae		
Pasteurella spp		
Salmonella spp		
Shigella spp		
Staphylococcus aureus (MSSA, MRSA, VISA, VRSA)		
Streptococcus pneumoniae		
Ureaplasma urealyticum		
Viridans group Streptococci		

ANTIMICROBIAL SPECTRUM OF ACTIVITY†

TRIMETHOPRIM-SULFAMETHOXAZOLE (TMP/SMX)		
Predictable Activity	Unpredictable Activity	No/Insufficient Activity
Actinobacillus spp	Actinobaculum spp	Aerococcus urinae
Acinetobacter spp	Aeromonas spp	Arcanobacterium haemolyticum
Achromobacter spp	β-haemolytic Streptococci (Group C,G)	Bacillus spp
Aerococcus spp (other than A. urinae)	Bergeyella spp	Bordetella pertussis
Aggregatibacter spp	Burkholderia spp	Capnocytophaga spp (human source)
Alcaligenes spp	Capnocytophaga spp (canine source)	Enterococcus spp
Bordetella bronchoseptica	Campylobacter spp	Erysipelothrix rhusiopathiae
Brevundimonas spp	Chryseobacterium spp	Gardnerella vaginalis
Coagulase negative Staphylococci (CoNS)	Corynebacterium spp	Helicobacter pylori
Comamonas spp	Coryneform bacteria	Listeria monocytogenes*
Eikenella corrodens	Escherichia coli	Neisseria gonorrhoeae
Enterobacteriaceae (other than specified under	Kingella spp	Pseudomonas aeruginosa
Unpredictable Activity)	Morganella spp	Roseomonas spp
Haemophilus influenzae/H. parainfluenzae	Nocardia spp	Streptococcus pyogenes (Group A
Moraxella catarrhalis	Rhizobium spp	Streptococci)
Neisseria spp (other than N. gonorrhoeae)	Rhodococcus equi	Streptococcus agalactiae (Group B
Ochrobactrum spp	Salmonella spp	Streptococci)
Oligella spp	Shigella spp	
Pasteurella spp	Streptococcus pneumoniae	
Plesiomonas spp	Viridans group Streptococci	
Pseudomonas spp (other than P. aeruginosa)		
Ralstonia spp		
Shewanella spp		
Shingobacterium spp		
Staphylococcus aureus (MSSA, MRSA)		
Staphylococcus lugdunensis		
Stenotrophomonas maltophilia		
Weeksella spp		

* Has good in vitro activity but monotherapy not recommended.

ANTIMICROBIAL SPECTRUM OF ACTIVITY[†]

VANCOMYCIN IV

Predictable Activity	Unpredictable Activity	No/Insufficient Activity
Anaerobic cocci/bacilli	Actinomyces spp	Erysipelothrix spp
β-haemolytic Streptococci (Group A,B,C,G)	Lactobacillus spp	Gram negative organisms (aerobic & anaerobic)
Bacillus spp	Rhodococcus spp	Leuconostoc spp
Clostridium spp		Listeria monocytogenes
Coagulase negative Staphylococci (CoNS)		Pediococcus spp
Corynebacterium spp		Weissella confusa
Enterococcus spp (except VRE)		
Propionibacterium spp		
Staphylococcus aureus (MSSA, MRSA)		
Streptococcus pneumoniae		
Viridans group Streptococci		

VANCOMYCIN PO - NB: This drug is not absorbed and must NEVER be used to treat systemic infections. This drug is used solely for the treatment of C. difficile infection.

Predictable Activity		
C. difficile		

ANTIMICROBIAL SPECTRUM OF ACTIVITY[†]

ANTIFUNGALS

AMPHOTERICIN B		
Predictable Activity	**Unpredictable Activity**	**No/Insufficient Activity**
Agents of zygomycosis (e.g. Mucor, Rhizopus, Rhizomucor, Absidia, Cunninghamella spp)	Candida glabrata	Aspergillus lentulus
Aspergillus spp (other than A. terreus, A. ustus, A. lentulus)	Candida krusei	Aspergillus terreus
Blastomyces spp		Aspergillus ustus
Candida spp (other than those listed under Unpredictable or No Activity)		Candida guilliermondii
Coccidioides immitis		Candida lusitaniae
Cryptococcus neoformans		Pseudallescheria boydii (Scedosporium apiospermum)
Fusarium spp		Scedosporium prolificans
Histoplasma spp		Trichosporon spp
Malassezia spp		
Microsporum		
Paracoccidioides brasiliensis		
Rhodotorula spp		
Sporothrix schenckii		
Trichophyton		

ANTIMICROBIAL SPECTRUM OF ACTIVITY[†]

ANIDULAFUNGIN

Predictable Activity	Unpredictable Activity	No/Insufficient Activity
Aspergillus spp	Candida famata	Agents of zygomycosis (e.g. Mucor, Rhizopus,
Candida albicans	Candida guilliermondii	Rhizomucor, Absidia, Cunninghamella spp)
Candida dubliniensis	Candida parapsilosis	Blastomyces spp
Candida glabrata	Paecilomyces variotii	Coccidioides spp
Candida kefyr	Pseudoallescheria boydii (Scedosporium	Cryptococcus spp
Candida krusei	apiospermum)	Fusarium spp
Candida lusitaniae	Sporothrix schenckii	Histoplasma spp
Candida tropicalis		Paecilomyces lilacinus
		Rhodotorula spp
		Scedosporium prolificans
		Trichosporon asahii

ANTIMICROBIAL SPECTRUM OF ACTIVITY[†]

CASPOFUNGIN		
Predictable Activity	Unpredictable Activity	No/Insufficient Activity
Aspergillus spp	Candida famata	Agents of zygomycosis (e.g. Mucor, Rhizopus,
Candida albicans	Candida guilliermondii	Rhizomucor, Absidia, Cunninghamella spp)
Candida dubliniensis	Candida parapsilosis	Blastomyces spp
Candida glabrata	Paecilomyces variotii	Coccidioides spp
Candida kefyr	Pseudoallescheria boydii (Scedosporium	Cryptococcus spp
Candida krusei	apiospermum)	Fusarium spp
Candida lusitaniae	Sporothrix schenckii	Histoplasma spp
Candida tropicalis		Paecilomyces lilacinus
		Rhodotorula spp
		Scedosporium prolificans
		Trichosporon asahii

ANTIMICROBIAL SPECTRUM OF ACTIVITY[†]

FLUCONAZOLE IV/PO

Predictable Activity	Unpredictable Activity	No/Insufficient Activity
Candida albicans Candida guilliermondii Candida lusitaniae Candida parapsilosis Candida pseudotropicalis Candida tropicalis Cryptococcus spp Malassezia spp Trichosporon spp	Blastomyces spp Candida dubliniensis Candida glabrata Candida inconspicua Candida norvegensis Candida rugosa Coccidioides spp Histoplasma spp Sporothrix schenckii	Agents of zygomycosis (e.g. Mucor, Rhizopus, Rhizomucor, Absidia, and, Cunninghamella spp) Aspergillus spp Candida krusei Fusarium spp Pseudoallescheria spp (Scedosporium spp) Rhodotorula spp	

ITRACONAZOLE

Predictable Activity	Unpredictable Activity	No/Insufficient Activity
Aspergillus spp Blastomyces spp Candida spp (other than C. glabrata and C. krusei) Cryptococcus spp Histoplasma spp Malassezia spp Sporothrix schenckii	Absidia spp Candida glabrata Coccidioides spp Rhizomucor spp Rhodotorula spp spp Scedosporium apiospermum	Candida krusei Fusarium spp Mucor spp Rhizopus spp Scedosporium prolificans	

ANTIMICROBIAL SPECTRUM OF ACTIVITY[†]

MICAFUNGIN		
Predictable Activity	Unpredictable Activity	No/Insufficient Activity
Aspergillus spp Candida albicans Candida dubliniensis Candida glabrata Candida kefyr Candida krusei Candida lusitaniae Candida tropicalis	Candida famata Candida guilliermondii Candida parapsilosis Paecilomyces variotii Pseudoallescheria boydii (Scedosporium apiospermum) Sporothrix schenckii	Agents of zygomycosis (e.g. Mucor, Rhizopus, Rhizomucor, Absidia, Cunninghamella spp) Blastomyces spp Coccidioides spp Cryptococcus spp Fusarium spp Histoplasma spp Paecilomyces lilacinus Rhodotorula spp Scedosporium prolificans Trichosporon asahii

ANTIMICROBIAL SPECTRUM OF ACTIVITY†

POSACONAZOLE PO

Predictable Activity	Unpredictable Activity	No/Insufficient Activity
Agents of zygomycosis (e.g. Mucor, Rhizopus, Rhizomucor, Absidia, Cunninghamella spp)	Fusarium moniliforme	Fusarium solani
Aspergillus spp	Fusarium oxysporum	Fusarium verticillioides
Blastomyces spp	Rhodotorula spp	
Candida spp	Saccharomyces cerevisiae	
Coccidioides spp	Scedosporium prolificans	
Cryptococcus spp	Trichosporon spp	
Exophiala spp		
Fonsecaea pedrosoi		
Histoplasma spp		
Paecilomyces spp		
Paracoccidioides spp		
Pseudallescheria boydii (Scedosporium apiospermum)		
Sporothrix schenckii		

ANTIMICROBIAL SPECTRUM OF ACTIVITY[†]

VORICONAZOLE IV/PO		
Predictable Activity	Unpredictable Activity	No/Insufficient Activity
Aspergillus spp	Fusarium moniliforme	Agents of zygomycosis (e.g. Mucor, Rhizopus,
Blastomyces spp	Fusarium oxysporum	Rhizomucor, Absidia, Cunninghamella spp)
Candida albicans*	Malassezia spp	Fusarium solani
Candida dubliniensis**	Paecilomyces lilacinus	Fusarium verticillioides
Candida glabrata*	Rhodotorula spp	
Candida guilliermondii	Scedosporium prolificans	
Candida krusei**	Trichosporon asahii	
Candida lusitaniae		
Candida parapsilosis		
Candida tropicalis*		
Coccidioides spp		
Cryptococcus spp		
Histoplasma spp		
Paecilomyces variotti		
Pseudallescheria boydii (Scedosporium apiospermum)		
Sporothrix schenckii		
Trichosporon beigelii		

* < 30% of fluconazole-resistant strains are susceptible to voriconazole.
** ≥ 75% of fluconazole-resistant strains are susceptible to voriconazole [J Clin Micro 2007;45:1735-45].

PHARMACODYNAMICS OF ANTIMICROBIALS

Pharmacodynamic parameters predictive of outcome for the various classes of antimicrobials:

T > MIC	Cmax:MIC	AUC$_{24}$:MIC
Time-dependent antibacterial activity; dosing should aim to maximize time that the free drug concentration is above the MIC of the pathogen(s)	Concentration-dependent antibacterial activity; dosing should aim to achieve high peak serum drug concentration relative to the MIC of the pathogen(s), e.g. extended-interval AG dosing	Concentration-dependent with time dependence; dosing should aim to maximize amount of drug relative to the MIC of the pathogen(s); this can be achieved by increasing the dose and/or giving more frequently
Penicillins[1]	Aminoglycosides (AG)[2]	Fluoroquinolones[3]
Cephalosporins[1]	Fluoroquinolones[2,3]	Azithromycin
Carbapenems[1]	Metronidazole (vs anaerobes)	Clarithromycin
Aztreonam[1]	Amphotericin B	Clindamycin
Erythromycin	Daptomycin	Tetracyclines
Flucytosine	Anidulafungin	Linezolid
	Caspofungin	Vancomycin
	Micafungin	Tigecycline
		Colistin
		Fluconazole
		Itraconazole
		Posaconazole
		Voriconazole

T > MIC = time that the free drug concentration is above the MIC
MIC = minimum inhibitory concentration
Cmax = peak free drug concentration
AUC$_{24}$ = 24h area under the free drug concentration-time curve

1. ß-lactams exhibit time-dependent bactericidal activity, whereby bacterial killing is highly correlated with the percentage of the dosing interval that free drug concentrations are above the minimum inhibitory concentration ((fT>MIC). For penicillins and cephalosporins, the fT>MIC that is required for maximal bacterial killing is at least 50% while for carbapenems it is 40% fT>MIC.
2. Aim for Cmax:MIC ratio of 10-12.
3. As concentration-dependent antibacterials, the efficacy of fluoroquinolones has been shown to correlate with the ratio of the peak serum concentration to the MIC of the organism (Cmax:MIC), as well as the ratio of the 24 hour area under the plasma concentration curve (AUC$_{24}$:MIC). Optimizing the AUC$_{24}$/MIC ratio can result in better clinical outcomes and limit the development of resistance. Various AUC$_{24}$/MIC target ratios have been proposed in the literature but no firm recommendations can be made as these ratios are dependent on multiple factors including:
   - antibiotic
     - total vs free drug concentration (takes into account protein binding)
     - bacteriostatic vs bactericidal activity
   - organism
     - Gram positive or Gram negative (higher AUC$_{24}$/MIC ratio generally required for Gram negative infections)
     - MIC
     - inoculum at site of infection
   - immune status of the host (higher AUC$_{24}$/MIC ratio required in immuno-compromised patients).

ADULT ANTIMICROBIAL DOSING GUIDE AND DAILY COSTS

Antimicrobial	Normal Adult Dose[1]	Cost ($)/Day[2]
Penicillins		
amoxicillin	500mg PO tid	1.03
amoxicillin-clavulanate	875mg PO bid or	1.67
	500mg PO tid	2.00
ampicillin	1-2g IV/IM q6h	19.80-39.60
penicillin VK	300mg PO qid	0.28
penicillin G Na	3-4MU IV/IM q4-6h	14.79-29.58
cloxacillin	500mg PO qid	2.66
	1-2g IV/IM q4-6h[3]	27.09-53.03
piperacillin	4g IV/IM q6h[4]	116.20
piperacillin-tazobactam	3.375g IV q6h[4]	57.67
	HAP/VAP: 4.5g IV q6h	76.90
	IAI: 4.5g IV q8h[4]	57.68
ticarcillin-clavulanate	3.1g IV q4-6h	42.37-63.56
Carbapenems		
doripenem	500mg IV q8h	73.50
ertapenem	1g IV/IM daily	49.95
imipenem	500mg IV q6h	97.52
meropenem	500mg IV q6h[5] or	101.04
	1g IV q8h[5]	151.56
Cephalosporins		
cephalexin	500mg PO qid	1.80
cefazolin	1-2g IV/IM q8h	11.25-22.50
cefoxitin	1-2g IV/IM q6-8h	31.80-85.00
cefuroxime axetil	500mg PO bid	2.87
cefuroxime	0.75-1.5g IV/IM q8h	59.68-119.36
cefixime	400mg PO daily	3.54
cefotaxime	1-2g IV/IM q6-8h[3]	28.74-76.72
ceftriaxone	1-2g IV/IM q12-24h[3]	23.80-58.63
ceftazidime	1-2g IV/IM q8h	67.76-133.23
cefepime	1-2g IV/IM q8-12h	33.49-67.28
Aminoglycosides[6]		
amikacin[6]	15mg/kg IV daily or	73.82
	5-7.5mg/kg IV/IM q8h	73.82-110.72
gentamicin[6]	5-7mg/kg IV daily or	24.13-33.79
	1.5-2mg/kg IV/IM q8h	21.72-28.96
tobramycin[6]	5-7mg/kg IV daily or	26.13-36.58
	1.5-2mg/kg IV/IM q8h	23.51-31.35

ADULT ANTIMICROBIAL DOSING GUIDE AND DAILY COSTS

Antimicrobial	Normal Adult Dose[1]	Cost ($)/Day[2]
Macrolides		
erythromycin	250-500mg PO qid	0.73-1.46
	0.5-1g IV q6h	65.77-108.79
azithromycin PO	500 mg PO first day, then 250mg PO daily x 4 days or	1.89 (250mg)
	500 mg PO daily	3.78 (500mg)
azithromycin IV	500 mg IV daily	14.56
clarithromycin	250-500mg PO bid	1.18-3.26
	XL 1000mg PO daily	5.03
Quinolones		
ciprofloxacin	500-750mg PO bid	2.10-3.85
	UTI: 250-500mg PO bid or XL 500-1000mg PO daily	1.86-2.10 3.24
	200-400mg IV q12h	23.96-47.82
levofloxacin	500-750mg PO daily[7]	2.11-4.85
	500-750mg IV daily[7]	23.80-30.97
moxifloxacin	400mg PO daily	5.94
	400mg IV daily	35.02
norfloxacin	400mg PO bid	1.53
Tetracyclines/Glycylcycline		
tetracycline	250-500mg PO qid	0.26-0.53
doxycycline	100mg PO daily-bid	0.59-1.17
	100mg IV daily-bid[8]	-
tigecycline	100mg IV x 1 dose	160.50
	then 50mg IV q12h	160.50
Other		
aztreonam[8]	1-2g IV/IM q8-12h	58.00-174.00
	Meningitis/CNS infections/ P. aeruglnosa: 2g IV/IM q6-8h	174.00-232.00
colistin	2.5-5mg colistin base/ kg/day IV/IM div q8h[9,10]	38.44-76.87
clindamycin	150-450mg PO qid	1.42-4.25
	600mg IV/IM q8h	39.90
metronidazole	500mg PO bid[11]	0.24
	500mg IV q12h	4.80

ADULT ANTIMICROBIAL DOSING GUIDE AND DAILY COSTS

Antimicrobial	Normal Adult Dose[1]	Cost ($)/Day[2]
Other (cont'd)		
trimethoprim-sulfamethoxazole (TMP/SMX)	1 D.S. tab PO bid	0.24
	160-240mg TMP (10-15mL) IV q6, 8, or 12h	26.48-79.43
	PCP: 15-20mg TMP/kg/day div q6-8h	86.88-115.84
trimethoprim	100mg PO bid	0.51
fosfomycin	3g PO once	22.59
nitrofurantoin macrocrystal or macrocrystal/micro crystal	50-100mg PO qid	0.67-0.89
nitrofurantoin monohydrate/macrocrystal	100mg PO bid	1.45
vancomycin IV[12]	15mg/kg IV q8-12h	123.88-185.82
vancomycin PO	CDI only: 125mg PO qid	30.23
fidaxomicin	200mg PO bid	231.00
linezolid	600mg PO bid	144.25
	600mg IV q12h	200.69
daptomycin	SSTI: 4mg/kg IV daily[13]	97.44
	Bacteremia/endocarditis: 6 mg/kg IV daily[13]	146.16

ADULT ANTIMICROBIAL DOSING GUIDE AND DAILY COSTS

Antimicrobial	Normal Adult Dose[1]	Cost ($)/Day[2]
Antiviral		

acyclovir   HSV
                        VZV
                        HSVE
	400mg PO tid
	800mg PO 5x/day
	10mg/kg[9] IV q8h
		3.81
		8.92
		408.41

famciclovir
                        HSV
                        VZV
	250mg PO tid
	500mg PO tid
		8.16
		12.68

ganciclovir	<u>Induction</u> 5mg/kg IV q12h <u>Maintenance</u> 5mg/kg IV daily	58.85 29.43

valacyclovir
                        HSV
                        VZV
	500mg-1g PO bid
	1g PO tid
		2.55-6.11
		9.16

valganciclovir	<u>Induction</u> 900mg PO bid <u>Maintenance</u> 900mg PO daily	91.43 45.72
amantadine	<u>Prophylaxis & Treatment</u> **< 64 years old:** 100mg PO bid **≥ 65 years old:** 100mg PO daily	1.04 0.52
oseltamivir	<u>Prophylaxis</u> 75mg PO daily <u>Treatment</u> 75mg PO bid	3.90 7.80
zanamivir	<u>Prophylaxis</u> 10mg inhaled orally daily <u>Treatment</u> 10mg inhaled orally bid	18.27 36.54

ADULT ANTIMICROBIAL DOSING GUIDE AND DAILY COSTS

Antimicrobial	Normal Adult Dose[1]	Cost ($)/Day[2]
Antifungal		
amphotericin B	0.5-1mg/kg[14] IV daily	50.75-101.49
amphotericin B, lipid-complexed	5mg/kg[14] IV daily	682.50
amphotericin B, liposomal	3-5mg/kg[14] IV daily	508.20-847.00
flucytosine	100-150mg/kg/day PO div q6h	38.50-57.75
anidulafungin	200mg IV once then 100mg IV daily	411.30 205.65
caspofungin	70mg IV once then 50mg IV daily	222.00 222.00
micafungin	100mg IV daily	98.00
fluconazole	400-800mg PO daily 400-800mg IV daily	12.94-25.88 63.74-127.48
ketoconazole	200-400mg PO daily	0.94-1.88
itraconazole	100-200mg PO daily	7.83-15.66 (oral solution)
posaconazole	400mg PO bid with meals 200mg PO qid if NPO	188.20 188.20
voriconazole	6mg/kg IV q12h x 2 doses then 4mg/kg IV q12h ≥ 40kg: 400mg PO q12h x 2 doses then 200mg PO q12h < 40kg: 200mg PO q12h x 2 doses then 100mg PO q12h	600.35 400.24 199.63 99.81 99.81 49.93

1. Based on a 70kg adult with normal renal and hepatic function. For disease-specific dosing, see also Recommended Empiric Therapy in Adult Patients and/or Recommended Therapy of Culture-Directed Infections in Adult Patients.
2. Based on Alberta Health Drug Benefit List (AH DBL) price, September 2012, or manufacturer's list price or wholesale price if drug not on AH DBL. Prices in the hospital setting may be significantly different due to contract pricing. Check with pharmacy for actual prices. Does not include administration, supplies, or serum level costs.
3. For central nervous system infections or endophthalmitis, higher dose should be used.
4. For infections with <u>documented</u> Pseudomonas aeruginosa, increase dose to 3g IV q4h (piperacillin)/4.5g IV q6h (piperacillin-tazobactam).
5. Recommend meropenem 2g IV q8h in cystic fibrosis, central nervous system and ophthalmological infections.

6. See extended interval or conventional aminoglycoside dosing guidelines.
7. While 250mg IV/PO daily is the approved levofloxacin dosage for UTI/pyelonephritis, the authors do not advocate the use of levofloxacin for these indications, preferring to reserve levofloxacin for use in RTIs.
8. Available through the TPD Special Access Program (Emergency Release). Contact pharmacy for assistance when ordering.
9. Dose based on IBW or ABW, whichever is less.
10. 2.5-5mg colistin base/kg/day = 6.7-13.3mg colistimethate sodium (CMS)/kg/day. Each vial contains 150mg colistin base or 400mg CMS.
11. For antibiotic associated colitis use 250mg PO qid.
12. See vancomycin dosing guidelines.
13. Dose based on ABW; do not round dose to nearest 500mg.
14. If obese, base dose on IBW.

ABW	= actual body weight	PCP	= Pneumocystis pneumonia
CDI	= Clostridium difficile infection	RTI	= respiratory tract infection
HAP	= hospital-acquired pneumonia	SSTI	= skin/soft tissue infections
HSV	= Herpes simplex virus	VAP	= ventilator-associated pneumonia
HSVE	= Herpes simplex virus encephalitis		
IAI	= intra-abdominal infection	VZV	= Varicella zoster virus
IBW	= ideal body weight		

PAEDIATRIC ANTIMICROBIAL DOSING GUIDE AND DAILY COSTS

Antimicrobial	Recommended Paediatric Dose[1,2]	Cost ($) / Day[3,4]
Penicillins		
amoxicillin	40mg/kg/d PO div tid	0.86
	90mg/kg/d PO div bid-tid (see otitis media, sinusitis)	1.94
	90mg/kg/d PO div tid (see CAP)	1.94
amoxicillin-clavulanate	40mg amox./kg/d PO div tid (4:1)	1.39
	45-90mg amox./kg/d[5] PO div bid (7:1) (see otitis media, sinusitis, CAP)	3.10-6.19
ampicillin	100-200mg/kg/d IV div q6h	9.90-19.80
	300-400mg/kg/d IV div q4-6h for meningitis/CNS infections/ endocarditis	29.70-39.60
penicillin VK	25-50mg/kg/d PO div tid-qid	1.07-2.14
penicillin G Na	100,000-250,000 units/kg/d IV div q6h	5.80-14.50
	250,000-400,000 units/kg/d IV div q4h for severe infections	14.50-23.20
cloxacillin PO	40-50mg/kg/d PO div qid	2.87-3.59
	100mg/kg/d PO div qid[6]	2.66[4a]-7.18[4b]
cloxacillin IV	100-200mg/kg/d IV div q4-6h	22.04-44.08
piperacillin	200-300mg/kg/d IV div q4-6h	29.05-43.58
piperacillin-tazobactam	240-300mg piperacillin/kg/d IV div q6-8h	23.07-28.84
ticarcillin-clavulanate	200-300mg ticarcillin/kg/d IV div q4-6h	14.12-21.18
Carbapenems		
ertapenem	30 mg/kg/d IV div q12h	29.97
imipenem	60-100mg/kg/d IV div q6h	62.59-104.32
meropenem	60mg/kg/d IV div q6-8h (max 3g/day)	60.62
	120mg/kg/d IV div q8h (max 6g/day) for meningitis/CNS infections/cystic fibrosis	121.25
Cephalosporins		
cephalexin	40mg/kg/d PO div qid	2.22
	100mg/kg/d PO div qid[6]	1.80[4a]-5.56[4b]
cefazolin	75-100mg/kg/d IV div q8h	7.50-10.00
cefoxitin	80-160mg/kg/d IV div q6h	16.96-33.92
cefuroxime axetil	20-30mg/kg/d PO div bid	2.80-4.20
cefuroxime	100-150mg/kg/d IV div q8h	53.04-79.56
cefixime	8mg/kg/d PO div q12-24h	3.33

PAEDIATRIC ANTIMICROBIAL DOSING GUIDE AND DAILY COSTS

Antimicrobial	Recommended Paediatric Dose[1,2]	Cost ($) / Day[3,4]
Cephalosporins (cont'd)		
cefotaxime	100-200mg/kg/d IV div q6-8h 300mg/kg/d IV div q6h for meningitis/CNS infections	24.36-48.72 73.08
cefprozil	15-30mg/kg/d PO div bid	0.74-1.48
ceftriaxone	50-100mg/kg/d IV div q12-24h 100mg/kg/d IV div q12h for meningitis/CNS infections	23.80-47.60 47.60
ceftazidime	100-150mg/kg/d IV div q8h[7]	45.18-67.76
cefepime	100-150mg/kg/d IV div q8h[7]	33.50-50.25
Aminoglycosides[8]		
amikacin	15mg/kg IV daily[8] **or** 15-22.5mg/kg/d IV div q8h	21.09 21.09-31.64
gentamicin	7-9mg/kg IV daily[8] **or** 5-7.5mg/kg/d IV div q8h	9.65-12.41 6.89-10.34
tobramycin	7-9mg/kg IV daily[8] **or** 5-7.5mg/kg/d IV div q8h	10.45-13.44 7.47-11.20
Macrolides		
erythromycin	40mg/kg/d PO div qid 40mg/kg/d IV div q6h	2.03 26.30
azithromycin	10mg/kg PO first day, then 5mg/kg PO daily x 4 days 10mg/kg IV first day, then 5 or 10mg/kg IV daily	1.45 (5mg/kg PO) 5.82 (10mg/kg IV)
clarithromycin	15mg/kg/d PO div bid	3.40
Other		
aztreonam	90-120mg/kg/d IV div q6-8h 150-200mg/kg/d IV div q6-8h (max 8g/day) for cystic fibrosis	52.20-69.60 87.00-116.00
colistin	2.5-5mg colistin base/kg/d IV/IM div q6-12h 5-8mg colistin base/kg/d IV/IM div q8h for cystic fibrosis	10.98-21.96 21.96-35.14
clindamycin	10-40mg/kg/d PO div tid-qid 20-40mg/kg/d IV div q6-8h	1.66-6.63 8.87-17.73
metronidazole	15-30mg/kg/d PO div bid 30mg/kg/d IV div q8-12h[7]	0.07-0.14 2.88
trimethoprim-sulfamethoxazole (TMP/SMX)	8-12mg TMP/kg/d PO div bid PCP: 20mg TMP/kg/d IV/PO div q6h Severe infections: 15-20mg TMP/kg/d IV div q6-8h	1.91-2.86 4.77 (PO) 24.82-33.10 (IV)

PAEDIATRIC ANTIMICROBIAL DOSING GUIDE AND DAILY COSTS

Antimicrobial	Recommended Paediatric Dose[1,2]	Cost ($)/ Day[3,4]
Others (cont'd)		
trimethoprim	4-10mg/kg/d PO div bid	0.21-0.51
doxycycline[9]	2-4mg/kg/d PO div q12-24h	0.23-0.46
	2-4mg/kg/d IV div q12-24h[10]	-
nitrofurantoin	5-7mg/kg/d PO div qid	0.22-0.31
vancomycin	60mg/kg/d IV div q6h	74.52
linezolid	<u>< 5 y.o.:</u> 30mg/kg/d IV/PO div q8h	100.35/73.50[4b]
	<u>5-11 y.o.:</u> 20mg/kg/d IV/PO div q12h	66.90/49.00[4b]
	<u>≥ 12 y.o.:</u> 600mg IV/PO q12h	200.69/144.25[4a]
daptomycin	<u>2-6 y.o.:</u> 10mg/kg IV daily	69.60
	<u>> 6 y.o.:</u> 4-6mg/kg IV daily	27.84-41.76
Antiviral		
acyclovir HSV	40-60mg/kg/d PO div 2-5x/d	5.11-7.67
VZV	80mg/kg/d PO div 4-5x/d	10.23
HSVE	<u>≤ 12 y.o.:</u> 60mg/kg/d IV div q8h	233.38
	<u>> 12 y.o.:</u> 30mg/kg/d IV div q8h	116.69
VZV immuno- compromised	30-60mg/kg/d IV div q8h	116.69-233.38
Neonatal HSV	60mg/kg/d IV div q8h	233.38
valacyclovir	60mg/kg/d PO div q8h	3.06
amantadine	**Treatment & Prophylaxis of influenza A ONLY** <u>1-9 y.o. and/or < 40kg:</u> 5mg/kg/d PO div bid (max 150mg/day)	1.01[4b]
	<u>≥ 10 y.o. and ≥ 40kg:</u> 100mg PO bid	1.04[4a]

PAEDIATRIC ANTIMICROBIAL DOSING GUIDE AND DAILY COSTS

Antimicrobial	Recommended Paediatric Dose[1,2]	Cost ($)/ Day[3,4]
Antiviral (cont'd)		
oseltamivir	**Treatment of influenza A & B** <u>1-12 y.o.:</u> ≤ 15kg: 30mg PO bid > 15-23kg: 45 mg PO bid > 23-40kg: 60mg PO bid > 40kg: 75mg PO bid <u>≥ 13 y.o.:</u> 75mg PO bid **Prophylaxis of influenza A & B** <u>1-12 y.o.:</u> ≤ 15kg: 30mg PO daily > 15-23kg: 45 mg PO daily > 23-40kg: 60mg PO daily > 40kg: 75mg PO daily <u>≥ 13 y.o.:</u> 75mg PO daily	 3.06[4b] 4.60[4b] 6.12[4b] 7.66[4b] 7.80[4a] 1.53[4b] 2.30[4b] 3.06[4b] 3.83[4b] 3.90[4a]
zanamivir	<u>≥ 7 y.o.:</u> **Treatment of influenza A & B** 10mg inhaled orally bid **Prophylaxis of influenza A & B** 10mg inhaled orally daily	 36.54 18.27
Antifungal		
amphotericin B	0.25-1.5mg/kg IV daily	7.25-43.50
amphotericin B, lipid-complexed	5mg/kg IV daily	195.00
amphotericin B, liposomal	3-5mg/kg IV daily	145.20-242.00
flucytosine	50-150mg/kg/d PO div q6h	5.50-16.50
caspofungin	Neonates: 1-2mg/kg/day <u>2-11 y.o.:</u> 70mg/m^2/day IV (max 70mg) day 1, then 50mg/m^2/day IV (max 50mg) ≥ 12 y.o.: use adult dosing	- 177.60 177.60 (0.8m^2)
micafungin	Neonates: 10-15mg/kg IV daily <u>Infants/children < 40 kg:</u> 2-4mg/kg IV daily > 40kg: use adult dosing	- 39.20-78.40
ketoconazole	3.3-6.6 mg/kg/d PO once daily	0.31-0.62
fluconazole	3-12mg/kg/d PO div q24h 3-12mg/kg/d IV div q24h	5.94-23.76 9.56-38.24

PAEDIATRIC ANTIMICROBIAL DOSING GUIDE AND DAILY COSTS

Antimicrobial	Recommended Paediatric Dose[1,2]	Cost ($)/ Day[3,4]
Antifungal (cont'd)		
itraconazole	5-10mg/kg/d PO div q12-24h	7.83-15.66
nystatin	400,000-600,000 units tid-qid	0.62-1.25
voriconazole PO	16mg/kg/d PO div q12h (max. 400mg/dose) x 2 doses, then	77.68
	14mg/kg/d PO div q12h (max. 200mg/dose)	67.97
	≥ 12 y.o.: use adult dosing	
voriconazole IV	12-16mg/kg/d IV div q12h (max. 400mg/dose) x 2 doses, then	171.53-228.71
	14mg/kg/d IV div q12h (max. 200mg/dose)	200.12
	≥ 12 y.o.: use adult dosing	

1. Mg/kg/d = milligrams per kilogram per day. Usual doses for paediatric patients with normal renal and hepatic function. Paediatric dose should not exceed recommended adult dose. For disease-specific dosing, see Recommended Empiric Therapy in Neonatal/Paediatric Patients.
2. These doses do not apply to neonates, except where noted.
3. Based on a 20kg child.
4. Based on Alberta Health Drug Benefit List price, September 2012, or manufacturer's list price or wholesale price if drug not on AH DBL. Prices in the hospital setting may be significantly different due to contract pricing. Check with pharmacy for actual prices. Does not include preparation, administration, supplies, or serum level costs.
   a. price for tablet/capsule
   b. price for suspension (if compounded, only drug costs are included; not diluents)
5. This high dose of clavulanate (12.9mg/kg/day) may lead to unacceptably high incidence of diarrhea; alternative is to combine 45mg/kg/day div bid of amoxicillin-clavulanate (7:1) with 45mg/kg/day div bid of amoxicillin.
6. For completion of therapy of bone & joint infections.
7. For meningitis and other CNS infections, higher end of the dosage listed should be used.
8. See Extended Interval Aminoglycoside Dosing/Monitoring Guidelines.
   Gentamicin/tobramycin is used at 10mg/kg/day for infections in cystic fibrosis patients.
9. Children > 8 years old.
10. Doxycycline IV is available through the TPD Special Access Program (Emergency Release). Contact pharmacy for assistance when ordering.

y.o.	=	years old
CAP	=	community-acquired pneumonia
CNS	=	central nervous system
HSV	=	Herpes simplex virus
HSVE	=	Herpes simplex virus encephalitis
PCP	=	Pneumocystis pneumonia
TMP	=	trimethoprim
VZV	=	Varicella zoster virus

HIGH DOSE EXTENDED INTERVAL AMINOGLYCOSIDE DOSING/MONITORING GUIDELINES

Studies indicate that high dose extended interval dosing (HDEID) of aminoglycosides (AGs) results in at least comparable efficacy as conventional dosing, decreased or equal nephrotoxicity and comparable ototoxicity, and requires less serum level monitoring.

1. **Contraindications/Precautions to HDEID of AGs**

   Contraindications
   - pediatric patients with renal dysfunction at baseline (serum creatinine higher than normal limits for age) or ≥ 30% increase from baseline while on AG (consider alternate antibiotic)
   - patients requiring hemodialysis, hemoperfusion or peritoneal dialysis
   - patients with Gram positive infections where AG is used for synergy (use conventional dosing)
   - patients with rapid clearance of drug (e.g. burns > 20% BSA)
   - endocarditis
   - surgical prophylaxis (use conventional dosing)

   Precautions
   - patients with chronic ascites or serious liver disease
   - patients with known auditory or vestibular disease or pre-existing impairment
   - pregnancy/postpartum (altered volume of distribution)

2. **Recommended Gentamicin/Tobramycin† Dose**
   † For amikacin, use 15 mg/kg. Round dose to nearest 50mg.

   a) Pediatric patients
   - 1 month - < 9 years of age: 7-9 mg/kg based on **actual** body weight [ABW][†]
   - ≥ 9 years of age: 7mg/kg based on ABW[†]
   - Cystic fibrosis: 10mg/kg based on ABW[†]
   - Round dose to nearest 5mg
   - Administer over 60 minutes

     [†] If ABW > 25% above IBW, use dosing weight (DW)
     $$DW = 0.4 (ABW - IBW) + IBW$$

   b) Adult patients
   - 5-7 mg/kg based on **ideal** body weight (IBW)*. Use 7mg/kg for serious infections.
   - Round dose to nearest 20mg
   - Administer over 60 minutes

HIGH DOSE EXTENDED INTERVAL AMINOGLYCOSIDE
DOSING/MONITORING GUIDELINES

Ideal body weight (IBW)*
IBW (females) = 45.5kg + (2.3 x inches > 5 feet)**
IBW (males)   = 50kg + (2.3 x inches > 5 feet)**

* Malnourished: If ABW < IBW, use ABW
  Obese: If ABW > 20% above IBW or BMI ≥ 30kg/m^2,
         use dosing weight (DW)
         DW = 0.4 (ABW - IBW) + IBW
**or (0.92 x cm > 150cm)

3. **Dosing Interval Determination for Gentamicin/Tobramycin/Amikacin**

   a) Pediatric patients - give q24h. If serum level is necessary (see 4b), adjust
      interval of subsequent doses, if need be, as follows:
      - if interval level drawn - adjust interval according to the Hartford
        nomogram (see 5a), or
      - if trough level drawn and > 0.5-1mg/L - lengthen dosing interval or
        consider alternate antibiotic.

   b) Adult patients - calculate creatinine clearance (Clcr); determine dosing interval
      according to chart below.

      i) **Calculated creatinine clearance (mL/min)**

         Clcr (females) = $\dfrac{(140 - age) \times IBW*}{Scr\ (\mu mol/L)}$

         Clcr (males)   = Clcr (female) x 1.2

         * If ABW < IBW, use ABW in Clcr calculations
           If obese (ABW > 20% above IBW), use dosing weight (DW)
           DW = 0.4 (ABW - IBW) + IBW

Calculated Clcr (mL/min)	Dosing Interval
≥ 60	q24h
40 - 59	q36h
20 - 39	q48h
< 20	Obtain pharmacist consult

4. **Monitoring**

   a) **Serum creatinine**

      - Baseline
      - Two – three times weekly

HIGH DOSE EXTENDED INTERVAL AMINOGLYCOSIDE
DOSING/MONITORING GUIDELINES

b) Aminoglycoside serum concentrations

- DO NOT ORDER serum peak concentrations
- Interval or trough level recommended in patients:
    i.   receiving > 3-5 days of aminoglycoside therapy
    ii. with renal dysfunction and/or significant changes in renal function
    iii. with a large volume of distribution (e.g. third spacing, ascites)
    iv. > 65 years of age
    v.   concurrent nephrotoxic drugs (e.g. amphotericin B, cyclosporine)

- If levels are indicated, order an 8 hour interval level after first dose (if using Hartford nomogram), or a trough level at the end of the dosing interval. Repeat level at least once weekly. (May need more frequently if patient has renal dysfunction, i.e. requires q36h or q48h dosing; if renal function changing; or patient on concurrent nephrotoxic drugs.)

c) Aminoglycoside Therapeutic Drug Monitoring[‡] & Interpretation

Antibiotic	Specimen	Order on Requisition	Sampling Times	Interpretation
Gentamicin and Tobramycin and Amikacin	8 hour interval* OR 6-14 hour interval*	Interval - 8h after dose **start** Amikacin – select "random" Other	7-9 hours after START of infusion[†] 6-6.9 or 9.1-14 hours after START of infusion[†]	* Interpret in conjunction with Hartford Nomogram (next page)
	trough level OR	Trough	At the end of the dosing interval, i.e. 0-60 minutes before next dose	AG trough level > 0.5-1mg/L suggests accumulation; lengthen dosing interval, or consider alternative antibiotic.

[†] DO NOT collect < 6 hours or > 14 hours after START of infusion. Result will be uninterpretable.

[‡] Other methods of monitoring may be used at some centres; refer to local guidelines.

HIGH DOSE EXTENDED INTERVAL AMINOGLYCOSIDE DOSING/MONITORING GUIDELINES

d) **Ototoxicity** – may be irreversible
- Patients should be advised to watch for and report signs & symptoms of cochlear (e.g. tinnitus, sense of fullness in ears, loss of hearing) and/or vestibular (e.g. dysequilibrium, oscillopsia, cognitive dysfunction, visual sensitivity, nausea/vomiting, vertigo, headache, nystagmus) toxicity. AG should be discontinued immediately if any signs/symptoms of toxicity develop.
- Audiometry and vestibular testing recommended for patients receiving ≥ 7 days of aminoglycoside therapy, or at any time if ototoxicity suspected. Contact Audiology.

5. **Interpretation of Aminoglycoside Interval level – Hartford nomogram**
- Plot aminoglycoside concentration on following nomogram (Hartford Nomogram: Antimicrob Agents Chemother 1995; 39(3): 650-5):

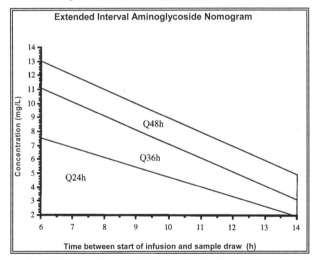

Extended Interval Aminoglycoside Nomogram

- **This nomogram applies only with doses of 7mg/kg. If other dose used - consult pharmacist.**
- **This nomogram assumes volume of distribution (Vd) of 0.3 L/kg. If patient's estimated Vd different, consult pharmacist.**
- **For amikacin, divide measured serum level by 2 and plot on the nomogram**

HIGH DOSE EXTENDED INTERVAL AMINOGLYCOSIDE DOSING/MONITORING GUIDELINES

- If the interval level falls in the areas marked as q24h, q36h, or q48h, the dosing interval should be every 24, 36, 48h respectively
- If the interval level falls on one of the sloping lines, choose the longer interval
- If above the q48h dosing interval area, DISCONTINUE extended interval dosing and switch to conventional dosing of aminoglycosides (See Conventional Aminoglycoside Dosing Guidelines on next page or consult pharmacist.)
- If below the nomogram (i.e. < 2 mg/L), aminoglycoside dosing/therapy should be reassessed if patient not improving. A pharmacist consult is suggested.

CONVENTIONAL AMINOGLYCOSIDE DOSING/MONITORING GUIDELINES

A. ADULTS

Loading Dose

Antibiotic	Loading Dose mg/kg (IBW*)
Gentamicin	2
Tobramycin	2
Amikacin	7.5

Maintenance Dose

Antibiotic	Maintenance Dose mg/kg (IBW*) per dose
Gentamicin	1.5 - 2
Tobramycin	1.5 - 2
Amikacin	5 - 7.5

Synergy Dose – Gentamicin & Tobramycin: 1mg/kg (IBW*)

- Round doses to nearest 20mg (Gentamicin/Tobramycin)/nearest 25mg (Amikacin).
- Administer over 30 minutes

    Ideal body weight (IBW)*
    IBW (females) = 45.5kg + (2.3 x inches > 5 feet)**
    IBW (males)   = 50kg + (2.3 x inches > 5 feet)**

    * Malnourished: If actual body weight (ABW) < IBW, use ABW
    Obese: If ABW > 20% above IBW or BMI ≥ 30kg/m²,
                use dosing weight (DW)
                DW = 0.4 (ABW - IBW) + IBW

    **or (0.92 x cm > 150cm)

Creatinine Clearance (Clcr)

a) Calculated creatinine clearance (mL/min)

$$Clcr \text{ (females)} = \frac{(140 - age) \times IBW^*}{Scr \text{ (}\mu mol/L)}$$

Clcr (males) = Clcr (female) x 1.2

* If ABW < IBW, use ABW in Clcr calculations
* If obese (ABW > 20% above IBW or BMI ≥ 30kg/m²), use dosing weight (DW)
  DW = 0.4 (ABW - IBW) + IBW

CONVENTIONAL AMINOGLYCOSIDE
DOSING/MONITORING GUIDELINES

Dosing Interval Determination for Gentamicin/Tobramycin/Amikacin

Calculated Clcr (mL/min)	Dosing Interval
≥ 80	q8h
50 - 79	q12h
20 - 49	q24h
< 20	Use serum levels to adjust dosing

B. PAEDIATRICS
- **Neonates ≤ 44 weeks post-conceptional age (PCA):** Refer to local guidelines for dosing & monitoring.
- **Infants > 44 weeks PCA & children:** 2.5mg/kg (IBW) q8h
- **Cystic Fibrosis:** 2.5-3.3 mg/kg (IBW) q6-8h
- **Synergy:** 1mg/kg (IBW) q8h

Monitoring

a) Serum creatinine
- Baseline
- Two - three times weekly

b) Aminoglycoside serum concentrations
- Order pre (trough) and post (peak) levels at steady state (usually after 3-4 doses in patients with normal renal function)
- If using gentamicin for synergy in the treatment of gram-positive infections (e.g. endocarditis), recommend trough*** level monitoring only in patients:
  - ⇒ with poor renal function
  - ⇒ on concurrent nephrotoxic drugs
  - ⇒ receiving prolonged therapy (> 5 days).
- *** These patients do not need peak (post) level; only a trough (pre) level is needed to rule out toxicity.

CONVENTIONAL AMINOGLYCOSIDE
DOSING/MONITORING GUIDELINES

c) **Aminoglycoside Therapeutic Drug Monitoring – Adults, Infants > 44 weeks PCA & Children**

Antibiotic	Specimen	Order on Requisition	Sampling Times	Notes
Gentamicin and Tobramycin and Amikacin	Pre (trough) **AND** Post (peak)	Pre (trough)	0-60 minutes before dose	DO NOT collect DURING infusion.
		Post (0.5-1h after dose **end**)	30-60 minutes after END of IV infusion At least 60 minutes post IM injection	DO NOT collect sooner than 30 minutes after END of infusion. Result will be uninterpretable.

Desired Serum Levels

Infection	Desired Peak (mg/L)	Desired Trough (mg/L)
Gentamicin/Tobramycin		
Synergy for Gram positive infections (e.g. endocarditis)		< 1
Lower UTI	3 - 4	< 1
PID/chorioamnionitis Pyelonephritis Peritonitis Soft tissue infections	6 - 7	< 2
Sepsis Neutropenia Burns Pneumonia Pseudomonas (non-urinary) infections	8 - 11	< 2
Cystic Fibrosis	12 - 15	< 2
Amikacin		
Moderate infections	20 - 25	< 4
Severe Infections	25 - 30	< 8

CONVENTIONAL AMINOGLYCOSIDE
DOSING/MONITORING GUIDELINES

Frequency of Serum Levels

- Once weekly (may need more frequently if renal function changing or concurrent nephrotoxic drugs)
- If creatinine changes (increase of > 40µmol/L, or 50% of baseline), draw trough aminoglycoside level to assess need for dosing change.

d) Ototoxicity – may be irreversible

- Patients should be advised to watch for and report signs & symptoms of cochlear (e.g. tinnitus, sense of fullness in ears, loss of hearing) and/or vestibular (e.g. dysequilibrium, oscillopsia, cognitive dysfunction, visual sensitivity, nausea/vomiting, vertigo, headache, nystagmus) toxicity. AG should be discontinued immediately if any signs/symptoms of toxicity develop.
- Audiometry and vestibular testing recommended for patients receiving ≥ 7 days of aminoglycoside therapy, or at any time if ototoxicity suspected. Contact Audiology.

VANCOMYCIN DOSING GUIDELINES

Recommended Initial Dose and Dosing Interval

A. Paediatrics
- Neonates ≤ 44 weeks post-conceptional age:
  - 15mg/kg/dose q8-24h depending on gestational age, post-natal age, and/or post-conceptional age. Refer to local guidelines.
  - if renal dysfunction (serum creatinine > 65µmol/L or urine output < 1mL/kg/h), extend dosing interval and adjust based on trough levels.
- Children > 44 weeks up to 12 years:
  - 60mgkg/day divided q6-8h
  - if renal dysfunction (serum creatinine higher than normal limits for age), extend dosing interval and adjust based on trough levels.
- Administration: ≤ 1g   – infuse over 60 minutes
                   > 1g – 1.5g   – infuse over 90 minutes
                   > 1.5g   – infuse over 120 minutes

B. Adults
1. Dose:
   i) Loading dose:
      - recommended in:
        - severe infections where rapid attainment of target trough level of 15-20mg/L is desired, e.g. vertebral osteomyelitis, MRSA pneumonia, epidural abscess, septic shock
        - patients with significant renal dysfunction in order to decrease time to target trough level
      - 25-30mg/kg (based on actual body weight (ABW); no maximum dose) single dose followed by maintenance dose (separated by dosing interval as recommended in 2 below).

   ii) Maintenance dose:
      - 15mg/kg (based on ABW)/dose (maximum of 2g/dose)
        - Doses > 500mg - round off to nearest 250mg
        - Doses < 500mg - round off to nearest 50mg

   iii) Dosing in Dialysis:
      - Peritoneal dialysis (PD) or low flux intermittent hemodialysis (IHD) – consider loading dose of 25-30 mg/kg. Subsequent doses should be based on vancomycin levels and usually given every 7-10 days.
      - High flux IHD – consider loading dose of 25-30 mg/kg (maximum of 2g/dose). Subsequent doses: either 500mg or 750mg infused in the last 60-120 minutes of each dialysis run:
        - 500mg if target vancomycin trough 10-15mg/L or patient weight < 60kg
        - 750mg if target vancomycin trough 15-20mg/L (unless weight < 60kg)

        Adjustment of high flux IHD dose based on levels:
        - < 10mg/L – increase dose by 50% (round to nearest 250mg)
        - > 20mg/L – decrease dose by 50% (round to nearest 250mg)

VANCOMYCIN DOSING GUIDELINES

- Administration: ≤ 1g   – infuse over 60 minutes
                > 1g – 1.5g   – infuse over 90 minutes
                > 1.5g   – infuse over 120 minutes

2. Dosing interval:

   i) Estimate creatinine clearance (Clcr):

      a. Calculated creatinine clearance (mL/min)

      $$\text{Clcr (females)} = \frac{(140 - \text{age}) \times \text{IBW*}}{\text{Scr } (\mu\text{mol/L})}$$

      Clcr (males)   = Clcr (females) x 1.2

      * IBW (females) = 45.5 kg + (2.3 x inches > 5 feet)[†]
         IBW (males)   = 50 kg + (2.3 x inches > 5 feet)[†]
         [†] or (0.92 x cm > 150 cm)

      If ABW < IBW, use ABW in Clcr calculations.
      If obese (ABW > 20% above IBW), use dosing weight (DW)
         DW = 0.4 (ABW - IBW) + IBW

   ii) Choose dosing interval based on chart:

Calculated Clcr (mL/min)	Dosing Interval for trough 10-20mg/L	Dosing Interval for trough 15-20mg/L
≥ 80	q12h	q8h
40 - 80	q24h	q12h
20 - 40	q36h	q24h
10 - 20	q48h	q48h
< 10	Consider loading dose. Obtain pharmacist consult.	Consider loading dose. Obtain pharmacist consult.

VANCOMYCIN MONITORING GUIDELINES

- Routine monitoring of vancomycin levels is NOT recommended because there is:
  - little literature evidence to support it
  - no clear evidence that nephrotoxicity and ototoxicity associated with vancomycin can be prevented by strict adherence to specific concentration ranges.

- Peak (post) levels are NOT needed because:
  - vancomycin does not exhibit concentration-dependent killing; AUC_{24h}/MIC correlates best with clinical outcome and bacterial eradication
  - vancomycin has slow distribution into peripheral tissues making it difficult to identify the true peak
  - they have not been correlated with improvements in clinical outcome.

1. Criteria for Vancomycin Serum Trough Concentration Monitoring

- deteriorating/unstable renal function (increase in baseline Scr of ≥ 40 µmol/L, or 50% of baseline)
- morbidly obese patients [≥ 190% IBW or BMI ≥ 40kg/m^2]
- patients with anticipated therapy ≥ 7 days
- patients who are severely ill (i.e. sepsis) and/or require target trough of 15-20mg/L (e.g. osteomyelitis, pneumonia, central nervous system infections, endocarditis, bacteremia, serious MRSA infections).
- patients with altered volume of distribution or clearance of vancomycin (e.g. cystic fibrosis, pediatrics, elderly > 60 years, cancer, burns > 20% BSA)
- selected dialysis patients [e.g. high flux and continuous hemodialysis/filtration (CAVH, CVVH, CVVHDF)]

2. Monitoring

a) Serum creatinine (Scr)
- Baseline
- Once weekly (more frequently if renal function changing or if concurrent nephrotoxic drugs)
- If creatinine changes (increase in Scr of ≥ 40 µmol/L, or 50% of baseline), draw vancomycin trough level to assess need for dosing change

b) Complete blood count with differential
- baseline
- once weekly

c) Peak (post) vancomycin levels are NOT RECOMMENDED.

d) Vancomycin trough level
- Order only if patient meets inclusion criteria above
- Collect serum specimen 30 minutes or less before next dose

Pediatrics:
- first level at steady state and after at least 2 doses (~ 24 hours if normal renal function)
  - neonates, GFR < 80mL/min/1.73m^2, and/or concomitant nephrotoxic medications: consider drawing first level sooner to ensure level is not above target
- subsequent levels every 5-7 days

Adults:
- first level at steady state and after at least 2 maintenance doses (~ 30 hours if normal renal function)
  - vancomycin clearance is enhanced in obesity. For morbidly obese patients (> 190% IBW or BMI ≥ 40kg/m^2) consider drawing first level sooner (e.g. before 2nd or 3rd dose)
- subsequent levels every 7-10 days (may need more frequently if renal function changing or concurrent nephrotoxic drugs)

Intermittent hemodialysis (IHD) with high flux filters:
- Draw pre-dialysis serum vancomycin level before 3rd and 4th dialysis runs. If within target range, do levels weekly (or less often if stable). If dosage change required, repeat levels before 3rd and 4th dialysis runs following dosage change until target trough achieved.

3. Desired Trough Level

Infection	Desired Trough Level (mg/L)
Osteomyelitis	15-20
Pneumonia	
Central nervous system infections	
Endocarditis	
Bacteremia	
Serious MRSA infections	
Other infections	10-20

ADULT DOSING RECOMMENDATIONS IN RENAL IMPAIRMENT*

Antimicrobial	Normal Adult Dose	Dose & Interval Adjustment for Renal Impairment		
		Creatinine Clearance (mL/min)**		
		>50	10-50	<10 (Anuric)
Penicillins				
Amoxicillin	500mg PO q8h	q8h	q8-12h	q12-24h
Amoxicillin-clavulanate	500mg PO q8h	q8h	10-30mL/min: q12h	q24h
Amoxicillin-clavulanate	875mg PO q12h	> 30 mL/min: NO CHANGE NEEDED		≤ 30 mL/min: Do not use 875mg tab; use 500mg tab (see recommendations above)
Ampicillin	1-2g IV q6h	q6h	q6-12h	q12-24h
Penicillin VK	300mg PO q6h	q6h	q8h	q12h
Penicillin G Na	3-4MU IV q4-6h	q6h	q8h	q12h
Cloxacillin	500mg PO q6h	NO CHANGE NEEDED		
Cloxacillin	1-2g IV q4-6h	NO CHANGE NEEDED		
Piperacillin	4g IV q6h	q6h	q6-8h	q8h
Piperacillin-tazobactam	3.375g IV q6h	3.375g q6h	2.25g q6h	2.25g q8h
Piperacillin-tazobactam	4.5g IV q8h	≥ 20 mL/min: NO CHANGE NEEDED		<20 mL/min: 4.5g q12h
Piperacillin-tazobactam	4.5g IV q6h	q6h	3.375g q6h	2.25g q6h
Ticarcillin-clavulanate	3.1g IV q4-6h	q4-6h	2.067-3.1g q6-8h	2.067g q12h
Carbapenems				
Doripenem	500mg IV q8h	q8h	30-50mL/min: 250mg q8h 10-29mL/min: 250mg q12h	unknown
Ertapenem	1g IV daily	1g daily	≤ 30mL/min: 500mg daily	
Imipenem	500mg IV q6h	q6h	q8-12h	250-500mg q12h
Meropenem	500mg IV q6h	q6h	26-50mL/min: q8h 10-25mL/min: q12h	q24h
Meropenem	1-2g IV q8h	q8h	q12h	500mg q24h
Cephalosporins				
Cephalexin	500mg PO q6h	q6h	q8-12h	q12-24h
Cefazolin	1-2g IV q8h	q8h	q8-12h	q24h
Cefoxitin	1-2g IV q8h	q8h	q8-12h	q24h
Cefuroxime axetil	500mg PO q12h	NO CHANGE NEEDED		250mg q24h
Cefuroxime	0.75-1.5g IV q8h	q8h	q8-12h	q24h
Cefixime	400mg PO daily	NO CHANGE NEEDED		200mg daily
Cefotaxime	1-2g IV q6-8h	q6-8h	q8-12h	q24h
Ceftriaxone	1-2g IV q12-24h	NO CHANGE NEEDED		
Ceftazidime	1-2g IV q8h	q8-12h	q12-24h	q24-48h
Cefepime	1-2g IV q8-12h	q8-12h	q12-24h	q24h
Aminoglycosides	See Aminoglycoside Dosing Guidelines, Conventional or Extended Interval.			

ADULT DOSING RECOMMENDATIONS IN RENAL IMPAIRMENT*

Antimicrobial	Normal Adult Dose	Dose & Interval Adjustment for Renal Impairment		
		Creatinine Clearance (mL/min)**		
		>50	10-50	<10 (Anuric)
Macrolides				
Erythromycin	250-500mg PO q6h	NO CHANGE NEEDED		50-75% dose q6h
Erythromycin	0.5-1g IV q6h	NO CHANGE NEEDED		50-75% dose q6h
Azithromycin	250-500mg PO daily	NO CHANGE NEEDED		unknown
Azithromycin	500mg IV daily	NO CHANGE NEEDED		unknown
Clarithromycin	250-500mg PO q12h	q12h	q12-24h	q24h
Clarithromycin XL	XL 1000mg PO daily	< 30 mL/min: NO CHANGE NEEDED		< 30 mL/min: 500mg daily
Quinolones				
Ciprofloxacin	250-750mg PO q12h	q12h		< 30mL/min: q24h
Ciprofloxacin	200-400mg IV q12h	q12h		< 30mL/min: q24h
Levofloxacin	500mg PO/IV daily	q24h	500mg once then 250mg q24h	500mg once then 250mg q48h
Levofloxacin	750mg PO/IV daily	q24h	750mg q48h	750mg once then 500mg q48h
Moxifloxacin	400mg PO/IV daily	NO CHANGE NEEDED		
Norfloxacin	400mg PO q12h	q12h	q12-24h	q24h
Other				
Aztreonam	1-2g IV q8h	q8h	50-75% dose	25% dose
Colistin	5mg colistin base/kg/day IV div q8h	> 70mL/min: NO CHANGE NEEDED	10-70mL/min: q8-12h	< 10mL/min: q12h
Doxycycline	100mg PO/IV q12-24h	NO CHANGE NEEDED		
Tigecycline	100mg IV x 1 dose then 50mg IV q12h	NO CHANGE NEEDED		
Clindamycin	150-450mg PO q6h	NO CHANGE NEEDED		
Clindamycin	600mg IV q8h	NO CHANGE NEEDED		
Metronidazole	500mg PO/IV q12h	NO CHANGE NEEDED		
Trimethoprim-sulfamethoxazole	1DS tab PO q12h	q12h	15-25mL /min: 50% dose	< 15mL/min: DO NOT USE
Trimethoprim-sulfamethoxazole	160-240mg TMP (10-15mL) IV q6, 8, or 12h	q6-12h	15-25mL/min: 50% dose	< 15mL/min: DO NOT USE
Trimethoprim	100mg PO q12h	> 30mL/min: NO CHANGE NEEDED	15-30mL/min: 50mg PO q12h	< 15mL/min: DO NOT USE
Fosfomycin	3g PO once	NO CHANGE NEEDED		
Nitrofurantoin	50-100mg PO q6h	< 60mL/min: CONTRAINDICATED - DO NOT USE		
Nitrofurantoin (MacroBID)	100mg PO q12h	< 60mL/min: CONTRAINDICATED - DO NOT USE		
Vancomycin	15mg/kg IV q12h	q12-24h	q24-72h	use serum levels to assist dosing
Vancomycin	125mg PO qid	NO CHANGE NEEDED†		
Linezolid	600mg PO/IV q12h	NO CHANGE NEEDED		
Daptomycin	4-6mg/kg IV q24h	q24h		< 30mL/min: q48h

† If patient has significant renal impairment and colitis, clinically important serum concentrations may result. Trough vancomycin level to rule out toxicity should be considered.

ADULT DOSING RECOMMENDATIONS IN RENAL IMPAIRMENT*

Antimicrobial	Normal Adult Dose	Dose & Interval Adjustment for Renal Impairment		
		Creatinine Clearance (mL/min)**		
		>50	10-50	<10 (Anuric)
Antiviral				
Acyclovir	400mg PO tid	NO CHANGE NEEDED		q12h
Acyclovir	5-10mg/kg IV q8h	q8h	25-50mL/min: q12h 10-25mL/min: q24h	50% dose q24h
Amantadine	100mg PO bid or 100mg PO daily	See Prophylaxis for Influenza A.		
Famciclovir	500mg PO tid	q8h	q12-24h	250mg q24h
Ganciclovir	Induction 5mg/kg IV q12h	q12h	1.25-2.5mg/kg q24h	1.25mg/kg 3x/week
	Maintenance 5mg/kg IV q24h	2.5-5mg/kg q24h	0.625-1.25mg/kg q24h	0.625mg/kg 3x/week
Oseltamivir	Treatment 75mg PO bid	> 60mL/min: NO CHANGE NEEDED	> 30-60mL/min: 30mg PO bid 10-30mL/min: 30mg PO daily	USE WITH CAUTION: 75mg PO once only
	Prophylaxis 75mg PO daily	> 60mL/min: NO CHANGE NEEDED	> 30-60mL/min: 30mg PO daily 10-30mL/min: 30mg PO q2days	USE WITH CAUTION: 30mg PO once only
Valacyclovir	1g PO tid	q8h	q12-24h	500mg q24h
Valganciclovir	Induction 900mg PO bid	q12h	450mg daily-q2days	DO NOT USE
	Maintenance 900mg PO daily	daily	450mg q2days-2x/week	DO NOT USE
Zanamivir	10mg inhaled orally daily-bid	NO CHANGE NEEDED		
Antifungal				
Amphotericin B	0.5-1mg/kg IV daily	q24h	q24h	q24-36h
Anidulafungin	200mg IV once then 100mg IV daily	NO CHANGE NEEDED		
Caspofungin	50mg IV daily	NO CHANGE NEEDED		
Fluconazole	400mg PO/IV daily	q24h	q24-48h	q48-72h
Flucytosine	37.5mg/kg PO q6h	q12h	q12-24h	q24h
Itraconazole	100-200mg PO daily	NO CHANGE NEEDED		
Ketoconazole	200-400mg PO daily	NO CHANGE NEEDED		
Micafungin	100mg IV daily	NO CHANGE NEEDED		
Posaconazole	400mg PO bid	NO CHANGE NEEDED		
Voriconazole	4mg/kg IV q12h	NO CHANGE NEEDED	Accumulation & resultant toxicity of the diluent can occur if Clcr < 50mL/min. Use oral voriconazole at normal doses.	
Voriconazole	200mg PO q12h	NO CHANGE NEEDED		

ADULT DOSING RECOMMENDATIONS IN RENAL IMPAIRMENT*

Antimicrobial	Normal Adult Dose	Dose & Interval Adjustment for Renal Impairment		
		Creatinine Clearance (mL/min)**		
		>50	10-50	<10 (Anuric)
Antituberculous Agents				
Ethambutol	15-25mg/kg PO daily	q24h	q24-36h	q48h
Isoniazid	5mg/kg PO daily	NO CHANGE NEEDED		
Pyrazinamide	20-25mg/kg PO daily	NO CHANGE NEEDED		50-100% dose q24h
Rifampin	10mg/kg PO daily	NO CHANGE NEEDED		

* For dosage adjustment in hepatic impairment, see Adult Dosing Recommendations in Hepatic Impairment.
** > 50mL/min = > 0.83mL/s; 10-50mL/min = 0.17-0.83mL/s; < 10mL/min = < 0.17mL/s

ADULT DOSING RECOMMENDATIONS IN HEPATIC IMPAIRMENT*

- The effect of hepatic dysfunction on drug clearance depends on several factors: degree of protein binding, hepatic blood flow, hepatic extraction ratio, whether the drug undergoes Phase I or Phase II metabolism, and degree to which other routes of metabolism/elimination compensate.
- Unless otherwise stated, recommendations are for dosage adjustments in cases of severe hepatic dysfunction caused by cirrhosis.

Antimicrobial	Dosage Adjustment
Penicillins	
Amoxicillin	No change necessary
Amoxicillin-clavulanate	No change necessary
Ampicillin	No change necessary
Penicillin	No change necessary
Cloxacillin	Consider dosage reduction in combined renal and hepatic impairment. No specific dosing information available.
Piperacillin	No change necessary
Piperacillin-tazobactam	No change necessary
Ticarcillin-clavulanate	No change necessary
Carbapenems	
Doripenem	Has not been studied in patients with hepatic impairment but since doripenem does not undergo hepatic metabolism, the pharmacokinetics of doripenem are not expected to be affected by hepatic impairment.
Ertapenem	No change necessary
Imipenem	No change necessary
Meropenem	No change necessary
Cephalosporins	
Cephalexin	No change necessary
Cefazolin	No change necessary
Cefoxitin	No change necessary
Cefuroxime	No change necessary
Cefixime	No change necessary
Cefotaxime	No change necessary
Ceftriaxone	Dosage reduction recommended in combined renal and hepatic impairment
Ceftazidime	No change necessary
Cefepime	No change necessary

ADULT DOSING RECOMMENDATIONS IN HEPATIC IMPAIRMENT*

Antimicrobial	Dosage Adjustment
Aminoglycosides	
Amikacin Gentamicin Tobramycin	**Monitoring is strongly recommended as patients may be more prone to nephro- or ototoxicity.** See conventional/extended interval* aminoglycoside (AG) dosing/monitoring guidelines. An increase in dose may be required to compensate for increased volume of distribution (V_d) because of ascites. *** Cannot use extended interval AG nomogram to interpret levels in these patients due to higher V_d.**
Macrolides	
Erythromycin	Lengthen dosing interval to q12h. **Avoid estolate salt in patients with hepatic dysfunction.**
Azithromycin	Use with caution.
Clarithromycin	No change necessary
Quinolones	
Ciprofloxacin	No change necessary
Levofloxacin	No change necessary
Moxifloxacin	No change necessary in patients with mild to moderate (Child Pugh A or B) impairment. No information available for patients with more severe (Child Pugh C) hepatic impairment.
Norfloxacin	No change necessary
Ofloxacin	Lengthen dosing interval to once daily
Tetracyclines/Glycylcycline	
Doxycycline	No change necessary
Minocycline	Significant excretion via biliary tract. No accumulation noted with hepatic impairment. No change necessary
Tetracycline	Do not use with severe hepatic impairment
Tigecycline	No change necessary in patients with mild to moderate (Child Pugh A or B) impairment. Severe (Child Pugh C) hepatic impairment: 100mg IV x 1 dose then 25mg IV q12h.
Other	
Aztreonam	Reduce dose 25% when used chronically at high doses
Colistin	No change necessary
Chloramphenicol	Lengthen dosing interval to q12-24h. Monitor serum levels to maintain between 5-20 mg/L.
Clindamycin	Lengthen dosing interval to q12h

ADULT DOSING RECOMMENDATIONS IN HEPATIC IMPAIRMENT*

Antimicrobial	Dosage Adjustment
Other (cont'd)	
Metronidazole	Lengthen dosing interval to q12-24h
Trimethoprim-sulfamethoxazole	Use with caution in hepatic impairment
Trimethoprim	No change necessary
Fosfomycin	No change necessary
Nitrofurantoin	No change necessary
Vancomycin	**Monitoring of trough levels is strongly recommended.** See Vancomycin Monitoring Guidelines.
Linezolid	No change necessary in patients with mild to moderate (Child Pugh A or B) impairment. No information available for patients with severe (Child Pugh C) hepatic impairment.
Daptomycin	No change necessary in patients with mild to moderate (Child Pugh A or B) impairment. No information available for patients with severe (Child Pugh C) hepatic impairment.
Antivirals	
Acyclovir	No change necessary
Amantadine	No change necessary
Famciclovir	No change necessary
Ganciclovir	No change necessary
Oseltamivir	Has not been studied in patients with hepatic impairment.
Valacyclovir	No change necessary
Valganciclovir	Has not been studied in patients with hepatic impairment.
Zanamivir	No change necessary
Antituberculous Agents	
Ethambutol	No change necessary
Isoniazid	**Genetic predisposition (slow/fast acetylation) is more important in determining clearance than hepatic disease.** Consider lengthening dosing interval to q48h or deferral of isoniazid therapy in patients with acute liver disease.
Pyrazinamide	Dosage reduction recommended
Rifampin	Lengthen dosing interval to q48h. **Consider deferral of rifampin therapy in patients with jaundice.**

ADULT DOSING RECOMMENDATIONS IN HEPATIC IMPAIRMENT*

Antimicrobial	Dosage Adjustment
Antifungals	
Amphotericin B	No change necessary
Flucytosine	No change necessary
Anidulafungin	No change necessary
Caspofungin	Reduce maintenance dose from 50 mg daily to 35 mg daily in patients with moderate (Child Pugh B) hepatic impairment. No information available for patients with severe (Child Pugh C) hepatic impairment.
Micafungin	No change necessary in patients with mild to moderate (Child Pugh A or B) impairment. No information available for patients with severe (Child Pugh C) hepatic impairment.
Fluconazole	No change necessary
Ketoconazole	Dosage reduction recommended
Itraconazole	No change necessary
Terbinafine	Reduce dosage by 50% and monitor liver function tests.
Voriconazole	Use standard loading dose followed by half the standard maintenance dose in patients with mild to moderate hepatic impairment (Child Pugh A and B). No data is available for patients with severe hepatic impairment (Child-Pugh C). Additional monitoring of liver function tests is recommended in patients with any degree of abnormal liver function.

* For dosage adjustment in renal impairment, see Adult Dosing Recommendations in Renal Impairment.

Child-Pugh Grading of Chronic Liver Disease

Score	1	2	3
Bilirubin (μmol/L)	17.1-34.2	34.2-51.3	> 51.3
Albumin (g/L)	> 35	28-35	< 28
Ascites	none	mild	moderate
Encephalopathy (grade)	none	1 or 2	3 or 4
Prothrombin time (seconds prolonged)	1-4	4-6	> 6

Grade A < 7 points, Grade B 7-9 points, Grade C 10-15 points
Modified from DiPiro et al. Pharmacotherapy 6th edition.

ANTIMICROBIAL GENERIC/TRADE NAME LISTING

Generic Name	Common Trade Name(s)*
Penicillins	
amoxicillin	Amoxil
amoxicillin-clavulanate	Clavulin
ampicillin PO	Teva-Ampicillin Nu-Ampi
ampicillin IV	Ampicin
cloxacillin PO	Orbenin
cloxacillin IV	Orbenin Tegopen
penicillin VK	Apo-Pen VK Nu-Pen-VK Teva-Penicillin-VK
penicillin G Na IV	Crystapen
piperacillin	Pipracil
piperacillin-tazobactam	Tazocin
ticarcillin-clavulanate	Timentin
Carbapenems	
doripenem	Doribax
ertapenem	Invanz
imipenem	Primaxin
meropenem	Merrem
Cephalosporins	
1st generation cephalexin	Keflex
cefazolin	Ancef Kefzol
2nd generation cefoxitin	Mefoxin
cefprozil	Cefzil
cefuroxime axetil	Ceftin
cefuroxime IV	Kefurox Zinacef
3rd generation cefixime	Suprax
cefotaxime	Claforan
ceftriaxone	Rocephin
ceftazidime	Fortaz

ANTIMICROBIAL GENERIC/TRADE NAME LISTING

Generic Name	Common Trade Name(s)*
Cephalosporins (cont'd)	
4th generation	
cefepime	Maxipime
Aminoglycosides	
amikacin	Amikin
gentamicin	Garamycin
tobramycin	Tobrex
Macrolides	
azithromycin PO/IV	Zithromax
clarithromycin	Biaxin
erythromycin base PO	Erybid
	Eryc
erythromycin estolate PO	Ilosone
erythromycin ethylsuccinate PO	EES
erythromycin lactobionate IV	Erythrocin
Quinolones	
ciprofloxacin IV/PO	Cipro
levofloxacin IV/PO	Levaquin
moxifloxacin IV/PO	Avelox
norfloxacin	Noroxin
Tetracyclines	
doxycycline PO	Doxycin
	Doxytec
	Vibra-tabs
doxycycline IV**	Vibramycin
minocycline	Minocin
tetracycline	Tetracyn
Glycylcycline	
tigecycline	Tygacil
Other	
aztreonam**	Azactam
clindamycin	Dalacin C
colistin, colistimethate	Coly-Mycin M
daptomycin	Cubicin
fidaxomicin	Dificid
fosfomycin	Monurol
linezolid IV/PO	Zyvoxam
metronidazole	Flagyl

ANTIMICROBIAL GENERIC/TRADE NAME LISTING

Generic Name	Common Trade Name(s)*
Other (cont'd)	
nitrofurantoin macrocrystal/ microcrystal	Nitrofurantoin [AA Pharma]
nitrofurantoin macrocrystal	Macrodantin, Teva-Nitrofurantoin
nitrofurantoin monohydrate/ macrocrystal	MacroBID
trimethoprim	Proloprim
trimethoprim/sulfamethoxazole, co-trimoxazole	Bactrim Septra
vancomycin PO/IV	Vancocin
Antivirals	
acyclovir IV/PO	Zovirax
amantadine	Symmetrel
famciclovir	Famvir
foscarnet**	Foscavir
ganciclovir IV	Cytovene
oseltamivir	Tamiflu
ribavirin IV	Virazole
valacyclovir	Valtrex
valganciclovir	Valcyte
zanamivir	Relenza
Antifungals	
amphotericin B	Fungizone
amphotericin B, lipid-complexed	Abelcet
amphotericin B, liposomal	AmBisome
anidulafungin	Eraxis
caspofungin	Cancidas
fluconazole PO/IV	Diflucan
flucytosine	Ancobon
itraconazole	Sporanox
ketoconazole	Nizoral
micafungin	Mycamine
posaconazole	Posanol
terbinafine	Lamisil
voriconazole IV/PO	Vfend

* Trade names are listed for information/product recognition only. Trade name or
  equivalent generic product may be dispensed.
**SAP= TPD Special Access Program (Emergency Release)

IV to PO SWITCH RECOMMENDATIONS

Parenteral Regimen [1]	Cost ($)/ Day [2,3]	Oral Regimen [1]	Cost ($)/ Day [2]	Bioavail-ability (%)
Azithromycin 500mg daily	3.78	Azithromycin 250mg daily	1.89	37
Cefazolin 1g q8h	11.25	Cephalexin 500mg q6h[4]	1.80	90
Cefuroxime 0.75-1.5g q8h	59.68-119.36	Cefuroxime axetil 0.5-1g q12h	2.87-5.73	52
Genitourinary tract infections:				
Ciprofloxacin 200mg q12h	23.96	Ciprofloxacin 250-500mg q12h	1.86-2.10	70
Nosocomial pneumonia, Gram negative bone/joint infections:				
Ciprofloxacin 400mg q12h	47.82	Ciprofloxacin 500-750mg q12h	2.10-3.85	70
Clindamycin 600mg q8h	39.90	Clindamycin 300mg q6h *Bone/joint infections:* 450mg q6h	2.83 4.25	90
Fluconazole 400mg daily	63.74	Fluconazole 400mg daily	12.94	90
Levofloxacin 250-750mg daily	12.60-30.97	Levofloxacin 250-750mg daily	1.87-4.85	99
Linezolid 600mg q12h	200.69	Linezolid 600mg q12h	144.25	100
Metronidazole 500mg q12h	4.80	Metronidazole 500mg q12h	0.24	100
Moxifloxacin 400mg daily	35.02	Moxifloxacin 400mg daily	5.94	89
Trimethoprim-sulfamethoxazole 160/800mg q8h	39.72	Trimethoprim-sulfamethoxazole 1 DS tab q12h	0.24	85
Voriconazole 400mg q12h x 2 doses then 200mg q12h	571.77 285.88	Voriconazole 400mg q12h x 2 doses then 200mg q12h	199.63 99.81	96

1. Usual adult dose in patients with normal renal and hepatic function.
2. Based on Alberta Health Drug Benefit List (AH DBL) price, September 2012, or manufacturer's list price or wholesale price if drug not on AH DBL. Prices in the hospital setting may be significantly different due to contract pricing. Check with pharmacy for actual prices.
3. Drug cost only. Does not include administration, supplies, or serum level costs.
4. Can switch to cephalexin for Gram positive infections if organism susceptible to cefazolin; for Gram negative urinary tract infections ONLY can switch to cephalexin if susceptible to cephalothin/ cephalexin.

CSF PENETRATION OF ANTIMICROBIALS

- Ability of antimicrobials to penetrate into CSF is dependent on:
    - ⇒ age of patient (better in infants and older persons than in children and young adults)
    - ⇒ degree of meningeal inflammation (↑ inflammation → ↑ penetration)
    - ⇒ lipid solubility (↑ lipid solubility → ↑ penetration)
    - ⇒ degree of ionization (↑ ionization → ↓ penetration)
    - ⇒ molecular weight (↑ molecular weight → ↓ penetration)
    - ⇒ protein binding (↑ protein binding → ↓ penetration)
    - ⇒ susceptibility to active transport systems (which pump antibiotics out of the CSF)
- Bactericidal effect maximal when CSF antibiotic concentration exceeds in vitro MIC of the pathogen by 10 - 20 times.

Table 1: Antimicrobial Penetration into Cerebrospinal Fluid (CSF)

Class	Excellent Penetration	Good Penetration	Poor Penetration
Antibiotics	Chloramphenicol Ciprofloxacin[1, 4] Cycloserine Isoniazid Linezolid Metronidazole Minocycline Moxifloxacin[1, 4] Pyrazinamide Trimethoprim-sulfamethoxazole	Aztreonam Cefepime[1] Cefotaxime[2] Ceftazidime Ceftriaxone[2] Cloxacillin Doxycycline Ertapenem[1] Meropenem[1] Rifampin Tetracycline Vancomycin[5,9]	Amikacin[3,9] Ampicillin[1] Azithromycin Cefazolin Cefoxitin Cefuroxime Clarithromycin Clindamycin Colistin[9] Daptomycin[8,9] Doripenem[8] Erythromycin Ethambutol Gentamicin[3,9] Imipenem[1] Levofloxacin[1] Norfloxacin Ofloxacin Penicillin[1] Piperacillin[1] +/- tazobactam Polymyxin B Streptomycin[3,9] Ticarcillin[1] +/- clavulanate Tigecycline[8] Tobramycin[3,9]
Antivirals		Acyclovir Famciclovir Ganciclovir[8] Valacyclovir	Other antivirals

CSF PENETRATION OF ANTIMICROBIALS

Table 1: Antimicrobial Penetration into Cerebrospinal Fluid (CSF)

Class	Excellent Penetration	Good Penetration	Poor Penetration
Antifungals	Flucytosine Fluconazole Voriconazole	Itraconazole[6]	Amphotericin B[7,9] Anidulafungin[8] Caspofungin[8] Micafungin[8] Ketoconazole Posaconazole

Footnotes:
1. Penetration may be enhanced with meningeal inflammation. Use optimal doses.
2. CSF concentration adequate for most susceptible organisms, except certain Gram negative bacilli, such as Acinetobacter, Flavobacterium, and Enterobacteriaceae producing inducible (*Enterobacter spp, Citrobacter freundii complex, Serratia spp, Morganella spp, Providencia spp, Proteus vulgaris, Proteus penneri, and some Hafnia spp*) and extended-spectrum ß-lactamases. Ceftriaxone achieves sustained reliable bactericidal activity within the CSF despite its high protein binding. Agents of choice for penicillin-intermediate S. pneumoniae.
3. Monotherapy not recommended. Difficult to achieve adequate CSF concentrations with IV dosing alone. Extended interval dosing increases CSF penetration. Acidic nature of purulent CSF decreases antimicrobial activity of aminoglycosides. For CNS infections, concomitant intrathecal / intraventricular* preservative-free aminoglycoside may be required (see Table 2 for pediatric and adult dosing information).
4. CSF concentrations inadequate for streptococci. Ciprofloxacin may be useful for meningitis due to multi-resistant Gram negative organisms and as an alternative to β-lactams (ceftazidime, cefepime, meropenem) for P. aeruginosa meningitis, and moxifloxacin for M. tuberculosis CNS infections.
5. Maintain trough serum concentration at 15 – 20 mg/L. If not responding to optimal IV doses, may have to use intrathecal / intraventricular* administration along with IV (see Table 2 for pediatric and adult dosing information).
6. Achieves therapeutic concentrations for cryptococcal meningitis. Not recommended for other CNS fungal infections.
7. Achieves therapeutic concentrations for cryptococcal meningitis despite penetration of the blood brain barrier being marginal. Can be administered intrathecal* for other mycoses – see Table 2 for pediatric and adult dosing information.
8. Based on limited human and/or animal data.
9. See Table 2 for pediatric and adult dosing information for intrathecal and intraventricular administration.

* **Intrathecal and Intraventricular administration**
  * These modes of administration are seldom necessary given the systemic antimicrobials currently available.
  * Concomitant systemic therapy recommended whenever possible.
  * Intrathecal administration is unlikely to provide therapeutic concentrations in the ventricles due to the unidirectional flow of CSF. Intraventricular administration is preferred for this reason; however, this mode of administration requires the placement of an Ommaya or Rickham reservoir.

CSF PENETRATION OF ANTIMICROBIALS

Table 2: Intrathecal and/or Intraventricular Doses
Adapted from Clin Microbiol Rev 2010; 23: 858-83.

Drug	Doses	Reported severe adverse effects
Amikacin	Intrathecal / intraventricular: Adults: 20 – 30 mg q24h	Transient hearing loss, seizures, aseptic meningitis, and eosinophilic CSF pleocytosis.
Amphotericin B	Intrathecal: Neonates/ children: 0.025 – 0.1 mg q48-72h. May increase to 0.5 mg as tolerated. Adults: 0.2 – 0.5 mg q24-48h	
Colistin	Intrathecal / intraventricular: Adults: 5 – 20 mg colistin base/ day, in 1 or 2 divided doses NB: 5-20mg colistin base/day = 13.3-53.4mg colistimethate sodium (CMS)/ kg/day. Each vial contains 150mg colistin base or 400mg CMS.	Meningeal inflammation. High doses can cause seizures, anorexia, agitation, eosinophilia, edema, pain, and albuminuria.
Daptomycin	Intraventricular: Adults: 5 – 10 mg q72h	Fever
Gentamicin	Intrathecal / intraventricular: Newborns: 1 mg q24h. More than 3 months old: 1 – 2 mg q24h. Adults: 5 – 10 mg q24h	Transient hearing loss, seizures, aseptic meningitis, and eosinophilic CSF pleocytosis.
Streptomycin	Intraventricular: Adults: Up to 1 mg/kg q24 - 48h.	Transient hearing loss, seizures, radiculitis, transverse myelitis, arachnoiditis, and paraplegia.
Tobramycin	Intrathecal / intraventricular: Adults: 5 – 10 mg q24h	Transient hearing loss, seizures, aseptic meningitis, and eosinophilic CSF pleocytosis.
Vancomycin	Intrathecal / intraventricular: Pediatrics: 5 – 10 mg q24h. Adults: 10 – 20 mg q24h.	Transient hearing loss.

β-LACTAM ALLERGY

Incidence:
- 1-10% of patients treated with penicillin will have an adverse reaction, including allergy.
  - 0.01-0.02% of patients treated with parenteral penicillin experience life-threatening anaphylactic reactions to penicillin with a fatality rate of 0.0015-0.02%.
- 1-3% of patients treated with cephalosporins will have an allergic reaction.

History of Penicillin Allergy:
- It is very important to determine:
  - the nature of the patient's reaction, in order to differentiate between allergic and other adverse reactions (e.g. diarrhea, nausea, vomiting, headache), and
  - the onset of the allergic reaction, which will help to classify the reaction (see below). This will help determine whether β-lactam antibiotics can be used. Non-β-lactam alternatives are available for most indications however they may be less effective, more toxic, more broad spectrum, and/or more expensive.
- Less than 10% of patients who report a penicillin allergy actually have an IgE-mediated allergy (skin test positive).
- Mild rash due to aminopenicillins (ampicillin, amoxicillin, pivampicillin) is often caused by a drug-viral interaction, e.g. mononucleosis (Epstein-Barr virus) and is not IgE-mediated.
- 50% and 80% of penicillin allergic patients lose their sensitivity to penicillin after 5 and 10 years, respectively.
  - Positive penicillin skin tests decrease by ~10% per year.
  - ~80-90% of patients with a history of penicillin allergy may no longer react to penicillin.
Therefore, if a patient with a past history of penicillin allergy requires penicillin, skin testing should be considered to determine allergy status. If skin testing is not available:
  - patients with a distant (longer than 10 years) or questionable (e.g. vague childhood rash) reaction history may be candidates to receive penicillin via graded challenge*.
  - patients with a convincing/definite history of an IgE-mediated reaction to penicillin, particularly if recent, should receive alternate non-β-lactam antibiotics, or if alternate antibiotic not available/suitable, penicillin desensitization should be performed prior to penicillin administration.

---

* **Graded challenge**: administration of 1/100 of the therapeutic dose; if no reaction, then 30-60 minutes later give 1/10 of the therapeutic dose, and if no reaction, then 30-60 minutes later, give full therapeutic dose.

β-LACTAM ALLERGY

Classification of β-lactam Allergic Reactions:

Type of Reaction	Clinical Manifestations	Usual Onset
I **Immediate** (IgE-mediated) upon repeat exposure	Anaphylaxis, hypotension, bronchoconstriction, allergic rhinitis, early onset urticaria (hives), laryngeal edema, angioedema	within 1 hour (anaphylaxis) - up to 72 hours
II **Cytotoxic** (IgG, IgM mediated)	Hemolytic anemia, agranulocytosis, leukopenia, thrombocytopenia	> 72 hours
III **Immune Complex**	Serum sickness (cefaclor, cefprozil), drug-induced fever, allergic vasculitis, interstitial nephritis	7-14 days
IV **T - cell mediated** (delayed)	Contact dermatitis, exfoliative dermatitis, maculopapular or morbilliform drug eruptions	> 72 hours

Risk Factors for Penicillin Allergy:

- History of previous reaction to penicillin – Patients are six times more likely to react on subsequent exposure than patients with a negative history.
- Route of administration - More likely with the parenteral route than with the oral route.
- Age - Most common in patients between 20 and 49 years. True penicillin allergy is uncommon in the pediatric population.

NB: Anaphylaxis to β-lactam antibiotics is not genetic, i.e. it does not run in families.

Cross Reactivity:

- Cephalosporins - The incidence of cross reactivity between penicillins and cephalosporins in patients who report a penicillin allergy is ~ 1% (2.55% in those with a confirmed penicillin allergy) and:
  - mostly between penicillins and first-generation cephalosporins, and
  - negligible between penicillins and second-generation (other than cefaclor or cefprozil) and all third and fourth generation cephalosporins.
- Third- and fourth-generation cephalosporins - Less cross reactivity with penicillin than with first and second generation cephalosporins because of their structural (side chain) differences.
- Carbapenems - Cross reactivity with penicillins ~ 1% [Ann Pharmacother 2009; 43:304-15].
- Aztreonam (not commercially available in Canada) – minimal cross reactivity except with ceftazidime and perhaps cefprozil (common side chain).
- The degree of cross reactivity among cephalosporins, and between cephalosporins and carbapenems, is unknown but is thought to be low.

β-LACTAM ALLERGY

- Cross reactivity between β-lactams is related to the similarity of the side chain structure. Each column below represents a group of β-lactams with similar side chains:

amoxicillin	ampicillin	cefprozil	cefotaxime	penicillin G
cefadroxil	cephalexin	aztreonam	ceftriaxone	cefoxitin
cefprozil	cefaclor	ceftazidime	cefepime	

Management of β-Lactam Allergy:

- Avoid all β-lactams (penicillins, cephalosporins, carbapenems) in patients with a documented severe non-IgE-mediated reaction to penicillin such as:
    o interstitial nephritis
    o hepatitis
    o hemolytic anemia
    o serum sickness
    o severe cutaneous reactions (e.g. Stevens-Johnson syndrome (SJS), toxic epidermal necrolysis (TEN), exfoliative dermatitis, acute generalized exanthematous pustulosis (AGEP), drug rash with eosinophilia and systemic symptoms (DRESS)).
- Avoid penicillins and first- (cefadroxil, cephalexin but NOT cefazolin) and second- (cefaclor, cefprozil but NOT cefuroxime) generation cephalosporins in patients with a documented severe IgE-mediated reaction to penicillin, such as:
    o urticaria (hives)
    o laryngeal edema, angioedema.
- Treatment options include:
    1. Alternate non-β-lactam antibiotic
    2. Administration of a third- or fourth-generation cephalosporin or carbapenem via graded challenge*
    3. Administration of a third- or fourth-generation cephalosporin or carbapenem after drug desensitization.

Penicillin administration to patients with a history of cephalosporin allergy:

- In patients with IgE-mediated/immediate-type reaction to a cephalosporin, perform penicillin skin testing if available.
    o if test results are negative, patient may safely receive penicillin
    o if test results are positive, use alternate non-β-lactam antibiotic or perform penicillin desensitization.
  If penicillin skin testing not available, use alternate non-β-lactam antibiotic, or if alternate antibiotic not available/suitable, could consider giving penicillin via graded challenge*.
- In patients with history of non-IgE-mediated reaction to cephalosporin other than severe reaction (interstitial nephritis, hepatitis, hemolytic anemia, serum sickness, cutaneous reactions (e.g. SJS, TEN, exfoliative dermatitis, AGEP, DRESS)), give penicillin via graded challenge*.

Penicillin Skin Testing:

- Indicated in patients who have a reaction history consistent with a possible IgE-mediated mechanism.

β-LACTAM ALLERGY

- 99% effective in predicting penicillin allergic reactions if both the major and minor determinants are used. The major determinant (benzylpenicilloyl-polylysine [PRE-PEN] is commercially available. The minor determinant mixture (penicilloate and penilloate) needed for the test is available via TPD Special Access Program. However, skin testing has several limitations to its use:
  - Only predictive of IgE-mediated allergic reactions to penicillin (not cephalosporins).
  - Skin testing with major determinant and penicillin G 10,000units/mL only may miss up to 20% of allergic patients.
  - Although usually safe, fatalities have occurred when done improperly. Therefore, **penicillin skin testing should only be performed and interpreted by a qualified allergist**.
- Skin testing should NOT be performed for patients with a history of:
  - severe cutaneous reactions (e.g. SJS, TEN, exfoliative dermatitis, AGEP, DRESS)
  - hepatitis
  - hemolytic anemia
  - interstitial nephritis.
- Patients with negative skin test results to penicillin major and minor determinants may receive penicillin with minimal risk of an IgE-mediated reaction.
- Patients with a history of penicillin allergy but negative skin test results are NOT at increased risk for cephalosporin allergy and so may receive these drugs.

Desensitization (temporary induction of drug tolerance):

- Indicated when the patient has a history of IgE-mediated penicillin allergy and/or is skin test positive, and has a serious infection where alternatives to penicillin are not suitable, e.g. syphilis in pregnancy.
- Will **not** prevent non-IgE-mediated reactions.
- Desensitization should never be attempted in patients with a history of reactions involving major organs (e.g. interstitial nephritis, hepatitis, hemolytic anemia, serum sickness, or severe cutaneous reactions (e.g. SJS, TEN, exfoliative dermatitis, AGEP, DRESS).
- Once complete, treatment with penicillin must be started immediately and must not be interrupted.
- **Usually lost within two days after cessation of penicillin therapy**. If penicillin is needed again in the future, desensitization must be repeated, i.e. patient still has an IgE-mediated allergy.
- **Desensitization Protocols:**
  - Oral method of penicillin desensitization (see Wendell GD, et al. N Engl J Med 1985;312:1229-32).
  - Intravenous method of ceftazidime desensitization (see Castells M. Curr Opin Allergy Clin Immunol 2006;6:476-81).
  - Rapid intravenous cephalosporin desensitization (see Win PH, et al. J Allergy Clin Immunol 2005;116:225-8).
  - Intravenous method of meropenem desensitization (see Wilson DL, et al. Ann Pharmacother 2003;37:1424-8).
  - Rapid intravenous method of imipenem desensitization (see Gorman SK, et al. Ann Pharmacother 2003;37:513-6).

RECOMMENDED EMPIRIC THERAPY OF SELECTED INFECTIONS IN NEONATAL/PAEDIATRIC PATIENTS[A]

Infection	Usual Pathogens	Recommended Empiric Therapy	Recommended Dose[B]	Recommended Duration	Comments

Skin & Soft Tissue

Community-associated methicillin-resistant S. aureus (CA-MRSA)

- Incidence of CA-MRSA is significant and in many locations in Canada constitutes > 20% of S. aureus isolates.

- **Screening:**
  Community - nares
  - Active screening to identify MRSA carriers in the community is NOT warranted except in:
    - individuals with recurrent S. aureus skin infections (≥2 episodes in 6 months) despite enhanced hygiene measures, and in whom eradication is being considered.
    - closed community or family setting with recurrent infection despite enhanced hygiene measures.

  Institution - nares and groin
  Controversy exists as to whether to screen select high risk patient groups versus high risk settings (presurgical, ICU, hemodialysis). Regardless, the benefit of active screening and isolation is of unproven benefit without strict adherence to hand hygiene and consistent use of contact precautions.

- **Decolonization:**
  - Decolonization regimens of limited success as recolonization is frequent (up to 75% at one year post decolonization).
  - Success of decolonization is much less if extranasal colonization, presence of active skin infection, or presence of indwelling catheters/tubes.
  - Prolonged/repeated use of mupirocin has led to significant mupirocin resistance.
  Therefore decolonization should only be considered in the following circumstances:
    - recurrent CA-MRSA skin infections (≥ 2 episodes in 6 months) despite enhanced hygiene measures and with no evidence of re-exposure.
    - outbreaks in selected closed communities or family settings despite enhanced hygiene measures
  - Recommended decolonization regimen (only for infants > 1 month old and children):

Mupirocin 2%	bid-tid intranasally	7 days
Chlorhexidine 2-4%	full body wash daily	7 days
2 active systemic antibiotics:		
rifampin	20mg/kg/d PO div bid	7 days
TMP/SMX	6-10mg TMP/kg/d PO div bid	7 days

RECOMMENDED EMPIRIC THERAPY OF SELECTED INFECTIONS IN NEONATAL/PAEDIATRIC PATIENTS[A]

Infection	Usual Pathogens	Recommended Empiric Therapy	Recommended Paediatric Dose[B]	Recommended Duration	Comments
Skin & Soft Tissue					
Impetigo*	*- Superficial non-follicular pustules*				
	Bullous S. aureus Nonbullous, honey crust lesions Group A Streptococci	Limited involvement/ disease **Mupirocin 2%** or **Fusidic acid 2%** Unresponsive to topical or indication for systemic antibiotic** **Cloxacillin** or **Cephalexin** β-lactam allergy **Erythromycin** or **Clindamycin**	 tid topically tid-qid topically 40-50mg/kg/d PO div qid 40mg/kg/d PO div qid 40mg/kg/d PO div qid 20mg/kg/d PO div qid	 7 days 7 days 7 days 7 days 7 days 7 days	- No evidence that disinfecting solutions are of any value. * Epidemics must be reported to Public Health. **Systemic antibiotics recommended if: • < 1 month old • multiple/extensive/recurrent lesions • fever/constitutional symptoms/ lymphadenopathy • immunocompromised • valvular heart disease.
Folliculitis/ Furunculosis	*- Folliculitis - superficial inflammation/infection of hair follicle.* *- Furunculosis - deep infection of multiple hair follicles leading to boils (furuncles).*				
	S. aureus	Hot compresses + Antiseptic cleanser Unresponsive to above or extensive **Mupirocin 2%** or **Fusidic acid 2%**	 tid topically tid-qid topically	 7 days 7 days	- Usually self-limiting. - Recommend incision and drainage of pus, probing cavities to break up loculations, and covering with dry dressing. - Systemic antibiotics recommended if scalp folliculitis (see Carbuncles). - Unresolving furunculosis - consider mycobacterial infections.
Whirlpool/hot tub	Pseudomonas aeruginosa	Hot compresses + Antiseptic cleanser			- Self-limiting in immunocompetent individuals.

- 92 -

RECOMMENDED EMPIRIC THERAPY OF SELECTED INFECTIONS IN NEONATAL/PAEDIATRIC PATIENTS[A]

Infection	Usual Pathogens	Recommended Empiric Therapy	Recommended Paediatric Dose[B]	Recommended Duration	Comments
Skin & Soft Tissue					
Recurrent furunculosis	S. aureus	<u>Consider decolonization:</u> **Mupirocin 2%**	bid intranasally	5 days. Repeat monthly for 1st 5 days/mo x 6-12 mos	- Success rate is low as recolonization is common. May require consultation with Infectious Diseases/ Dermatology.
Carbuncles	S. aureus	<u>Limited disease</u> Hot compresses + Antiseptic cleanser <u>Unresponsive to above or indication for systemic antibiotic*</u> **Cloxacillin** or **Cephalexin** β-lactam allergy **TMP/SMX** (if > 1 month old) or **Clindamycin** MRSA suspected** **TMP/SMX** (if > 1 month old) or **Doxycycline** (if > 8 y.o.)	 40-50mg/kg/d PO div qid 40mg/kg/d PO div qid 8-12mg TMP/kg/d PO div bid 20mg/kg/d PO div qid 8-12mg TMP/kg/d PO div bid 2-4mg/kg/d PO div bid	 7 days 7 days 7 days 7 days 7 days 7 days	- Recommend incision and drainage of pus, probing cavities to break up loculations, and covering with dry dressing. * Systemic antibiotics recommended if: • neonates • immunosuppression/diabetes/ concurrent malignancy • surrounding cellulitis/septic phlebitis. • fever/constitutional symptoms • located in area difficult to drain (face, genitalia). **Increased incidence of community-associated MRSA. Incision and drainage may be all that is required. If antibiotic therapy is deemed necessary, cultures recommended. Check susceptibility of MRSA. Do not use clindamycin empirically for MRSA as significant resistance.

RECOMMENDED EMPIRIC THERAPY OF SELECTED INFECTIONS IN NEONATAL/PAEDIATRIC PATIENTS[A]

Infection	Usual Pathogens	Recommended Empiric Therapy	Recommended Paediatric Dose[B]	Recommended Duration	Comments
Skin & Soft Tissue					
Vesicular lesions Chickenpox	- Notify Public Health. - For contact prophylaxis recommendations, see Prophylaxis for Contacts of Communicable Diseases.				
Immuno-competent	Varicella zoster	≤12 years old See comments >12 years old **Acyclovir**	80mg/kg/d PO div qid	5 days	- Therapy not recommended unless: • chronic cutaneous or pulmonary disorder • long term salicylate therapy • short, intermittent or aerosolized courses of corticosteroids. - Most benefit if initiate acyclovir within 24h of rash onset. - For encephalitis, hepatitis, pneumonitis, use acyclovir **IV** for all ages.
Immunocom-promised	Varicella zoster	**Acyclovir**	30mg/kg/d IV div q8h	7-10 days	
		Disseminated or central nervous system disease **Acyclovir**	60mg/kg/d IV div q8h	7-14 days	

RECOMMENDED EMPIRIC THERAPY OF SELECTED INFECTIONS IN NEONATAL/PAEDIATRIC PATIENTS[A]

Infection	Usual Pathogens	Recommended Empiric Therapy	Recommended Paediatric Dose[B]	Recommended Duration	Comments
Skin & Soft Tissue					
Vesicular lesions (cont'd) **Zoster (Shingles)**	— see below				

- Risk factors: maternal varicella during pregnancy, or primary varicella in first year of life.
- Herpes zoster ophthalmicus - involvement of cranial nerve V_1 occurs in 10-25% of herpes zoster (HZ) cases. Blisters on tip of nose may be seen. Consult ophthalmology.
- Ramsay-Hunt syndrome - severe ear pain, facial muscle weakness, and rash indicates infection of facial nerve. Consult otolaryngologist.
- Immunity is boosted once a person has herpes zoster, so recurrence is uncommon (≤ 5%) in immunocompetent persons.
- Direct contact with the skin lesions of a person with regional/limited herpes zoster, or via airborne route in disseminated zoster, can lead to varicella (chicken pox) in persons who have not had varicella or been immunized.

Infection	Usual Pathogens	Recommended Empiric Therapy	Recommended Paediatric Dose[B]	Recommended Duration	Comments

Immunocom-petent*	Varicella zoster	**Acyclovir***	80mg/kg/d PO div 5x/d	7 days**	- Topical therapy not recommended as ineffective.
					* Therapy recommended if:
					  • ophthalmic involvement
					  • Ramsay-Hunt syndrome
					  • disseminated beyond two dermatomes.
					- Therapy should be started within 72h of rash onset, or at any time if new vesicles forming or cutaneous/motor/neurologic/ocular complications.
					**Treat longer if:
					  • new vesicles forming
					  • cutaneous, motor, neurologic or ocular complications.

RECOMMENDED EMPIRIC THERAPY OF SELECTED INFECTIONS IN NEONATAL/PAEDIATRIC PATIENTS[A]

Infection	Usual Pathogens	Recommended Empiric Therapy	Recommended Paediatric Dose[B]	Recommended Duration	Comments
Skin & Soft Tissue					
Vesicular lesions (cont'd)					
Zoster (Shingles) (cont'd)					
Immunocom-promised	Varicella zoster	Mild **Acyclovir**	80mg/kg/d PO div 5x/d	7-10 days	- Therapy should be started within 72h of rash onset, or at any time if new vesicles forming or cutaneous/ motor/ neurologic/ocular complications.
		Moderate-severe/ Disseminated* **Acyclovir**	60mg/kg/d IV div q8h	7-10 days	* Disseminated herpes zoster: bilateral involvement, spread beyond contiguous dermatomes, or organ involvement (lung, liver, brain).

RECOMMENDED EMPIRIC THERAPY OF SELECTED INFECTIONS IN NEONATAL/PAEDIATRIC PATIENTS[A]

Infection	Usual Pathogens	Recommended Empiric Therapy	Recommended Paediatric Dose[B]	Recommended Duration	Comments
Skin & Soft Tissue					
Vesicular lesions (cont'd)					
Mucocutaneous					
Immunocompetent					
Primary (gingivo-stomatitis)	Herpes simplex	Mild None Severe **Acyclovir**	40-60mg/kg/d PO div 4-5x/d **or** 30mg/kg/d IV div q8h	5-10 days 5-10 days	- Therapy should be started within 72 hours of symptom onset, or at any time if new lesions forming. - Topical therapy not recommended as ineffective.
Recurrent (fever blisters, cold sores)	Herpes simplex	No therapy indicated unless recurrences are: • severe <u>and</u> • > 6 episodes/year can give suppressive therapy: **Acyclovir**	40-60mg/kg/d PO div bid-tid		
Immunocompromised	Herpes simplex	**Acyclovir**	40-60mg/kg/d PO div 5x/d or 30mg/kg/d IV div q8h	7-14 days 7-14 days	

RECOMMENDED EMPIRIC THERAPY OF SELECTED INFECTIONS IN NEONATAL/PAEDIATRIC PATIENTS[A]

Infection	Usual Pathogens	Recommended Empiric Therapy	Recommended Paediatric Dose[B]	Recommended Duration	Comments
Skin & Soft Tissue					

Cellulitis	Cellulitis includes:
	• erysipelas – acute, superficial, nonncrotizing infection of dermis/hypodermis typically caused by streptococci. Classically presents with well defined raised edge/erythematous plaque of sudden onset associated with pain, swelling and fever.
	• cellulitis - acute, subacute or chronic nonncrotizing infection of dermis/ hypodermis that extends into the subcutaneous/connective tissues with/without lymphadenopathy and/or abscess formation.
	Investigations:
	- Superficial skin cultures not recommended.
	  Exceptions
	    • if subcutaneous abscess present: incision and drainage with culture recommended.
	    • if toe web intertrigo: culture of fissures may yield pathogen (β-hemolytic strep/S. aureus/MRSA) to help guide treatment.
	      Also culture for dermatophytes and treat if positive as may be source of bacterial entry/recurrence.
	- Blood cultures recommended if septic, temp ≥ 38.5°C, immunocompromised, or diabetic.
	Management:
	  • Elevate affected area if possible (essential for lower limbs).
	  • If no response to initial antibiotic therapy in 3 days, consider other diagnoses (see Differential Diagnosis in Adult section) and/or change the antibiotic regimen.				

Neonates[†]	S. aureus Group B Streptococci Enterobacteriaceae Group A Streptococci	**Cefazolin** + **Gentamicin**	75mg/kg/d IV div q8h 4-5mg/kg IV q24h	10-14 days	- If meningitis is possible (e.g. fever, lethargy, or poor feeding), do a lumbar puncture and use meningitic doses of cloxacillin + [gentamicin or cefotaxime].
Omphalitis/ Funisitis[†]	S. aureus/MRSA* Group B Streptococci Enterobacteriaceae Group A Streptococci Anaerobes	**Cloxacillin** + **Cefotaxime** + **Metronidazole** MRSA suspected* **Vancomycin**[D] + **Cefotaxime** + **Metronidazole**	200mg/kg/d IV div q6h 200mg/kg/d IV div q6h 30mg/kg/d IV div q12h 60mg/kg/d IV div q6h 200mg/kg/d IV div q6h 30mg/kg/d IV div q12h	10-14 days 10-14 days	- Recommend blood culture. * If mother colonized or infected with MRSA.

† Neonatal doses listed are for term infants > 7 days old. For infants > 7 days old, refer to Neofax or Lexi-Comp or Pediatric Red Book, or consult pharmacy for dosing.
D. Desired vancomycin trough is 15-20mg/L. Monitor renal function closely. See Vancomycin Dosing & Monitoring Guidelines.

RECOMMENDED EMPIRIC THERAPY OF SELECTED INFECTIONS IN NEONATAL/PAEDIATRIC PATIENTS[A]

Infection	Usual Pathogens	Recommended Empiric Therapy	Recommended Paediatric Dose[B]	Recommended Duration	Comments
Skin & Soft Tissue					
Cellulitis (cont'd) **Children** • periorbital • orbital	See Recommended Empiric Therapy of Ophthalmic Infections				
• facial	Group A Streptococci S. aureus	Mild/Afebrile **Cephalexin**	40mg/kg/d PO div qid	7-10 days	
		Moderate-severe < 5 years old: **Cefuroxime**	100-150mg/kg/d IV div q8h	10 days	
	H. influenzae • if < 5 years old	> 5 years old: **Cefazolin**	75mg/kg/d IV div q8h	10 days	
		β-lactam allergy **Clindamycin IV/PO**[C*]	20-40mg/kg/d IV div q8h/ 20-40mg/kg/d PO div qid	7-10 days	* Significant Strep/Staph resistance. Monitor clinical response.
• extremities	Group A Streptococci S. aureus	Mild **Cephalexin**	40mg/kg/d PO div qid	7-10 days	** Extrapolated from adult data.
	For severe infections or those unresponsive to listed empiric therapy, assess for additional risk factors. See Recommended Empiric Therapy of Selected Infections in Adult Patients, Cellulitis, Extremities.	β-lactam allergy **Clindamycin**	20-40mg/kg/d PO div qid	7-10 days	†Give 30 minutes before cefazolin dose.
		Moderate-severe **Cefazolin** or **Clindamycin IV/PO**[C*]	75mg/kg/d IV div q8h 20-40mg/kg/d IV div q8h/ 20-40mg/kg/d PO div qid	10 days 10 days	- Switch to oral agent when: • resolution of systemic symptoms • no further progression of cellulitis.
		Outpatient IV Therapy > 2 years old** consider: **Cefazolin + Probenecid**	100mg/kg/d IV div q12h 40mg/kg/d PO div qid (max 500mg/dose)†	7-10 days	
		or **Ceftriaxone**	50-75mg/kg IV q24h	7-10 days	

- 99 -

RECOMMENDED EMPIRIC THERAPY OF SELECTED INFECTIONS IN NEONATAL/PAEDIATRIC PATIENTS[A]

Infection	Usual Pathogens	Recommended Empiric Therapy	Recommended Paediatric Dose[B]	Recommended Duration	Comments
Skin & Soft Tissue					
Cellulitis (cont'd) **Children** • **extremities** (cont'd)	Group A Streptococci S. aureus For severe infections or those unresponsive to listed empiric therapy, assess for additional risk factors. See Recommended Empiric Therapy of Selected Infections in Adult Patients, Cellulitis, Extremities.	**MRSA suspected/ purulent** Mild I&D if abscess* ± **Cephalexin** + [**TMP/SMX** (if > 1 month old) or **Doxycycline** (if >8 y.o.)] Moderate-Severe I&D if abscess + **Vancomycin**[D]	40mg/kg/d PO div qid 8-12mg TMP/kg/d PO div bid 2-4mg/kg/d PO div bid 60mg/kg/d IV div q6h	7-10 days 10-14 days	* I&D may be all that is required for mild cellulitis. - If systemic symptoms, do blood cultures.

D. Desired vancomycin trough is 15-20mg/L. Monitor renal function closely. See Vancomycin Dosing & Monitoring Guidelines.

RECOMMENDED EMPIRIC THERAPY OF SELECTED INFECTIONS IN NEONATAL/PAEDIATRIC PATIENTS[A]

Infection	Usual Pathogens	Recommended Empiric Therapy	Recommended Paediatric Dose[B]	Recommended Duration	Comments
Skin & Soft Tissue					
Peri-rectal cellulitis/abscess	Polymicrobial: • Group A Streptococci • S. aureus • Anaerobes • Enterobacteriaceae	Mild **Amoxicillin-clavulanate**	40mg/kg/d PO div tid	7-10 days	- Incision/drainage necessary for abscesses.
		Moderate-severe **Clindamycin**[C] + **Gentamicin**	20-40mg/kg/d IV/PO div q8h 7mg/kg IV q24h **or** 7.5mg/kg/d IV div q8h	10 days	
		or **Cefazolin** + **Metronidazole**	75mg/kg/d IV div q8h 30mg/kg/d IV/PO div q12h	10 days	
		MRSA suspected Mild **Amoxicillin-clavulanate** + **TMP/SMX** (if > 1 month old)	40mg/kg/d PO div tid 8-12mg TMP/kg/d PO div bid	7-10 days	
		Moderate-Severe **Vancomycin**[D] + **Ceftriaxone** + **Metronidazole**	60mg/kg/d IV div q6h 50-75mg/kg IV q24h 30mg/kg/d IV div q12h	10 days	

D. Desired vancomycin trough is 15-20mg/L. Monitor renal function closely. See Vancomycin Dosing & Monitoring Guidelines.

RECOMMENDED EMPIRIC THERAPY OF SELECTED INFECTIONS IN NEONATAL/PAEDIATRIC PATIENTS[A]

Infection	Usual Pathogens	Recommended Empiric Therapy	Recommended Paediatric Dose[B]	Recommended Duration	Comments
Skin & Soft Tissue					
Lymphadenitis, infectious Acute For complete list of infectious etiologies, see Recommended Empiric Therapy of Selected Infections in Adult Patients, Lymphadenitis	Cervical • S. aureus • Group A Streptococci • Anaerobes	Mild **Cephalexin**	40mg/kg/d PO div qid	10-14 days	- Surgical drainage of abscess may be required. Bacterial, mycobacterial and fungal cultures recommended.
		Alternative **Clindamycin** or **Amoxicillin-clavulanate**	20-40mg/kg/d PO div qid 40mg/kg/d PO div tid	10-14 days 10-14 days	
		Moderate-Severe **Cefazolin** or **Clindamycin IV/PO**[C]	75mg/kg/d IV div q8h 20-40mg/kg/d IV div q8h/ 20-40mg/kg/d PO div qid	10-14 days 10-14 days	

Animal bites	- If animal unknown or escaped, or unprovoked attack, contact local Public Health or local Medical Officer of Health re: risk/management of rabies.
	- Ensure tetanus status up to date.
	- Irrigation and debridement necessary.
	- Primary closure of wound(s) NOT recommended if: • puncture wounds
	                                                                                              • ≥ 12 hours post injury.
	- Amoxicillin-clavulanate is drug of choice.
	- Cloxacillin/cephalexin/cefazolin, clindamycin, and erythromycin NOT effective against Pasteurella spp or Eikenella spp.
	- Pus/deep wound cultures recommended in established infections.
	- For animal exposures below, consider also: • reptiles – Salmonella spp. Aeromonas spp
	                                                                          • marine animals - Vibrio spp
	
	Infectious Diseases consult recommended.				

RECOMMENDED EMPIRIC THERAPY OF SELECTED INFECTIONS IN NEONATAL/PAEDIATRIC PATIENTS[A]

Infection	Usual Pathogens	Recommended Empiric Therapy	Recommended Paediatric Dose[B]	Recommended Duration	Comments
Skin & Soft Tissue					
Animal bites					
Cats	Polymicrobial: • Pasteurella spp • Streptococcus spp • Staphylococcus spp/ MRSA • Anaerobes • Neisseria spp • Moraxella spp • Corynebacterium spp • Enterococcus spp • Bacillus spp • Bergeyella spp Rare: • Bartonella spp • Francisella tularensis • Yersinia pestis • Sporothrix schenckii	Prophylaxis* **Amoxicillin-clavulanate** Alternative **Cefuroxime axetil** +/- **Metronidazole** β-lactam allergy ≤ 8 years old: **Clindamycin** +/- **TMP/SMX** (if > 1 month old) > 8 years old: **Doxycycline** +/- **Metronidazole**	40mg/kg/d PO div tid 30mg/kg/d PO div bid 15-30mg/kg/d PO div bid 20mg/kg/d PO div tid 8-12mg TMP/kg/d PO div bid 2-4mg/kg/d PO div q12-24h 15-30mg/kg/d PO div bid	3-5 days 3-5 days 3-5 days 3-5 days 3-5 days	* Prophylaxis within 12 hours of bite is recommended for all significant cat bites because of high rate of infection (up to 80%).

RECOMMENDED EMPIRIC THERAPY OF SELECTED INFECTIONS IN NEONATAL/PAEDIATRIC PATIENTS[A]

Infection	Usual Pathogens	Recommended Empiric Therapy	Recommended Paediatric Dose[B]	Recommended Duration	Comments
Skin & Soft Tissue					
Animal bites (cont'd) **Cats** (cont'd)	Polymicrobial: • Pasteurella spp • Streptococcus spp • Staphylococcus spp/ MRSA • Anaerobes • Neisseria spp • Moraxella spp • Corynebacterium spp • Enterococcus spp • Bacillus spp • Bergeyella spp Rare: • Bartonella spp • Francisella tularensis • Yersinia pestis • Sporothrix schenckii	<u>Treatment</u> **Amoxicillin-clavulanate** <u>Alternative</u> **Cefuroxime axetil** +/- **Metronidazole** <u>β-lactam allergy</u> ≤ 8 years old: **Clindamycin** + **TMP/SMX** (if > 1 month old) > 8 years old: **Doxycycline** +/- **Metronidazole** Severe/Limb-threatening **Piperacillin-tazobactam** or **Imipenem**	40mg/kg/d PO div tid 30mg/kg/d PO div bid 15-30mg/kg/d PO div bid 20-40mg/kg/d PO div tid 8-12mg TMP/kg/d PO div bid 2-4mg/kg/d PO div q12-24h 15-30mg/kg/d PO div bid 240-300mg piperacillin/ kg/d IV div q6-8h 60mg/kg/d IV div q6h	7-10 days* 7-10 days* 7-10 days* 7-10 days* 10-14 days* 10-14 days*	* Prolonged therapy is required if associated osteomyelitis (4-6 weeks)/septic arthritis (3-4 weeks).

RECOMMENDED EMPIRIC THERAPY OF SELECTED INFECTIONS IN NEONATAL/PAEDIATRIC PATIENTS[A]

Infection	Usual Pathogens	Recommended Empiric Therapy	Recommended Paediatric Dose[B]	Recommended Duration	Comments
Skin & Soft Tissue					
Animal bites (cont'd) **Dogs**	Polymicrobial: • Pasteurella spp • Streptococcus spp • Staphylococcus spp/MRSA • Anaerobes • Capnocytophaga spp • Eikenella spp • Bergeyella spp • Neisseria spp • Moraxella spp • Corynebacterium spp • Enterococcus spp • Bacillus spp	<u>Prophylaxis*</u> **Amoxicillin-clavulanate** +/- <u>Alternative</u> **Cefuroxime axetil** +/- **Metronidazole** β-lactam allergy ≤ 8 years old: **Clindamycin** + **TMP/SMX** (if > 1 month old) > 8 years old: **Doxycycline** +/- **Metronidazole**	40mg/kg/d PO div tid 30mg/kg/d PO div bid 15-30mg/kg/d PO div bid 20mg/kg/d PO div tid 8-12mg TMP/kg/d PO div bid 2-4mg/kg/d PO div q12-24h 15-30mg/kg/d PO div bid	3-5 days 3-5 days 3-5 days 3-5 days	* Infection rate up to 20%. Prophylaxis within 12 hours of bite is recommended if: • moderate/severe • crush injury/edema • puncture wounds • bone/joint involvement • injuries to hand, foot, face, genitalia • splenectomized patients • immunocompromised patients.

RECOMMENDED EMPIRIC THERAPY OF SELECTED INFECTIONS IN NEONATAL/PAEDIATRIC PATIENTS[A]

Infection	Usual Pathogens	Recommended Empiric Therapy	Recommended Paediatric Dose[B]	Recommended Duration	Comments
Skin & Soft Tissue					
Animal bites (cont'd) **Dogs** (cont'd)	Polymicrobial: • Pasteurella spp • Streptococcus spp • Staphylococcus spp/MRSA • Anaerobes • Capnocytophaga spp • Eikenella spp • Bergeyella spp • Neisseria spp • Moraxella spp • Corynebacterium spp • Enterococcus spp • Bacillus spp	<u>Treatment</u> **Amoxicillin-clavulanate** <u>Alternative</u> **Cefuroxime axetil** +/- **Metronidazole** β-lactam allergy ≤ 8 years old **Clindamycin** + **TMP/SMX** (if > 1 month old) > 8 years old **Doxycycline** +/- **Metronidazole** <u>Severe/Limb-threatening</u> **Piperacillin-tazobactam** or **Imipenem**	40mg/kg/d PO div tid 30mg/kg/d PO div bid 15-30mg/kg/d PO div bid 20-40mg/kg/d PO div tid 8-12mg TMP/kg/d PO div bid 2-4mg/kg/d PO div q12-24h 15-30mg/kg/d PO div bid 240-300mg piperacillin/kg/d IV div q6-8h 60mg/kg/d IV div q6h	7-10 days* 7-10 days* 7-10 days* 7-10 days* 10-14 days* 10-14 days*	* Prolonged therapy is required if associated osteomyelitis (4-6 weeks)/septic arthritis (3-4 weeks).

RECOMMENDED EMPIRIC THERAPY OF SELECTED INFECTIONS IN NEONATAL/PAEDIATRIC PATIENTS[A]

Infection	Usual Pathogens	Recommended Empiric Therapy	Recommended Paediatric Dose[B]	Recommended Duration	Comments
Skin & Soft Tissue					

Human bites	- Irrigation and debridement necessary.
	- Immobilization and wound elevation, if possible, are beneficial.
	- HIV and Hepatitis B & C have very rarely been transmitted by human bites. Assessment of risk factors and relevant management should be considered.
	- Risk factors for developing osteomyelitis:
	  • delay in initial treatment
	  • inadequate debridement
	  • primary closure of wound.
	- Amoxicillin-clavulanate is drug of choice.
	- Cloxacillin/cephalexin/cefazolin, clindamycin, and macrolides NOT effective against Eikenella spp.
	- Pus/deep wound cultures recommended in established infections.				

	Polymicrobial: • Streptococcus spp • S. aureus/MRSA • Eikenella spp • Haemophilus spp • Anaerobes	Prophylaxis:* **Amoxicillin-clavulanate** Alternative **Cefuroxime axetil** +/- **Metronidazole** β-lactam allergy ≤ 8 years old: **Clindamycin** + **TMP/SMX** (if > 1 month old) > 8 years old: **Doxycycline** +/- **Metronidazole**	40mg/kg/d PO div tid 30mg/kg/d PO div bid 15-30mg/kg/d PO div bid 20mg/kg/d PO div tid 8-12mg TMP/kg/d PO div bid 2-4mg/kg/d PO div q12-24h 15-30mg/kg/d PO div bid	3-5 days 3-5 days 3-5 days 3-5 days	* Infection rate up to 50%. Prophylaxis within 12 hours of bite is recommended if: • moderate/severe • crush injury/edema • puncture wounds • bone/joint involvement • hand injuries.

RECOMMENDED EMPIRIC THERAPY OF SELECTED INFECTIONS IN NEONATAL/PAEDIATRIC PATIENTS[A]

Infection	Usual Pathogens	Recommended Empiric Therapy	Recommended Paediatric Dose[B]	Recommended Duration	Comments
Skin & Soft Tissue					
Human bites (cont'd)	Polymicrobial: • Streptococcus spp • S. aureus/MRSA • Eikenella spp • Haemophilus spp • Anaerobes	Treatment **Amoxicillin-clavulanate** Alternative **Cefuroxime axetil** +/- **Metronidazole** β-lactam allergy ≤ 8 years old: **Clindamycin** + **TMP/SMX** (if > 1 month old) > 8 years old: **Doxycycline** +/- **Metronidazole** Severe/Limb-threatening **Piperacillin-tazobactam** or **Imipenem**	40mg/kg/d PO div tid 30mg/kg/d PO div bid 15-30mg/kg/d PO div bid 20-40mg/kg/d PO div tid 8-12mg TMP/kg/d PO div bid 2-4mg/kg/d PO div q12-24h 15-30mg/kg/d PO div bid 240-300mg piperacillin/ kg/d IV div q6-8h 60mg/kg/d IV div q6h	7-10 days* 7-10 days* 7-10 days* 7-10 days* 10-14 days* 10-14 days*	* Prolonged therapy is required if associated osteomyelitis (4-6 weeks)/septic arthritis (3-4 weeks).

RECOMMENDED EMPIRIC THERAPY OF SELECTED INFECTIONS IN NEONATAL/PAEDIATRIC PATIENTS[A]

Infection	Usual Pathogens	Recommended Empiric Therapy	Recommended Paediatric Dose[B]	Recommended Duration	Comments
Skin & Soft Tissue					
Scabies	Sarcoptes scabiei (subsp hominis)	**Permethrin 5% cream** (Nix®)	<u>Infants</u> Apply on head and body, wash off in 8-14 hours <u>Children</u> Apply over entire body below the head, wash off in 8-14 hours	one application*	- Scabies can affect the head/scalp of infants and young toddlers. - Treatment of entire household recommended. - Wash clothes and bedding. Use hot water (> 50°C) and dry on hot cycle. If item cannot be washed, store in plastic bags for 3-7 days. Vacuum mattresses. * Pruritus may persist for several weeks even with successful treatment. Retreat after 1 week if no clinical improvement. - Lindane has been discontinued from the Canadian market (Feb 2012) as it is a persistent organic pollutant. **Must be obtained through the TPD Special Access Program (Emergency Release). Contact pharmacy for assistance in ordering.
		<u>Alternative</u> **Crotamiton 10% cream** or	Apply hs for 2 nights, wash off 24 hours after last application	two applications*	
		Ivermectin**	200µg/kg PO	1 dose. May be repeated in 2 weeks.	

RECOMMENDED EMPIRIC THERAPY OF SELECTED INFECTIONS IN NEONATAL/PAEDIATRIC PATIENTS[A]

Infection	Usual Pathogens	Recommended Empiric Therapy	Recommended Paediatric Dose[B]	Recommended Duration	Comments
Skin & Soft Tissue					
Lice	- Hair length, hair hygiene, socioeconomic status, and overall personal hygiene have little impact on risk of lice infestation. - Shaving the head is not generally recommended. - Children can attend school after their first shampoo treatment.				
	Pediculus humanus capitis	**Permethrin 1% creme rinse** (Nix®) *Alternative* **Isopropyl myristate 50%*** (Resultz®) or **Dimeticone 50%*** (NYDA®) or **Pyrethrin 0.33%-piperonyl butoxide 3% shampoo** (R&C®) *Treatment failure* Reapply shampoo treatment making sure to carefully follow product directions.	Apply, wash off after 10 minutes. Apply, wash off after 10 minutes. Apply, after 30 minutes, comb hair with lice comb and allow solution to dry on hair for at least 8 hours and then wash off. Apply, wash off after 10 minutes.	Apply on day 1 and day 8 Apply on day 1 and day 8 Apply on day 1 and day 8 Apply on day 1 and day 8	- Lindane has been discontinued from the Canadian market (Feb 2012) as it is a persistent organic pollutant. - Wash clothes, bedding, toys that are slept with, and fomites in hot water (>50°C) and dry on hot cycle. If item can not be washed, store in plastic bags for 7 days. Only items that have been in contact with the head of the person with lice within 24-48 hours prior to treatment need to be cleaned. Vacuum mattresses. * Not recommended for children < 2 years old. - In recalcitrant cases, mechanical removal may be only option.

RECOMMENDED EMPIRIC THERAPY OF SELECTED INFECTIONS IN NEONATAL/PAEDIATRIC PATIENTS[A]

Infection	Usual Pathogens	Recommended Empiric Therapy	Recommended Paediatric Dose[B]	Recommended Duration	Comments
Skin & Soft Tissue					
Post-operative wounds		- Fever in first 48 hours post-op unlikely to represent wound infection. Most important therapy for surgical site infections (SSIs) is to open the incision, drain pus, and continue dressing changes until wound heals by secondary intention. There is little evidence to support the use of antibiotics in mild SSIs. - Cellulitis within 24 hours postoperatively usually due to Group A streptococci or Clostridium spp.			
Involving trunk, neck, head, extremity	S. aureus/MRSA Group A Streptococci	**Mild*** - temp < 38.5°C and pulse < 100/min: **Local management** **No antibiotics required.** - temp > 38.5°C or pulse > 100/min: **Cephalexin****			* Minimal erythema/ induration **If previous (prior 12 months)/current MRSA colonization or infection, or high endemic rate of MRSA, add TMP/SMX (if > 1 month old). ***Switch to oral therapy after 48-72h if clinical improvement.
			40mg/kg/d PO div qid	24-48 hours	
		β-lactam allergy **Clindamycin****	20mg/kg/d PO div qid	24-48 hours	
		Moderate-severe* **Cefazolin**	75mg/kg/d IV div q8h	7-10 days	
		β-lactam allergy/MRSA suspected **Vancomycin**[D]	60mg/kg/d IV div q6h	7-10 days	

D. Desired vancomycin trough is 15-20mg/L. Monitor renal function closely. See Vancomycin Dosing & Monitoring Guidelines.

RECOMMENDED EMPIRIC THERAPY OF SELECTED INFECTIONS IN NEONATAL/PAEDIATRIC PATIENTS[A]

Infection	Usual Pathogens	Recommended Empiric Therapy	Recommended Paediatric Dose[B]	Recommended Duration	Comments
Skin & Soft Tissue					
Post-operative wounds (cont'd) **Involving perineum, GI tract, female genital tract, axilla**	Polymicrobial: • S. aureus/MRSA • Group A Streptococci • Enterobacteriaceae • Anaerobes Occasionally: • Enterococcus spp • Pseudomonas spp	Mild **Amoxicillin-clavulanate***	40mg/kg/d PO div tid	10-14 days	- Surgical drainage may be indicated. - Anaerobic coverage is recommended. - **Cephalosporins and clindamycin do not cover Enterococcus spp.** * If previous (prior 12 months)/current MRSA colonization or infection, or high endemic rate of MRSA, add TMP/SMX (if > 1 month old).
		Moderate-severe* **Clindamycin**[C] +/- **Gentamicin**	20-40mg/kg/d IV div q8h 7mg/kg IV q24h **or** 7.5mg/kg/d IV div q8h	10-14 days	
		or **Cefazolin** + **Metronidazole**[C]	75mg/kg/d IV div q8h 30mg/kg/d IV div q12h	10-14 days	
		Severe **Piperacillin-tazobactam**	240-300mg piperacillin/ kg/d IV div q6-8h	10-14 days	
		Severe and MRSA suspected **Piperacillin-tazobactam** + **Vancomycin**[D]	240-300mg piperacillin/ kg/d IV div q6-8h 60mg/kg/d IV div q6h	10-14 days	

D. Desired vancomycin trough is 15-20mg/L. Monitor renal function closely. See Vancomycin Dosing & Monitoring Guidelines.

Infection	Usual Pathogens	Recommended Empiric Therapy	Recommended Dose[B]	Recommended Duration	Comments
Skin & Soft Tissue					
Rapidly progressive skin & soft tissue infections	Predisposing factors • trauma/surgery • immunosuppression/malignancy • diabetes • chronic renal/hepatic disease • chicken pox • IVDU Clinical Findings Early: • pain out of proportion to appearance • swelling • cellulitis • fever • tachycardia • induration • areas of anaesthesia in affected skin Late: • severe pain • skin discoloration (purple or black) • blistering • hemorrhagic bullae • crepitus • "dishwater" gray drainage • systemic inflammatory response syndrome (SIRS)/sepsis • multi-organ failure/shock Management - Surgical debridement and irrigation are essential. Send specimens for culture. - Infectious Diseases consult strongly recommended. - Duration of therapy (IV/PO) dependent on clinical picture.				

RECOMMENDED EMPIRIC THERAPY OF SELECTED INFECTIONS IN NEONATAL/PAEDIATRIC PATIENTS[A]

Infection	Usual Pathogens	Recommended Empiric Therapy	Recommended Paediatric Dose[B]	Recommended Duration	Comments
Skin & Soft Tissue					
Rapidly progressive skin/soft tissue infections (cont'd)	S. pyogenes (Group A Strep) Rare: • S. agalactiae (Grp B Strep) • Grp C,G Streptococci • S. pneumoniae • S. aureus/MRSA • Clostridium spp • Mixed aerobic/anaerobic organisms • Vibrio vulnificus (salt water exposure) • Aeromonas hydrophila (fresh water exposure) • Enterobacteriaceae (chronic hepatic/renal disease) • P. aeruginosa (neutropenia, burns, IVDU)	**Clindamycin* + Ceftriaxone** <u>Polymicrobial or MRSA suspected</u> [**Linezolid***] or **Vancomycin**[D]] + **Piperacillin-tazobactam**	40mg/kg/d IV div q8h 100mg/kg IV q24h < 5 y.o.:30mg/kg/d IV/PO div q8h > 5 y.o.:20mg/kg/d IV/PO div q12h 60mg/kg/d IV div q6h 300mg piperacillin/kg/d IV div q6-8h	minimum 10 days minimum 10 days	- On initial presentation it may be difficult to determine etiologic agent(s). * Inhibits toxin production of Streptococcal spp, Staphylococcal spp and Clostridium spp.

D. Desired vancomycin trough is 15-20mg/L. Monitor renal function closely. See Vancomycin Dosing & Monitoring Guidelines.

RECOMMENDED EMPIRIC THERAPY OF SELECTED INFECTIONS IN NEONATAL/PAEDIATRIC PATIENTS[A]

Infection	Usual Pathogens	Recommended Empiric Therapy	Recommended Paediatric Dose[B]	Recommended Duration	Comments
Skin & Soft Tissue					
Rapidly progressive skin/soft tissue infections (cont'd) **Necrotizing fasciitis/ myositis**		- Use of IV immune globulin (1g/kg/day x 2 days) could be considered if streptococcal toxic shock also present.			
	S. pyogenes (Group A Strep)	**Clindamycin*** + **Penicillin**	40mg/kg/d IV div q8h 300,000 units/kg/d IV div q4h	minimum 10 days	- Invasive Group A Streptococci is reportable to Public Health. - Prophylaxis of contacts of invasive Group A Streptococci is recommended by most Public Health experts. See Prophylaxis for Contacts of Communicable Diseases. *Inhibits toxin production of Streptococcal spp.
	S. agalactiae (Group B Strep) Group C, G Strep S. pneumoniae	**Clindamycin*** + **Ceftriaxone**	40mg/kg/d IV div q8h 100mg/kg IV q24h	minimum 10 days	*Inhibits toxin production of Streptococcal spp. **If penicillin MIC ≤ 0.12 μg/mL, switch ceftriaxone to penicillin.
	Methicillin-susceptible S. aureus (MSSA)	**Clindamycin*** + **Cloxacillin**	40mg/kg/d IV div q8h 200mg/kg/d IV div q4h	minimum 10 days	*Inhibits toxin production of Staphylococcal spp.

RECOMMENDED EMPIRIC THERAPY OF SELECTED INFECTIONS IN NEONATAL/PAEDIATRIC PATIENTS[A]

Infection	Usual Pathogens	Recommended Empiric Therapy	Recommended Paediatric Dose[B]	Recommended Duration	Comments
Skin & Soft Tissue					
Rapidly progressive skin/soft tissue infections (cont'd)					
Necrotizing fasciitis/ myositis (cont'd)	MRSA	**Vancomycin**[D]	60mg/kg/d IV div q6h	minimum 10 days	[T] Clindamycin and linezolid inhibit toxin production of Staphylococcal spp. * Ensure MRSA is susceptible to clindamycin.
		<u>Alternative</u> **Linezolid**[T]	< 5 y.o.:30mg/kg/d IV/PO div q8h > 5 y.o.:20mg/kg/d IV/PO div q12h	minimum 10 days	
		or **Clindamycin**[*T]	40mg/kg/d IV div q8h	minimum 10 days	

D. Desired vancomycin trough is 15-20mg/L. Monitor renal function closely. See Vancomycin Dosing & Monitoring Guidelines.

RECOMMENDED EMPIRIC THERAPY OF SELECTED INFECTIONS IN NEONATAL/PAEDIATRIC PATIENTS[A]

Infection	Usual Pathogens	Recommended Empiric Therapy	Recommended Paediatric Dose[B]	Recommended Duration	Comments
Bone & Joint					

Osteomyelitis	Investigations:
	• Blood cultures recommended. If positive, repeat blood cultures to ensure clearance of bacteremia.
	• CBC and differential, serum creatinine.
	• ESR, CRP (may be useful to follow response but normal initial values do not exclude diagnosis).
	• Plain x-ray +/- MRI, or bone scan +/- WBC scan
	   o MRI superior to x-ray and bone scan for early diagnosis of bone/joint infections
	   o bone scan may be falsely positive if recent trauma/aspiration of joint/superficial infection
	Therapy:
	- Clindamycin achieves excellent bone penetration and is a good agent for osteomyelitis if organism susceptible. However due to high resistance rates, not recommended empirically.				

Neonates[†]	S. aureus Group A, B Strep Enterobacteriaceae	**Cloxacillin** + **Cefotaxime** <u>Neonate/mother colonized with MRSA</u> **Vancomycin**[D] + **Cefotaxime**	200mg/kg/d IV div q6h 200mg/kg/d IV div q6h 45mg/kg/d IV div q8h 200mg/kg/d IV div q6h	4-6 weeks 4-6 weeks	- Bone cultures recommended as occasionally other organisms may be involved. - If meningitis is possible (e.g. fever, lethargy, or poor feeding), recommend lumbar puncture.

† Neonatal doses listed are for term infants > 7 days old. For neonates outside of this range, refer to Neofax or Lexi-Comp or Pediatric Red Book, or consult pharmacy for dosing.
D. Desired vancomycin trough is 15-20mg/L. Monitor renal function closely. See Vancomycin Dosing & Monitoring Guidelines.

RECOMMENDED EMPIRIC THERAPY OF SELECTED INFECTIONS IN NEONATAL/PAEDIATRIC PATIENTS[A]

Infection	Usual Pathogens	Recommended Empiric Therapy	Recommended Paediatric Dose[B]	Recommended Duration	Comments
Bone & Joint					
Osteomyelitis (cont'd) **Children**	S. aureus/MRSA Others: • Group A Streptococci • S. pneumoniae • H. influenzae • Kingella spp (< 4 y.o.) • Anaerobes	**Cloxacillin** Stepdown **Cloxacillin** or **Cephalexin** If MRSA colonized **Vancomycin**[D] +/- **Rifampin**[‡]	200mg/kg/d IV div q6h 100mg/kg/d PO div q6h 100mg/kg/d PO div q6h 60mg/kg/d IV div q6h 10-20mg/kg/d PO div q12-24h	4-6 weeks to complete 4-6 weeks 4-6 weeks ‡ If no debridement, consider adding rifampin.	- Surgical debridement and drainage of associated soft tissue abscesses recommended. - If unresponsive to cloxacillin IV after 3-5 days, consider: • bone biopsy for pathology and cultures • Infectious Diseases consult. - Consider change to oral therapy if: ⇒ at least 5 days of IV antibiotics ⇒ clinically well ⇒ falling ESR or CRP ⇒ compliance of patient and parents guaranteed. - Clindamycin can be used if: • bacteremia cleared • no intravascular infection AND • documented susceptibility to clindamycin.
• with sickle cell anemia	S. aureus Salmonella spp	**Cloxacillin + Ceftriaxone***	200mg/kg/d IV div q6h 100mg/kg IV q24h	4-6 weeks	* Ceftriaxone preferred over cefotaxime for Salmonella infections.

D. Desired vancomycin trough is 15-20mg/L. Monitor renal function closely. See Vancomycin Dosing & Monitoring Guidelines.

RECOMMENDED EMPIRIC THERAPY OF SELECTED INFECTIONS IN NEONATAL/PAEDIATRIC PATIENTS[A]

Infection	Usual Pathogens	Recommended Empiric Therapy	Recommended Paediatric Dose[B]	Recommended Duration	Comments
Bone & Joint					
Osteomyelitis (cont'd)					
Post-operative	S. aureus/MRSA Group A Streptococci Occasionally: • Enterobacteriaceae	**Cefazolin** +/- **Gentamicin*** MRSA colonized or high endemic rate **Vancomycin**[D] +/- **Gentamicin**	100mg/kg/d IV div q8h 7mg/kg IV q24h **or** 7.5mg/kg/d IV div q8h 60mg/kg/d IV div q6h 7mg/kg IV q24h **or** 7.5mg/kg/d IV div q8h	6 weeks 6 weeks	- All require surgical debridement for therapy and C&S of bone. - Hardware should be removed if possible. If not possible, consider adding rifampin if S. aureus/MRSA. * Gentamicin recommended for empiric Gram negative coverage. Discontinue if Gram positive infection confirmed.
• spinal rods	S. aureus Coagulase negative Staph Group A Streptococcus Enterobacteriaceae P. aeruginosa	**Cefazolin** (pending cultures) + **Gentamicin** Severely ill **Piperacillin- tazobactam** +/- **Tobramycin** MRSA colonized Add **Vancomycin**[D] to above regimens	100mg/kg/d IV div q8h 7mg/kg IV q24h **or** 7.5mg/kg/d IV div q8h 240-300mg piperacillin/ kg/d IV div q6-8h 7mg/kg IV q24h **or** 7.5mg/kg/d IV div q8h 60mg/kg/d IV div q6h	6 weeks 6 weeks	

D. Desired vancomycin trough is 15-20mg/L. Monitor renal function closely. See Vancomycin Dosing & Monitoring Guidelines.

Infection	Usual Pathogens	Recommended Empiric Therapy	Recommended Paediatric Dose[B]	Recommended Duration	Comments
Bone & Joint					
Osteomyelitis					
Post-operative (cont'd)					
•**mediastinitis /sternotomy**	S. aureus Enterobacteriaceae Coagulase negative Staph Occasionally: • Candida spp • P. aeruginosa	**Cefazolin** (pending cultures) + **Gentamicin** Severely ill **Piperacillin/ tazobactam** +/- **Tobramycin** MRSA colonized Add **Vancomycin**[D] to above regimens	100mg/kg/d IV div q8h 7mg/kg IV q24h **or** 7.5mg/kg/d IV div q8h 240-300mg piperacillin/ kg/d IV div q6-8h 7mg/kg IV q24h **or** 7.5mg/kg/d IV div q8h 60mg/kg/d IV div q6h	≥ 4 weeks ≥ 4 weeks	
Post-nail puncture of foot	Pseudomonas aeruginosa S. aureus	Mild-moderate **Ciprofloxacin*** +/- **Clindamycin** Severe/systemic symptoms **Piperacillin-tazobactam**	20-30mg/kg/d PO div bid 30-40mg/kg/d PO div qid 240-300mg piperacillin/ kg/d IV div q6-8h	7-14 days 7-14 days	- All require surgical debridement for therapy and C&S. - Tetanus prophylaxis recommended. * Use ciprofloxacin alone if only P. aeruginosa cultured.

D. Desired vancomycin trough is 15-20mg/L. Monitor renal function closely. See Vancomycin Dosing & Monitoring Guidelines.

RECOMMENDED EMPIRIC THERAPY OF SELECTED INFECTIONS IN NEONATAL/PAEDIATRIC PATIENTS[A]

Infection	Usual Pathogens	Recommended Empiric Therapy	Recommended Paediatric Dose[B]	Recommended Duration	Comments
Bone & Joint					

Septic arthritis		*Investigations:*
		• Blood cultures recommended. If positive, repeat blood cultures to ensure clearance of bacteremia.
		• Synovial fluid for cell count and C&S (fluid can be injected into paediatric blood culture bottle). NB: Gram stain lacks sensitivity; whereas culture is more sensitive. Tailor antibiotics according to Gram stain and subsequent C&S results. Typical findings of septic arthritis: purulence, variable viscosity, WBC > 50 x 10⁹/L with > 75% neutrophils. NB: protein and glucose levels are not diagnostically useful.
		• CBC and differential, serum creatinine.
		• ESR, CRP - low sensitivity for diagnosis but if initially elevated, may be useful to monitor response.
		• Plain x-ray +/- bone scan/MRI
		   ○ MRI superior to x-ray and bone scan for early diagnosis of bone/joint infections
		   ○ Bone scan may be falsely positive if recent trauma/aspiration of joint/superficial infection
		- Drainage and/or debridement of the joint space recommended.
		- If fever, lethargy, or poor feeding in the neonate, recommend lumbar puncture to rule out meningitis.
		- Specialist consult is recommended.			

Neonates[†]	S. aureus Group B Streptococci Enterobacteriaceae	**Cloxacillin + Cefotaxime**	200mg/kg/d IV div q6h 200mg/kg/d IV div q6h	3-4 weeks	

[†] Neonatal doses listed are for term infants > 7 days old. For neonates outside of this range, refer to Neofax or Lexi-Comp or Pediatric Red Book, or consult pharmacy for dosing.

RECOMMENDED EMPIRIC THERAPY OF SELECTED INFECTIONS IN NEONATAL/PAEDIATRIC PATIENTS[A]

Infection	Usual Pathogens	Recommended Empiric Therapy	Recommended Paediatric Dose[B]	Recommended Duration	Comments
Bone & Joint					
Septic arthritis (cont'd) **Children**	S. aureus* Streptococcus spp Rare: • Haemophilus influenzae • Kingella kingae (< 2 y.o.)	<u>< 5 years old</u> **Cefuroxime** <u>> 5 years old</u> **Cloxacillin** or **Cefazolin** If MRSA colonized **Vancomycin**[D] +/- **Rifampin**	150mg/kg/d IV div q8h 200mg/kg/d IV div q6h 100mg/kg/d IV div q8h 60mg/kg/d IV div q6h 10-20mg/kg/d PO div q12-24h	3 weeks‡** 3 weeks‡* 3 weeks‡* 3-4 weeks‡	‡ Can switch to oral therapy with clinical improvement. * Consult Infectious Diseases if a shorter course of therapy (e.g. 10 days; 2-4 days IV, rest high dose oral) is being considered AND the following factors are present: • joint drainage has been performed • clinical improvement • resolution of fever • normalization of CRP • known organism and susceptibility • compliance of patient and parents guaranteed.
• **Sexually active**	S. aureus Streptococcus spp N. gonorrhoeae*	**Ceftriaxone** + **Cloxacillin**	50mg/kg IV q24h 200mg/kg/d IV div q6h	3 weeks if Staph/Strep** 7 days if gonococcal tenosynovitis/ dermatitis/ polyarthralgia syndrome** 7-14 days for purulent arthritis**	* Testing for HIV and syphilis recommended. Consider concomitant therapy for Chlamydia trachomatis. **Can switch to oral therapy with clinical improvement.

D. Desired vancomycin trough is 15-20mg/L. Monitor renal function closely. See Vancomycin Dosing & Monitoring Guidelines.

RECOMMENDED EMPIRIC THERAPY OF SELECTED INFECTIONS IN NEONATAL/PAEDIATRIC PATIENTS[A]

Infection	Usual Pathogens	Recommended Empiric Therapy	Recommended Paediatric Dose[B]	Recommended Duration	Comments
Bone & Joint					

Septic bursitis	- Absence of pain with joint movement may help differentiate septic bursitis from septic arthritis.
	- Recommend:
	  • Blood cultures if systemically ill
	  • Baseline and follow-up x-rays to rule out bone or joint involvement
	  • Aspirate fluid initially for drainage and C&S, and aspirate daily until fluid sterile and no longer accumulating				

	S. aureus/MRSA*
	Group A Streptococci
		Mild
		Cephalexin or
		Cloxacillin
		
		MRSA suspected*
		TMP/SMX (if > 1 month old)
		+
		[**Cephalexin** or
		Cloxacillin]
		
		Moderate-severe
		Cefazolin
		or
		Cloxacillin
		
		β-lactam allergy/
		MRSA suspected*
		Vancomycin[D]
			100mg/kg/d PO div qid
			100mg/kg/d PO div qid
			
			8-12mg TMP/kg/d PO div q12h
			
			100mg/kg/d PO div qid
			100mg/kg/d PO div qid
			
			100mg/kg/d IV div q8h
			
			150-200mg/kg/d IV div q6h
			
			60mg/kg/d IV div q6h
				All regimens:
				10 days or until 5 days after sterilization of bursa**
					* MRSA risk factors:
					  • recent hospitalization
					  • recent antibiotic use
					  • previous (prior 12 months) MRSA infection/ colonization
					  • household contact of patient with MRSA infection
					  • involvement in contact sports
					  • aboriginal.
					**Longer therapy (2-3 weeks) if immunocompromised or initial symptoms >7 days. In patients who fail to respond to antibiotic therapy and percutaneous drainage, surgical drainage and/or bursectomy may be required.

D. Desired vancomycin trough is 15-20mg/L. Monitor renal function closely. See Vancomycin Dosing & Monitoring Guidelines.

RECOMMENDED EMPIRIC THERAPY OF SELECTED INFECTIONS IN NEONATAL/PAEDIATRIC PATIENTS[A]

Infection	Usual Pathogens	Recommended Empiric Therapy	Recommended Paediatric Dose[B]	Recommended Duration	Comments
Respiratory					

Pharyngitis					Etiology
					- **Majority of cases (> 70%) of pharyngitis are of viral etiology and do not require antimicrobial therapy.**
					- Group A Streptococcus (GAS) is most common bacterial cause of pharyngitis.
					- Occasionally pharyngitis is caused by Group C or G Streptococci, or Arcanobacterium haemolyticum. A. haemolyticum causes pharyngitis in young adults (12-30 years old); majority of patients have scarlatiniform rash most marked on the extremities. Notify laboratory if clinically suspected as culture requires prolonged incubation.
					- If sexually active, consider N. gonorrhoeae. For treatment, see Adult Empiric Therapy Recommendations, Pharyngitis.
					
					Clinical presentation
					- The following suggests a viral etiology: conjunctivitis, cough, hoarseness, rhinorrhea, and/or diarrhea. Patients with these symptoms should not have a throat swab taken for culture or rapid antigen-detection test (RADT).
					- Typical signs/symptoms of GAS pharyngitis:
					    • pharyngeal or tonsillar exudate
					    • fever
					    • tenderness/enlargement of anterior cervical lymph nodes
					    • absence of cough
					Increased risk if exposure to individual with strep throat in previous 2 weeks.
					- Infectious for 2-5 days prior to symptoms.
					- Uncommon in children < 3 years old. It is most common in children between 5-10 years old, and in fall and winter.
					- Consider Lemierre's syndrome (jugular vein suppurative phlebitis) in teenagers/young adults with pharyngitis, persistent fever, and neck pain. Recommend aerobic and anaerobic blood cultures and imaging of neck veins with ultrasound or CT.
					
					Diagnosis
					- Cannot diagnose GAS pharyngitis with symptoms alone (even if all 4 signs/symptoms listed above are present). **Throat swab for culture or rapid antigen-detection test recommended.**
					- Newer RADT have high specificity and much improved sensitivity therefore confirmatory throat culture may no longer be required for negative RADT results.

RECOMMENDED EMPIRIC THERAPY OF SELECTED INFECTIONS IN NEONATAL/PAEDIATRIC PATIENTS[A]

Infection	Usual Pathogens	Recommended Empiric Therapy	Recommended Paediatric Dose[B]	Recommended Duration	Comments
Respiratory					

Pharyngitis (cont'd)	Antibiotic therapy - Awaiting throat culture results before initiating antibiotic therapy remains a reasonable strategy as:
	  • Group A Strep pharyngitis is a self-limited disease (8-10 days)
	  • antibiotic therapy can be delayed for up to 9 days after onset of illness and still prevent acute rheumatic fever
	  • delay in antibiotic therapy may decrease reinfection rates
	  • unnecessary antibiotic use can be avoided in ~50% of patients.
	- Antibiotic therapy decreases: severity of symptoms, duration of symptoms by ~1 day, risk of transmission (after 24h of therapy), and likelihood of suppurative complications and of rheumatic fever.
	- Group A Streptococci:
	  • No in vitro resistance to penicillin
	  • Significant macrolide and clindamycin resistance
	  • TMP/SMX – no activity against Group A Streptococcus
	- Quinolones and broad spectrum cephalosporins NOT indicated in pharyngitis – too broad spectrum, potential to increase resistance.
	
	- **Follow up cultures are not routinely recommended** except if there is:
	  • history of rheumatic fever (increased risk for recurrence)
	  • persistent symptoms
	  • recurrent symptoms.			

RECOMMENDED EMPIRIC THERAPY OF SELECTED INFECTIONS IN NEONATAL/PAEDIATRIC PATIENTS[A]

Infection	Usual Pathogens	Recommended Empiric Therapy	Recommended Paediatric Dose[B]	Recommended Duration	Comments
Respiratory					
Pharyngitis (cont'd) **Acute**	Group A Streptococci	**Penicillin VK** Penicillin allergy **Cephalexin**** or **Clindamycin** or **Azithromycin** or **Clarithromycin**	40mg/kg/d PO div bid 40mg/kg/d PO div bid 20mg/kg/d PO div tid 20mg/kg PO daily 15mg/kg/d PO div bid	10 days* 10 days 10 days 3 days 10 days	* Meta-analysis indicates that 5 days of penicillin therapy is inferior to 10 days of therapy. - If treated empirically (**NOT recommended**), & 48 hour throat swab culture is negative, discontinue antibiotics. **Do not use if anaphylaxis/severe penicillin allergy.
Non-responders (after 72 hours of therapy*) or **Early relapse** (2-7 days post-therapy*)	Group A Streptococci	Non-responders* Change in antibiotic therapy may not be required. Early relapse*† **Clindamycin** or **Azithromycin** or **Clarithromycin**	 20mg/kg/d PO div tid 20mg/kg PO daily 15mg/kg/d PO div bid	 10 days 3 days 10 days	• Consider: • noncompliance • concurrent viral infection in a Group A Strep carrier • suppurative complication of Group A Strep pharyngitis (e.g. peritonsillar, tonsillar, or retropharyngeal abscess). †Early relapse: repeat throat swab necessary – only treat if culture positive for Group A Strep. - Group A Strep resistance to macrolides and clindamycin is significant.

- 126 -

RECOMMENDED EMPIRIC THERAPY OF SELECTED INFECTIONS IN NEONATAL/PAEDIATRIC PATIENTS[A]

Infection	Usual Pathogens	Recommended Empiric Therapy	Recommended Paediatric Dose[B]	Recommended Duration	Comments
Respiratory					
Pharyngitis (cont'd) **Late relapse** **or** **Recurrent***	* Late relapse or recurrence should be confirmed by culture. Consider: • concurrent viral infection in a Group A Strep carrier • new infections with Group A Strep. - **Continuous antibiotic propylaxis is not recommended.**				
	Group A Streptococci	**Clindamycin** or **Amoxicillin-clavulanate** or **Azithromycin** or **Clarithromycin** or **Penicillin VK****	20mg/kg/d PO div tid 40mg/kg/d PO div tid 20mg/kg PO daily 15mg/kg/d PO div bid 40mg/kg/d PO div bid	10 days 10 days 3 days 10 days 10 days	**Although Pen VK should be effective, there is some evidence that antibiotics with activity against β-lactamase producing organisms (e.g. anaerobes) may be superior.
Asymptomatic carrier	- Up to 20% of the paediatric population may carry Group A Strep asymptomatically. Carriage rate is much lower in older adolescents and adults (2.4-3.7%). - Chronic carriers are not significant in the spread of Group A Strep and are at little risk of rheumatic fever. These individuals do not need to be identified or treated.				

Infection	Usual Pathogens	Recommended Empiric Therapy	Recommended Paediatric Dose[B]	Recommended Duration	Comments
Respiratory					
Jugular Vein Septic Phlebitis (Lemierre's Syndrome)	Fusobacterium necrophorum* or Polymicrobial (1/3): • Oral anaerobes • Streptococcus spp	Surgical drainage as appropriate + **Penicillin** + **Metronidazole** β-lactam allergy **Clindamycin** + **Metronidazole*****	150,000-250,000 units/kg/d IV div q4-6h 30mg/kg/d IV div q8h** 30-40mg/kg/d IV div q8h** 30mg/kg/d IV div q8h**	6-12 weeks 6-12 weeks	- Suspect in teenagers with pharyngitis/fever and neck pain/swelling. - May occur as a rare complication of otitis media, tonsillitis, or dental infections. * Organism difficult to grow; notify lab if suspected. **May switch to oral therapy when clinically stable. ***Combination recommended due to increasing clindamycin resistance in oral anaerobes but need for aerobic Strep coverage with clindamycin.
Parapharyngeal space infections*	Polymicrobial: • Anaerobes • Streptococcus spp • Eikenella corrodens	Surgical drainage + **Penicillin** + **Metronidazole** β-lactam allergy **Clindamycin**	150,000-250,000 units/kg/d IV div q4-6h 30mg/kg/d IV div q12h** 30-40mg/kg/d IV div q8h**	10-14 days 10-14 days	- Consult ENT. * Includes sublingual, submandibular (Ludwig's angina), lateral pharyngeal, retropharyngeal, pretracheal infections. **May switch to oral therapy when clinically stable.
Odontogenic	See Recommended Empiric Therapy of Dental Infections				
Retropharyngeal abscess	Group A Streptococci S. aureus Haemophilus spp Anaerobes	**Cloxacillin** + **Ceftriaxone** + **Metronidazole**	200mg/kg/d IV div q6h 100mg/kg/d IV div q24h 30mg/kg/d IV div q12h	Duration dependent on extent and progression of disease.	- Most common in children < 6 years old. - Urgent ENT consult recommended. - May be complicated by progression to contiguous structures.

RECOMMENDED EMPIRIC THERAPY OF SELECTED INFECTIONS IN NEONATAL/PAEDIATRIC PATIENTS[A]

Infection	Usual Pathogens	Recommended Empiric Therapy	Recommended Paediatric Dose[B]	Recommended Duration	Comments
Respiratory					
Epiglottitis	Group A, B, C Streptococci S. pneumoniae S. aureus H. influenzae H. parainfluenzae N. meningitidis	**Ceftriaxone**	50-100mg/kg IV q24h	7-10 days	- If suspected, admit to hospital immediately, call ICU, anaesthesia, and ENT, without distressing the child. - Keep in position of comfort (usually sitting).
		β-lactam allergy **Levofloxacin**	10-20mg/kg/d IV div q12-24h	7-10 days	
Laryngitis	Viruses	**No antibiotic therapy recommended**			
Rhinitis	- Children can have 6-10 viral URTIs per year. - Up to 25% have purulent discolored nasal discharge for as long as 14 days. - Counsel parents/patients on: • importance of handwashing in preventing transmission of RTIs • washing toys that are shared frequently.				
	Viruses (up to 200 different viruses) or Allergic	No antibiotic therapy recommended. **Saline nasal irrigation***			* Saline solutions are available comercially, or can be made at home. Saline solution recipe 125 mL (4 oz or ½ cup) warm distilled or previously boiled/filtered water ¼ tsp non-iodinated salt +/- ¼ tsp baking soda. • Mix well. • Prepare fresh every day. • Position child so that head is slightly back. • Use a medicine dropper to instill 1-2 drops per nostril. • Repeat 4 to 5 times per day. - Decongestants may alleviate symptoms but will not shorten duration of symptoms.

RECOMMENDED EMPIRIC THERAPY OF SELECTED INFECTIONS IN NEONATAL/PAEDIATRIC PATIENTS[A]

Infection	Usual Pathogens	Recommended Empiric Therapy	Recommended Paediatric Dose[B]	Recommended Duration	Comments
Respiratory					

Otitis Media		- It is critical to distinguish between:
		   i) acute otitis media (AOM)
		   ii) myringitis
		   iii) otitis media with effusion (OME)
		
		AOM:
		- AOM is very common in young children. AOM presents with fever, irritability, and otalgia, with a bulging, inflamed tympanic membrane. (The redness and light reflex of a tympanic membrane are nonspecific and often misleading signs.) Acute inflammation with decreased mobility on pneumatoscopic exam confirms diagnosis of AOM. AOM does not always require antibiotics, providing good follow-up is provided.
		- Routine follow-up post-therapy is not necessary for asymptomatic patients. Three month follow-up post-AOM recommended to rule out persistent OME (occurs in 10% of children) and potential risk for hearing loss.
		
		OME:
		- OME is defined as fluid in the middle ear without signs or symptoms of acute inflammation of the eardrum.
		- OME is common. Up to 50% of children will have an effusion for 1 month post AOM. Antibiotic therapy is <u>not</u> required.
		
		- Prophylactic antibiotics not recommended for recurrent AOM.
		- Prevention:
		   • Handwashing
		   • Breastfeeding
		   • Avoidance of environmental tobacco smoke
		   • Avoidance of feeding in a supine, flat position
		   • Decrease pacifier use in children ≥ 6 months old.
		- Decongestants/antihistamines are not routinely recommended in the treatment of AOM (may be of benefit if allergic etiology).			

RECOMMENDED EMPIRIC THERAPY OF SELECTED INFECTIONS IN NEONATAL/PAEDIATRIC PATIENTS[A]

Infection	Usual Pathogens	Recommended Empiric Therapy	Recommended Paediatric Dose[B]	Recommended Duration	Comments
Respiratory					
Otitis Media (cont'd)		- Adequate coverage of S. pneumoniae in AOM is essential. Amoxicillin provides the best coverage of all oral agents used for AOM. Use of pneumococcal vaccines has shifted etiology of AOM such that H. influenzae and M. catarrhalis are more prevalent. Hence, if failure of therapy with amoxicillin, coverage of these organisms is recommended.			
		Antibiotic Therapy			
		Amoxicillin - Drug of choice in AOM as retains the best activity of all oral β-lactam agents against S. pneumoniae, even majority of penicillin-resistant strains. - No activity against β-lactamase (+) H. influenzae, M. catarrhalis			
		Amoxicillin-clavulanate - Drug of choice for failure of high-dose amoxicillin, and used in combination with amoxicillin for high risk patients and those who have failed low dose amoxicillin. - Activity against S. aureus, β-lactamase (+) H. influenzae and M. catarrhalis.			
		Doxycycline - Recommended agent for AOM in β-lactam allergic patients > 8 years of age. - Reasonable activity against S. pneumoniae, S. aureus, and Group A Streptococcus. - Good activity against H. influenzae and M. catarrhalis.			
		Cephalexin - Not recommended in AOM - Poor activity against Pen I/R S. pneumoniae. - No activity against Haemophilus/Moraxella spp.			
		Cefaclor - Not recommended in AOM. - No activity against Pen I/R S. pneumoniae. - Poor activity against Haemophilus influenzae, M. catarrhalis.			
		Cefuroxime axetil/Cefprozil - Not recommended in AOM. - Poor activity against Pen I/R S. pneumoniae and M. catarrhalis. - Increasing resistance of H. influenzae			

Infection	Usual Pathogens	Recommended Empiric Therapy	Recommended Paediatric Dose[B]	Recommended Duration	Comments
Respiratory					
Otitis Media (cont'd)	Antibiotic Therapy (cont'd)				
	Cefixime	- Option in AOM but only in combination with clindamycin. - No activity against Pen I/R S. pneumoniae. - Excellent activity against Haemophilus spp/M. catarrhalis.			
	Ceftriaxone	- May be an option in high risk patients with penicillin allergy, or neonates. NB: Ceftriaxone 50mg/kg IM/IV daily x 3 days recommended (single dose not as effective in eradicating penicillin resistant S. pneumoniae).			
	Clindamycin	- Option in AOM but only in combination with cefixime. - Reasonable activity against S. pneumoniae. - No activity against Haemophilus/Moraxella spp.			
	TMP/SMX	- Not recommended in AOM but may be considered for β-lactam allergic patients if local S. pneumoniae TMP/SMX resistance < 15%. - Significant TMP/SMX resistance in S. pneumoniae and H. influenzae. - No activity against Group A Strep.			
	Macrolides: **Azithromycin** **Clarithromycin** **Erythromycin**	- Not recommended in AOM but may be considered for β-lactam allergic patients if local S. pneumoniae macrolide resistance < 15%. - Poor activity against Haemophilus influenzae. - Significant macrolide resistance in S. pneumoniae and Group A Strep.			
	Levofloxacin	- Not approved for use in children nor recommended in AOM but may be only option in high risk patients with cephalosporin or severe penicillin allergy or patients who have failed amoxicillin plus amoxicillin-clavulanate regimen. - Good activity against most AOM pathogens. S. aureus coverage not optimal.			

RECOMMENDED EMPIRIC THERAPY OF SELECTED INFECTIONS IN NEONATAL/PAEDIATRIC PATIENTS[A]

Infection	Usual Pathogens	Recommended Empiric Therapy	Recommended Paediatric Dose[B]	Recommended Duration	Comments
Respiratory					
Otitis Media (cont'd) - **AOM - High risk***	S. pneumoniae Moraxella catarrhalis H. influenzae Occasionally: • Group A Streptococci • S. aureus	**Amoxicillin** + **Amoxicillin-clavulanate** <u>Penicillin allergy</u> **Ceftriaxone**	45mg/kg/d PO div bid-tid 45mg/kg/d PO div bid-tid *(7:1 - Clavulin-200 or -400)* 50mg/kg IM/IV daily	10 days 3 days	* High risk: <6 months old, immuno-compromised, cranio-facial abnormalities, chronic cardiac or pulmonary disease, Down syndrome, underlying hearing impairment, perforated tympanic membrane

- 133 -

Infection	Usual Pathogens	Recommended Empiric Therapy	Recommended Paediatric Dose[B]	Recommended Duration	Comments
Respiratory					
Otitis Media (cont'd) **AOM - Healthy child, ≥ 6 months old**	S. pneumoniae Moraxella catarrhalis H. influenzae Occasionally: • Group A Streptococci • S. aureus	<u>Mild[†]</u> **Acetaminophen** or **Ibuprofen** <u>Moderate-severe</u> **Amoxicillin** <u>Penicillin allergy ≤ 8 years old</u> **Clindamycin + Cefixime** <u>>8 years old</u> **Doxycycline** <u>Severe penicillin allergy or cephalosporin allergy AND local S. pneumoniae resistance < 15%</u> **Doxycycline** (>8 years old) or **TMP/SMX***** or **Azithromycin***** or **Clarithromycin*****	10-15mg/kg/dose PO q4h prn (max 75mg/kg/day) 10mg/kg/dose PO q6-8h prn (max 40mg/kg/day) Standard dose 40mg/kg/d PO div tid or High dose** 90mg/kg/d PO div bid-tid 20-30mg/kg/d PO div tid 8mg/kg/d PO div bid 4mg/kg/d PO div bid 4mg/kg/d PO bid 8-12mg TMP/kg/d PO div bid 10mg/kg PO daily 15mg/kg/d PO div bid	48 hours 48 hours 5 days* 5 days* 5 days* 5 days* 5 days* 5 days* 5 days* 3 days 5 days*	[†] Mild = nontoxic, temp. <39°C without antipyretics, mild otalgia. - In children ≥ 6 months old, consider withholding antibiotics 48-72 hours from symptom onset if symptoms are manageable with systemic analgesics providing adequate follow-up can be assured and no deterioration. - If symptoms worsen or fail to respond to symptomatic treatment after 48-72 hours, treat with antibiotics. * 10 days recommended if: • < 2 years old • perforated eardrum. **Higher amoxicillin dose recommended if: • < 2 years old and/or • recent (< 3 months) antimicrobial exposure and/or • day care centre attendance. ***Significant resistance in S. pneumoniae.

RECOMMENDED EMPIRIC THERAPY OF SELECTED INFECTIONS IN NEONATAL/PAEDIATRIC PATIENTS[A]

Infection	Usual Pathogens	Recommended Empiric Therapy	Recommended Paediatric Dose[B]	Recommended Duration	Comments
Respiratory					
Otitis Media (cont'd) **AOM - Healthy child, ≥ 6 months old** (cont'd)	S. pneumoniae Moraxella catarrhalis H. influenzae Occasionally: • Group A Streptococci • S. aureus	Moderate-severe (cont'd) Severe penicillin allergy or cephalosporin allergy AND local S. pneumoniae tetracycline/ macrolide/TMP/SMX resistance all > 15% **Levofloxacin**	10-20mg/kg/d PO div q12-24h	5 days*	* 10 days recommended if: • < 2 years old • perforated eardrum.

RECOMMENDED EMPIRIC THERAPY OF SELECTED INFECTIONS IN NEONATAL/PAEDIATRIC PATIENTS[A]

Infection	Usual Pathogens	Recommended Empiric Therapy	Recommended Paediatric Dose[B]	Recommended Duration	Comments
Respiratory					
Otitis Media (cont'd) **AOM – failure of first line agents:** • persistent (still symptomatic at 48 - 72 h)	S. pneumoniae Moraxella catarrhalis H. influenzae Occasionally: • Group A Streptococci • S. aureus	Second line agents: <u>Failure of standard dose amoxicillin*</u> **Amoxicillin PLUS Amoxicillin-clavulanate** (7:1 - Clavulin-200 or -400) <u>Failure of high dose amoxicillin</u> **Amoxicillin-clavulanate** (7:1 - Clavulin-200 or -400) Penicillin allergy **[Clindamycin + Cefixime]** or **Ceftriaxone** Severe penicillin allergy or cephalosporin allergy **Levofloxacin**	45mg/kg/d PO div bid-tid 45mg/kg/d PO div bid-tid 40mg/kg/d PO div bid 20-40mg/kg/d PO div tid 8mg/kg/d PO div bid 50mg/kg IM/IV daily 10-20mg/kg/d PO div q12-24h	10 days 10 days 10 days 10 days 3 days 10 days	* Combination of amoxicillin and amoxicillin-clavulanate recommended to provide high dose of amoxicillin (for pen-I/R S. pneumoniae) and regular dose of amoxicillin-clavulanate for coverage of ampicillin resistant H. influenzae and M. catarrhalis) without excessive clavulanate (> 10mg/kg/day) - which may lead to increased incidence of diarrhea.
AOM – failure of second line agents	S. pneumoniae Moraxella catarrhalis H. influenzae Occasionally: • Group A Strep • S. aureus				- Consider: • I.D. consult • tympanocentesis by an expert.

RECOMMENDED EMPIRIC THERAPY OF SELECTED INFECTIONS IN NEONATAL/PAEDIATRIC PATIENTS[A]

Infection	Usual Pathogens	Recommended Empiric Therapy	Recommended Paediatric Dose[B]	Recommended Duration	Comments
Respiratory					
Otitis Media (cont'd)					
AOM - complicated • mastoiditis • vertigo • facial paralysis	S. pneumoniae Moraxella catarrhalis H. influenzae Occasionally: • Group A Strep • S. aureus	**Early/mild** **Cefuroxime** **Moderate-severe** **Cloxacillin** + **Ceftriaxone**	150mg/kg/d IV div q8h 150-200mg/kg/d IV div q6h 100mg/kg IV daily	≥ 14 days ≥ 14 days	- ENT consult with tympanocentesis +/- more extensive drainage required. - Infectious Diseases consult is strongly recommended.
AOM - recurrent • ≥ 3 episodes in 6 months or • ≥ 4 episodes in 12 months	- Observation over time is reasonable because of a decreasing incidence of AOM with advancing age. - Antibiotic prophylaxis is NO longer recommended. - Consider ENT referral if: • OME for ≥ 3 months with hearing loss ≥ 40 dB • ≥ 3 episodes in 6 months • ≥ 4 episodes in 12 months • retracted tympanic membrane • cleft palate or craniofacial malformations.				
	S. pneumoniae Moraxella catarrhalis H. influenzae Occasionally: • Group A Streptococci • S. aureus	≥ 6 weeks from last episode See AOM – healthy child* < 6 weeks from last episode See AOM - failure of first line agents		10 days	* Use high dose amoxicillin x 10 days.

Infection	Usual Pathogens	Recommended Empiric Therapy	Recommended Paediatric Dose[B]	Recommended Duration	Comments
Respiratory					
Otitis Media (cont'd) **AOM with otorrhea through tympanostomy tubes***	S. pneumoniae H. influenzae S. aureus P. aeruginosa S. epidermidis M. catarrhalis	**Ciprofloxacin/ dexamethasone** (*Ciprodex*)	4 drops bid to affected ear(s)	7 days	* If significant systemic symptoms, add systemic antibiotic - see AOM, recurrent.
Otitis media with effusion (OME)	- Decongestants, antihistamines, corticosteroids, and antibiotics are NOT recommended in the treatment of OME. - Up to 50% of children will have an effusion 1 month post AOM. Further antibiotic therapy not required. Up to 10% of children will have an effusion 3 months post AOM. - Perform hearing test: • in children with OME ≥ 3 months, or • at any time, if speech or language delay, learning problems, significant hearing loss, or structural abnormalities of tympanic membrane, and refer to ENT if hearing loss: • hearing loss >20 dB: comprehensive audiologic evaluation. • hearing loss >40 dB: comprehensive audiologic evaluation + ENT consult. Duration of OME > 3 months and no hearing loss: Observation at 3-6 month intervals until resolution of effusion. **No antibiotics**.				

RECOMMENDED EMPIRIC THERAPY OF SELECTED INFECTIONS IN NEONATAL/PAEDIATRIC PATIENTS[A]

Infection	Usual Pathogens	Recommended Empiric Therapy	Recommended Paediatric Dose[B]	Recommended Duration	Comments
Respiratory					
Otitis externa					
Swimmer's ear		**Prevention** - Consider wearing earplugs during swimming. - After swimming, remove as much water from ears as possible by: • tilting head to allow water to drain from ears • using hair dryer set on low • **if intact eardrum and no ear tubes**, dry ears with a few drops of vinegar +/- rubbing alcohol in each ear after swimming.			
	Pseudomonas aeruginosa Enterobacteriaceae S. aureus[†]	**Aluminum acetate/ benzethonium** (*Buro-Sol*)	2-3 drops tid-qid	max. 7 days*	* If condition persists after 7 days, then re-assess. May require debridement. Consider referral to ENT specialist. **Corticosteroid-containing preparations are useful when there is underlying dermatitis Can use quinolone-containing ear drops in children as minimal systemic absorption. ***Risk of ototoxicity (hearing loss, tinnitus, vertigo, imbalance) if perforated eardrum, ear tubes, or > 7 days therapy. † If severe/acute onset, consider adding cloxacillin 40-50mg/kg/d PO div qid to cover methicillin-susceptible S. aureus or TMP/SMX 8-12mg/kg/d PO bid to cover methicillin-resistant S. aureus.
		Alternative **Gentamicin/betameth-asone** (*Garasone*)*** or	3-4 drops tid	max. 7 days*	
		Framycetin/gramicidin/ dexamethasone (*Sofracort*)*** or	2-3 drops tid-qid	max. 7 days*	
		Ciprofloxacin/dexa-methasone (*Ciprodex*) or	4 drops bid	max. 7 days*	
		Clioquinol/flumethasone (*Locacorten Vioform*)	2-3 drops bid	max. 7 days*	

- 139 -

RECOMMENDED EMPIRIC THERAPY OF SELECTED INFECTIONS IN NEONATAL/PAEDIATRIC PATIENTS[A]

Infection	Usual Pathogens	Recommended Empiric Therapy	Recommended Paediatric Dose[B]	Recommended Duration	Comments
Respiratory					
Otitis externa (cont'd) **Invasive otitis externa**	P. aeruginosa	Surgical debridement + **Piperacillin** + **Tobramycin** <u>Stepdown</u> **Ciprofloxacin**	200-300mg/kg/d IV div q4-6h 7mg/kg IV q24h **or** 7.5mg/kg IV div q8h 20-30mg/kg/d PO div bid	6-8 weeks (IV+PO)	- Most cases occur in diabetics. Extremely rare in children. - CT or MRI scan recommended.

RECOMMENDED EMPIRIC THERAPY OF SELECTED INFECTIONS IN NEONATAL/PAEDIATRIC PATIENTS[A]

Infection	Usual Pathogens	Recommended Empiric Therapy	Recommended Paediatric Dose[B]	Recommended Duration	Comments
Respiratory					

Pertussis (Whooping cough)	- Notify Public Health.
	- For contact prophylaxis recommendations, see Prophylaxis for Contacts of Communicable Diseases.
	
	- Persistent cough (≥ 6 days) in adolescents may indicate whooping cough in up to 32%.
	
	- Typical course of pertussis:
	  1) catarrhal phase - lasts 1-2 weeks; most contagious
	  2) paroxysmal phase - 3-6 weeks. Many children < 6 months of age do not develop paroxysmal cough or inspiratory whoop.
	  3) convalescent phase - > 6 weeks (mean duration of cough is 6 weeks).
	
	<u>Diagnosis</u>
	- cough present for up to 3 weeks - order culture and PCR of posterior nasopharynx (aspirate/swab).
	- cough present > 3 weeks - order PCR (beyond 4 weeks, PCR likely to be negative).
	
	<u>Antibiotic therapy</u>
	- Antibiotic therapy may reduce the duration or severity of symptoms (only if started in catarrhal phase) and limits transmission to susceptible contacts. Because viable organisms can be recovered from untreated patients for 3 weeks after onset of cough, a 5-7 day course of antibiotics is recommended during the first 4 weeks of illness. For individuals likely to be in contact with high risk contacts (infants, pregnant women in 3rd trimester, health care workers, child care workers who care for infants), a 5-7 day course of antibiotics is recommended during the 6-8 weeks after onset of illness.				

	Bordetella pertussis	<u>Treatment</u> **Azithromycin** or **Clarithromycin** or **Erythromycin estolate** <u>Alternative</u> **TMP/SMX** (if > 1 month old)**	10mg/kg PO daily 15mg/kg/d PO div bid 40mg/kg/d PO div qid 8mg TMP/kg/d PO div bid	5 days* 7 days* 7 days* 10 days*	* No longer infectious after 5 days of therapy. **Efficacy not established.

Infection	Usual Pathogens	Recommended Empiric Therapy	Recommended Paediatric Dose[B]	Recommended Duration	Comments
Respiratory					
Croup		- Illness of children younger than 6 years of age with peak incidence at 7-36 months. - Systemic/nebulized corticosteroids have been proven to lessen severity and duration of symptoms, and hospitalization. - Nebulized epinephrine is indicated in severe respiratory distress. - Give blow-by oxygen if hypoxia (O_2 sat < 92% on room air). - Antitussives and decongestants not indicated. Sedation contraindicated.			
	Viruses	**No antibiotic therapy recommended.** **Dexamethasone*** or **Budesonide***	0.6mg/kg PO/IM/IV 2mg in 4mL sterile water via nebulizer	Once. May repeat dose in 24h if symptoms recur.	*Budesonide should be reserved for patients who are vomiting or in severe respiratory distress as less convenient to administer and significantly more expensive than dexamethasone. **Duration of effect 2 hours; observe patient for at least 2 hours before discharge.
		Severe **Racemic epinephrine 2.25%** or **L-epinephrine**	0.5mL in 3mL NS or sterile water via nebulizer 1:1,000 solution - 5mL via nebulizer**	Repeat as necessary.	
Bacterial tracheitis	S. aureus Group A Streptococci H. influenzae	Ceftriaxone	100mg/kg IV q24h	10 days	- Uncommon. Presents as croup, but with more rapid onset and higher fever.

RECOMMENDED EMPIRIC THERAPY OF SELECTED INFECTIONS IN NEONATAL/PAEDIATRIC PATIENTS[A]

Infection	Usual Pathogens	Recommended Empiric Therapy	Recommended Paediatric Dose[B]	Recommended Duration	Comments
Respiratory					

Bronchitis		- Cough in absence of fever, tachypnea, and tachycardia suggests bronchitis rather than pneumonia.
		 - Bacterial bronchitis does NOT occur in children. Only occurs as a part of tracheobronchitis with viral infections.
		 - Green/yellow sputum production is indicative of inflammatory reaction and does not necessarily imply bacterial infection.
		 - Mycoplasma pneumoniae and Chlamydophila pneumoniae have been implicated but not fully established as pathogens in acute bronchitis. Empiric therapy for these organisms is not recommended.
		 - Viral URTI can result in cough >14 days in 20% of children. Prolonged (> 10-14 days) cough may be evaluated for Mycoplasma pneumoniae, Bordetella pertussis, or asthma.
		 - In most patients the respiratory exam is normal (few patients may have wheezes). Chest x-ray is indicated if there is any suspicion of pneumonia on history or physical exam.
		 - Follow-up not recommended unless:
		     • symptoms worsen or new symptoms develop (dyspnea, persistent fever, vomiting)
		     • cough not improving at 14 days or cough lasting > 1 month
		     • symptoms recur (> 3 episodes/year).			

	Viruses	**No antibiotic therapy recommended*** Management: • increased humidity • smoking cessation			* Meta-analyses have shown no benefit of antibiotics in patients with acute bronchitis. However a chronic (>4 weeks duration) wet cough may be indicative of a lower respiratory tract bacterial infection which may respond to antibiotic therapy [Pediatrics 2012;129:e364-9]. - Corticosteroids (inhaled/oral) are not recommended as there is insufficient evidence to support their use. - Expectorants are not recommended; good hydration more effective.

RECOMMENDED EMPIRIC THERAPY OF SELECTED INFECTIONS IN NEONATAL/PAEDIATRIC PATIENTS[A]

Infection	Usual Pathogens	Recommended Empiric Therapy	Recommended Paediatric Dose[B]	Recommended Duration	Comments
Respiratory					

Bronchiolitis	- Viral infection of children < 2 years of age (usually < 12 months of age).
	- Nasopharyngeal (NP) washing/swab for viral detection recommended only in hospitalized patients.
	- DDx includes:
	  • Chlamydia trachomatis (in ≤ 16 weeks old) (consider NP swab for Chlamydia)
	  • Pertussis (consider NP washing for pertussis culture or PCR)
	  • Secondary bacterial pneumonia unusual unless tachypnea and/or consolidation on chest x-ray.				

	Viruses: • RSV • Human meta-pneumovirus • Human bocavirus • Parainfluenza • Influenza • Adenovirus	**No antibiotic therapy recommended** (see Comments)			- Bronchodilators and corticosteroids not routinely recommended. - Ribavirin is NOT recommended.

RECOMMENDED EMPIRIC THERAPY OF SELECTED INFECTIONS IN NEONATAL/PAEDIATRIC PATIENTS[A]

Infection	Usual Pathogens	Recommended Empiric Therapy	Recommended Paediatric Dose[B]	Recommended Duration	Comments
Respiratory					
Sinusitis [Clin Infect Dis 2012;Mar.e1-41.]					- Most common predisposing factor is viral upper respiratory tract infection. Preschool and school age children can have 6-10 viral URTIs per year. Bacterial sinusitis complicates only <5% of these. - The role of Mycoplasma pneumoniae and Chlamydophila pneumoniae in acute sinusitis has been suggested but not substantiated. Empiric therapy for these organisms is not recommended. <u>Common presentation</u> - A bacterial etiology is more likely if: URTI symptoms persist for at least 10 days or worsen after 5-7 days with purulent nasal discharge +/- fever, cough, irritability, lethargy, facial pain. <u>Severe presentation</u> (uncommon) - Severely ill child with fever ≥ 39°C (unresponsive to appropriately dosed antipyretics) and purulent nasal discharge usually associated with facial swelling, sinus tenderness, headache. <u>Diagnosis</u> - The colour of nasal discharge/sputum should not be used to diagnose the sinusitis episode as bacterial since colour is related to presence of neutrophils, not bacteria. - Nasopharyngeal cultures are not helpful in identifying etiological sinus pathogen(s). - Sinus x-rays are not recommended as they will not differentiate between viral URTI and bacterial sinusitis. - CT scan is only recommended for complications of acute sinusitis, chronic sinusitis not responding to treatment, and/or severe presentations where hospitalization is required. - MRI not recommended due to poor bone definition. <u>Management</u> - Adjunctive therapy with short term topical or systemic decongestant in children > 2 years only and/or nasal irrigation with saline solution or steam inhalation may be helpful. Prolonged (> 5 days) use of topical decongestants should be avoided as it may lead to rebound symptoms. NB: Antihistamines and mucolytics have no role in the management of acute sinusitis. - The use of topical (intranasal) corticosteroids is controversial but may offer some benefit, especially in patients with allergic rhinosinusitis.

RECOMMENDED EMPIRIC THERAPY OF SELECTED INFECTIONS IN NEONATAL/PAEDIATRIC PATIENTS[A]

Infection	Usual Pathogens	Recommended Empiric Therapy	Recommended Paediatric Dose[B]	Recommended Duration	Comments
Respiratory					
Sinusitis (cont'd)	Antibiotic Therapy				

- The benefit of antibiotic therapy in sinusitis is controversial (~70% resolve spontaneously).
- Some guidelines recommend high-dose amoxicillin-clavulanate instead of amoxicillin for first line treatment of sinusitis because of high rates of penicillin-resistant S. pneumoniae and β-lactamase producing H. influenzae and M. catarrhalis.

- High-dose amoxicillin remains a reasonable first-line empiric option given:
  - the lower resistance rates in Canada
  - amoxicillin retains best coverage of all oral β-lactam agents against S. pneumoniae (even majority of penicillin-resistant strains)
  - higher incidence of adverse effects of amoxicillin-clavulanate
  - need to limit broad spectrum antibiotic use in order to minimize the development of antibiotic resistance.
- Use of pneumococcal vaccines has shifted etiology of sinusitis such that H. influenzae and M. catarrhalis are more prevalent. Hence, if failure of therapy with amoxicillin, coverage of these organisms is recommended.

- Macrolides, TMP/SMX, and oral cephalosporins are no longer recommended for empiric therapy of sinusitis due to unpredictable/ poor activity against S. pneumoniae and/or H. influenzae.

- Levofloxacin has good coverage of the pathogens involved. However because of its broad spectrum, potential for increasing resistance, and risk of C. difficile infection, it should be reserved for β-lactam allergic patients or patients who have failed first line antibiotic therapy.

Prevention:
- Handwashing
- Avoidance of environmental tobacco smoke
- Reduction of allergen exposure.

RECOMMENDED EMPIRIC THERAPY OF SELECTED INFECTIONS IN NEONATAL/PAEDIATRIC PATIENTS[A]

Infection	Usual Pathogens	Recommended Empiric Therapy	Recommended Paediatric Dose[B]	Recommended Duration	Comments
Respiratory (cont'd)					
Sinusitis **Acute** • symptoms < 4 weeks • ≤ 3 episodes per year	S. pneumoniae M. catarrhalis H. influenzae Occasionally: • S. aureus • Group A Streptococci • Anaerobes	**Amoxicillin***	<u>Standard dose</u> 40mg/kg/d PO tid <u>High dose*</u> 90mg/kg/d PO div bid-tid	10 days 10 days	*Higher amoxicillin dose recommended if: • < 2 years old and/or • recent (< 3 months) antimicrobial exposure and/or • day care centre attendance (extrapolated from AOM data). **Severe = high fever (≥ 39°C) and purulent nasal discharge or facial pain for 3-4 consecutive days.
		<u>Penicillin allergy</u> ≤ 8 years old **Clindamycin +** **Cefixime** > 8 years old **Doxycycline**	20-30mg/kg/d PO div tid 8mg/kg/d PO div bid 4mg/kg/d PO div bid	10 days 10 days	
		<u>Severe**/Immunocompromised</u> **Amoxicillin +** **Amoxicillin-clavulanate** *(7:1 - Clavulin -200 or -400)*	45mg/kg/d PO div bid-tid 45mg/kg/d PO div bid-tid	10 days	
		<u>Nonsevere β-lactam allergy</u> **Ceftriaxone**	100mg/kg IV daily	10 days	
		<u>Severe β-lactam allergy/ anaphylaxis</u> **Levofloxacin*****	10-20mg/kg/d IV/PO div q12-24h	10 days	***Levofloxacin use is justified in this setting as reliable therapeutic options limited.

- 147 -

RECOMMENDED EMPIRIC THERAPY OF SELECTED INFECTIONS IN NEONATAL/PAEDIATRIC PATIENTS[A]

Respiratory

Infection	Usual Pathogens	Recommended Empiric Therapy	Recommended Paediatric Dose[B]	Recommended Duration	Comments
Sinusitis (cont'd)					
Failure of first line agents: • no improvement or clinical deterioration after 72 hours of antibiotic therapy • recurrence within 3 months	S. pneumoniae M. catarrhalis H. influenzae Occasionally: • S. aureus • Group A Streptococci • Anaerobes	**Amoxicillin-clavulanate** *(7:1 - Clavulin-200 or -400)* +/- **Amoxicillin*** Penicillin allergy **[Clindamycin + Cefixime]** or **Ceftriaxone** Severe penicillin allergy or cephalosporin allergy **Levofloxacin**	45mg/kg/d PO div bid-tid 45mg/kg/d PO div bid-tid 20-30mg/kg/d PO div tid 8mg/kg/d PO div bid 100mg/kg IV daily 10-20mg/kg/d PO div q12-24h	10 days 10 days 10 days 10 days 10 days	- Need to consider resistant organisms, especially penicillin-resistant S. pneumoniae and ampicillin resistant H. influenzae. * If patient has failed high dose amoxicillin therapy, amoxicillin-clavulanate used alone is adequate to cover β-lactamase producing organisms.
Hospital acquired					
< 4 days hospitalization	See Sinusitis - Acute				

RECOMMENDED EMPIRIC THERAPY OF SELECTED INFECTIONS IN NEONATAL/PAEDIATRIC PATIENTS[A]

Infection	Usual Pathogens	Recommended Empiric Therapy	Recommended Paediatric Dose[B]	Recommended Duration	Comments
Respiratory					
Sinusitis (cont'd) **Hospital acquired** (cont'd) **≥ 4 days hospitalization**	- Majority of cases occur in second week of hospitalization. - Risk factors: • mechanical ventilation • facial/cranial fractures • nasal packing • nasogastric/nasoendotracheal tubes • otitis media post head trauma • corticosteroid therapy • prior antibiotic use. - Black, necrotic tissue or discharge in patients with poorly controlled diabetes/ketoacidosis, or with significant immunosuppression may indicate mucormycosis. Recommend urgent ENT/ID consult. - **Recommend:** • **Remove nasogastric/nasoendotracheal tube** • **Semi-recumbent (30-45°) positioning** • **Sinus aspiration for C&S:** ⇒ tailor antibiotics to C&S results ⇒ if Pseudomonas/Acinetobacter cultured, consider combination therapy with tobramycin.				
	S. aureus/MRSA* Enterobacteriaceae Occasionally: • Anaerobes • P. aeruginosa • Yeast	**Ceftriaxone + Gentamicin**	100mg/kg IV daily 7mg/kg IV q24h **or** 7.5mg/kg/d IV div q8h	7-10 days	- Surgical drainage usually needed. Consult ENT. * Add vancomycin if patient is colonized with MRSA or Gram stain is suggestive of Staph. **Consider combination empiric therapy with tobramycin if patient has received multiple courses of broad-spectrum antibiotic therapy.
		Severe** **Piperacillin-tazobactam**	240-300mg/kg/d IV div q6-8h	7-10 days	
		Facial fractures, head trauma, CNS infection/meningitis suspected **Meropenem**	120mg/kg/d IV div q8h	7-10 days	

- 149 -

RECOMMENDED EMPIRIC THERAPY OF SELECTED INFECTIONS IN NEONATAL/PAEDIATRIC PATIENTS[A]

Infection	Usual Pathogens	Recommended Empiric Therapy	Recommended Paediatric Dose[B]	Recommended Duration	Comments
Respiratory					
Cystic Fibrosis exacerbation	< 5 years old: • S. aureus • H. influenzae • Enterobacteriaceae	**Ceftriaxone***	100mg/kg IV q24h	10-14 days	* Choice of empiric therapy should be based on previous sputum/throat culture results. - Sputum culture recommended. Tailor therapy to C&S results.
	≥ 5 years old: • S. aureus • P. aeruginosa • Burkholderia cepacia • Alcaligenes spp • Achromobacter spp • Stenotrophomonas spp • Other non-fermenting Gram negative bacilli • Acinetobacter spp • Atypical mycobacteria • Fungi/yeast	**Piperacillin-tazobactam*** + **Tobramycin**	300mg/kg/d IV div q6-8h 10mg/kg IV q24h **or** 9mg/kg/d IV div q8h	14 days	
Pneumonia Neonates < 1 month[†]	Group B Streptococci Enterobacteriaceae Listeria monocytogenes Occasionally: • S. aureus	**Ampicillin** + **Gentamicin**	200mg/kg/d IV div q6h 4-5mg/kg IV q24h	10-14 days	- If sepsis/meningitis suspected (e.g. fever, lethargy, or poor feeding), strongly consider blood culture/ lumbar puncture.

† Neonatal doses listed are for term infants > 7 days old. For neonates outside of this range, refer to Neofax or Lexi-Comp or Pediatric Red Book, or consult pharmacy for dosing.

RECOMMENDED EMPIRIC THERAPY OF SELECTED INFECTIONS IN NEONATAL/PAEDIATRIC PATIENTS[A]

Infection	Usual Pathogens	Recommended Empiric Therapy	Recommended Paediatric Dose[B]	Recommended Duration	Comments
Respiratory					

Pneumonia (cont'd) **Infants 1-3 months**	- Hospitalization is recommended if:
	  • < 6 months old with suspected bacterial pneumonia
	  • respiratory distress and hypoxemia
	  • complicated pneumonia (parapneumonic effusions, multilobar disease, abscesses/cavities, necrosis, empyema, pneumothorax
	    or bronchopleural fistula, or hematogenously acquired pneumonia)
	  • suspected CA-MRSA
	  • careful observation/follow-up at home cannot be ensured.				

	Viral: • RSV • Parainfluenza • Human metapneumovirus • Influenza • Adenovirus	**None**			
	Bacterial: • Group A, B Streptococci • Enterobacteriaceae • S. pneumoniae • H. influenzae • S. aureus • Listeria monocytogenes • Chlamydia trachomatis	**Cefotaxime** +/- **Azithromycin** <u>Severely ill and meningitis possible</u> **Cloxacillin** + **Cefotaxime**	200mg/kg/d IV div q6h 10mg/kg IV/PO first day then 5mg/kg IV/PO daily x 4 days 200mg/kg/d IV div q4h 300mg/kg/d IV div q6h	10-14 days 5 days 10-14 days	

RECOMMENDED EMPIRIC THERAPY OF SELECTED INFECTIONS IN NEONATAL/PAEDIATRIC PATIENTS[A]

Infection	Usual Pathogens	Recommended Empiric Therapy	Recommended Paediatric Dose[B]	Recommended Duration	Comments
Respiratory					

Community acquired pneumonia (CAP)
 	
[Clin Infect Dis 2011; Aug: e1-52, and Thorax 2011;66:ii1-23]
	Diagnosis
	- Chest x ray recommended to confirm diagnosis whenever possible and if deterioration to rule out empyema.
	- S. pneumoniae is most common pathogen.
	Antibiotic therapy
	- Amoxicillin:
	  • provides the best coverage of all oral β-lactams against S. pneumoniae, even majority of penicillin-resistant strains.
	  • no activity against S. aureus, β-lactamase (+) H. influenzae, M. catarrhalis, M. pneumoniae, or C. pneumonia.
	
	- Macrolides:
	  • significant macrolide resistance in S. pneumoniae
	  • poor Haemophilus coverage
	  • recent (within previous 3 months) macrolide use may result in multidrug resistant S. pneumoniae
	  • monotherapy with macrolides has uncertain efficacy for pneumococcal bacteremia (clinical history of rigors/positive blood culture).
	
	- In sickle cell anemia, Mycoplasma common and can cause severe pneumonia; use ceftriaxone + macrolide.
	
	- Switch to oral therapy if:
	  • afebrile
	  • clinically improving
	  • tolerating oral intake
	  • no complications (e.g. empyema).				

> 3 months - 5 years	Viral: • RSV • Adenovirus • Bocavirus • Human metapneumovirus • Influenza • Parainfluenza • Coronavirus • Rhinovirus	**No antibiotic therapy recommended**			

RECOMMENDED EMPIRIC THERAPY OF SELECTED INFECTIONS IN NEONATAL/PAEDIATRIC PATIENTS[A]

Infection	Usual Pathogens	Recommended Empiric Therapy	Recommended Paediatric Dose[B]	Recommended Duration	Comments
Respiratory					
Community acquired pneumonia (CAP) (cont'd) > 3 months - 5 years (cont'd) [Clin Infect Dis 2011; Aug: e1-52, and Thorax 2011;66:ii1-23]	Diagnosis - Chest x ray recommended to confirm diagnosis whenever possible and if deterioration to rule out empyema.				
	Bacterial: • S. pneumoniae • H. influenzae • S. aureus/ MRSA* • Group A Streptococci • Mycoplasma pneumoniae • Chlamydophila pneumoniae	<u>Mild-moderate</u> **Amoxicillin** β-lactam allergy **Azithromycin**** or **Clarithromycin**** <u>Post-influenza</u> **[Cefuroxime** or **(Amoxicillin + Amoxicillin-clavulanate)** +/- **[Azithromycin** or **Clarithromycin]**	90mg/kg/d PO tid 10mg/kg PO first day, then 5mg/kg PO daily x 4 days 15mg/kg/d PO div bid 150mg/kg/d IV div q8h 45mg/kg/d PO div tid 45mg/kg/d PO div tid 10mg/kg PO first day, then 5mg/kg PO daily x 4 days 15mg/kg/d PO div bid	5-7 days[†] 5 days 5-7 days[†] 7 days[†] 5 days[†] 7 days[†]	* Consider adding vancomycin or linezolid‡ for CA-MRSA if: • rapid onset • necrotizing process on CXR • post-influenza • Gram positive cocci in clusters on Gram stain. ‡ Linezolid preferred over vancomycin if: • MRSA with vancomycin MIC ≥ 1.5µg/mL • concomitant nephrotoxic therapy • pre-existing renal dysfunction. Minimum 14 days for confirmed MRSA. **If local S. pneumoniae macrolide resistance > 15%, add clindamycin 20-40mg/kg/d PO div tid. † Treat for a minimum of 5 days and until afebrile for 48-72h.

RECOMMENDED EMPIRIC THERAPY OF SELECTED INFECTIONS IN NEONATAL/PAEDIATRIC PATIENTS[A]

Infection	Usual Pathogens	Recommended Empiric Therapy	Recommended Paediatric Dose[B]	Recommended Duration	Comments
Respiratory					
Community acquired pneumonia (CAP) (cont'd)					
> 3 months - 5 years (cont'd) [Clin Infect Dis 2011; Aug: e1-52, and Thorax 2011;66:ii1-23]	*Diagnosis* - Chest x ray recommended to confirm diagnosis whenever possible and if deterioration to rule out empyema.				
	Bacterial: • S. pneumoniae • H. influenzae • S. aureus/ MRSA* • Group A Streptococci • Mycoplasma pneumoniae • Chlamydophila pneumoniae	Hospitalized:** [**Ampicillin** or **Ceftriaxone**] +/- [**Azithromycin** or **Clarithromycin**] Severe/PICU admission **Ceftriaxone** + **Vancomycin**[D‡] +/- **Azithromycin**	 200mg/kg/d IV div q6h 100mg/kg IV q24h 10mg/kg PO first day, then 5mg/kg PO daily x 4 days 15mg/kg/d PO div bid 100mg/kg IV q24h 60mg/kg/d IV div q6h 10mg/kg IV/PO first day, then 5mg/kg IV/PO daily x 4 days	 5-10 days[†] 5-10 days[†] 5 days 5-10 days[†] 5-10 days[†] 5-10 days[†] 5 days	* Consider adding vancomycin or linezolid[‡] for CA-MRSA if: • rapid onset • necrotizing process on CXR • post-influenza • Gram positive cocci in clusters on Gram stain. ‡ Linezolid preferred over vancomycin if: • MRSA with vancomycin MIC ≥ 1.5µg/mL • concomitant nephrotoxic therapy • pre-existing renal dysfunction. Minimum 14 days for confirmed MRSA. † Treat for a minimum of 5 days and until afebrile for 48-72h.

D. Desired vancomycin trough is 15-20mg/L. Monitor renal function closely. See Vancomycin Dosing & Monitoring Guidelines.

RECOMMENDED EMPIRIC THERAPY OF SELECTED INFECTIONS IN NEONATAL/PAEDIATRIC PATIENTS[A]

Infection	Usual Pathogens	Recommended Empiric Therapy	Recommended Paediatric Dose[B]	Recommended Duration	Comments
Respiratory					

Community acquired pneumonia (CAP) (cont'd)
 	
[Clin Infect Dis 2011; Aug: e1-52, and Thorax 2011;66:ii1-23]
	Diagnosis
	- Chest x ray recommended to confirm diagnosis whenever possible and if deterioration to rule out empyema.
	Macrolides:
	• significant macrolide resistance in S. pneumoniae
	• poor Haemophilus coverage
	• recent (within previous 3 months) macrolide use may predispose to infection with multidrug resistant S. pneumoniae
	• monotherapy with macrolides has uncertain efficacy for pneumococcal bacteremia (clinical history of rigors/positive blood cultures).
	* Doxycycline:
	  • excellent activity against most CAP pathogens, including S. pneumoniae (increasing resistance), H. influenzae, M. catarrhalis, S. aureus, including MRSA, M. pneumoniae, C. pneumoniae, and Legionella spp.
	  • less doxycycline resistance than macrolide resistance in S. pneumoniae
	  • has not been associated with causing an increase in penicillin resistance among S. pneumoniae (macrolides have)
	  • excellent pharmacokinetics/dynamics (high serum and lung levels, concentration-dependent killing)
	  • less expensive than newer macrolides.				

Children > 5 years	Mycoplasma pneumoniae
	S. pneumoniae
	H. influenzae
	S. aureus/MRSA***
	(see next page)
	Group A Streptococci
	Chlamydophila pneumoniae
	Viruses
		Mild-moderate
		Amoxicillin
		
		PLUS if presumed atypical pneumonia**
		Azithromycin
		or
		Clarithromycin
		
		Penicillin allergy
		≤ 8 years old
		[**Azithromycin**
		or
		Clarithromycin]
		+/-
		Clindamycin[‡]
		> 8 years old
		Doxycycline*
			90mg/kg/d PO tid
			
			10mg/kg PO first day then 5mg/kg PO daily x 4 days
			15mg/kg/d PO div bid
			
			10mg/kg PO first day then 5mg/kg PO daily x 4 days
			15mg/kg/d PO div bid
			
			20-40mg/kg/d PO div tid
			
			4mg/kg/d PO div q12h
				5-7 days[†]
				
				5 days
				
				5-7 days
				
				5 days
				
				5-7 days[†]
				
				5-7 days[†]
				
				5-7 days[†]
					- In sickle cell anemia, Mycoplasma common and can cause severe pneumonia: use ceftriaxone + erythromycin.
					[†] Treat for a minimum of 5 days and until afebrile for 48-72h.
					**Features of atypical pneumonia:
					  • subacute onset
					  • prominent cough
					  • minimal leukocytosis
					  • nonlobar infiltrate.
					[‡]Add clindamycin if:
					  • lobar pneumonia with fever or rigors
					  • antibiotic therapy within previous 3 months
					  • local S. pneumoniae macrolide resistance > 15%.

RECOMMENDED EMPIRIC THERAPY OF SELECTED INFECTIONS IN NEONATAL/PAEDIATRIC PATIENTS[A]

Infection	Usual Pathogens	Recommended Empiric Therapy	Recommended Paediatric Dose[B]	Recommended Duration	Comments
Respiratory					
Community acquired pneumonia (CAP) Children > 5 years (cont'd)	Diagnosis - Chest x ray recommended to confirm diagnosis whenever possible and if deterioration to rule out empyema.				
	Mycoplasma pneumoniae S. pneumoniae H. influenzae S. aureus/MRSA[***] Group A Streptococci Chlamydophila pneumoniae Viruses	Post-influenza [Cefuroxime] or [Amoxicillin + Amoxicillin-clavulanate]] + [Azithromycin or Clarithromycin]	150mg/kg/d IV div q8h 45mg/kg/d PO div tid 45mg/kg/d PO div tid 10mg/kg PO first day then 5mg/kg PO daily x 4 days 15mg/kg/d PO div bid	7 days[†] 7 days[†] 7 days[†] 5 days 7 days[†]	- In sickle cell anemia, Mycoplasma common and can cause severe pneumonia; use ceftriaxone + erythromycin. † Treat for a minimum of 5 days and until afebrile for 48-72h. ***Consider adding vancomycin or linezolid for CA-MRSA if: • rapid onset • necrotizing process on CXR • post-influenza • Gram positive cocci in clusters on Gram stain. ‡ Linezolid preferred over vancomycin if: • MRSA with vancomycin MIC ≥ 1.5µg/mL • concomitant nephrotoxic therapy • pre-existing renal dysfunction. Minimum 14 days for confirmed MRSA. - Stepdown to oral therapy if: • afebrile • clinically improving • tolerating oral intake • no complications (e.g. empyema).
		Hospitalized[***‡] [Ampicillin or Ceftriaxone] + [Azithromycin or Clarithromycin]	200mg/kg/d IV div q6h 100mg/kg IV q24h 10mg/kg IV/PO first day then 5mg/kg IV/PO daily 15mg/kg/d PO div bid	5-10 days[†] 5-10 days[†] 5 days 5-10 days[†]	
		Severe/PICU admission Ceftriaxone + Vancomycin[D‡] + Azithromycin	100mg/kg IV q24h 60mg/kg/d IV div q6h 10mg/kg IV/PO first day then 5mg/kg IV/PO daily x 4 days	5-10 days[†] 5-10 days[†] 5 days	

D. Desired vancomycin trough is 15-20mg/L. Monitor renal function closely. See Vancomycin Dosing & Monitoring Guidelines.

RECOMMENDED EMPIRIC THERAPY OF SELECTED INFECTIONS IN NEONATAL/PAEDIATRIC PATIENTS[A]

Infection	Usual Pathogens	Recommended Empiric Therapy	Recommended Paediatric Dose[B]	Recommended Duration	Comments
Respiratory					
Influenza	Influenza A Influenza B	**- NB: It is essential to check resistance patterns of the current season's influenza strains.**			
Post-exposure Prophylaxis*		Oseltamivir	1-12 years old ≤15kg: 30mg PO daily >15-23kg: 45mg PO daily >23-40kg: 60mg PO daily >40kg: 75mg PO daily ≥ 13 years old 75mg PO daily	10 days**	- Vaccination is first line of defense. * Early therapy is preferred over post-exposure prophylaxis (PEP). PEP may be considered for: • exposures in closed institutional settings • selectively in family settings if individuals cannot be (reliably) protected by immunization, e.g. < 6 mos old, immunocompromised, or vaccine contraindicated.
				10 days**	
		or **Zanamivir**	≥ 7 years old 10mg inhaled by mouth once daily	10 days**	**Give for 10 days, or duration of outbreak, whichever is longer.
Treatment***		Oseltamivir	1-12 years old ≤15kg: 30mg PO bid >15-23kg: 45mg PO bid >23-40kg: 60mg PO bid >40kg: 75mg PO bid ≥ 13 years old 75mg PO bid	5 days	***Best efficacy of these agents if started within 48h of symptom onset. Consider even if after 48h of symptom onset if: • hospitalized patients • progressive, severe, or complicated illness.
				5 days	
		or **Zanamivir**	≥ 7 years old 10mg inhaled by mouth bid	5 days	

RECOMMENDED EMPIRIC THERAPY OF SELECTED INFECTIONS IN NEONATAL/PAEDIATRIC PATIENTS[A]

Infection	Usual Pathogens	Recommended Empiric Therapy	Recommended Paediatric Dose[B]	Recommended Duration	Comments
Respiratory					
Hospital acquired pneumonia (HAP)	- HAP = pneumonia that develops ≥ 48 hours after admission. - Blood cultures recommended. - For immunocompromised patients, recommend Infectious Diseases consult.				

Early onset (≤ 4 days hospitalization) or **Late onset** (> 4 days hospitalization) • non-ICU • no mechanical ventilation • no broad-spectrum antibiotics	S. pneumoniae
	S. aureus/MRSA
	H. influenzae
	Enterobacteriaceae
		<u>< 3 months old</u>
		Cefotaxime
		
		<u>≥ 3 months old</u>
		Ceftriaxone
		
		If MRSA suspected <u>add:</u>*
		Vancomycin[D]
		or
		
		Linezolid
			200mg/kg/d IV q6h
			
			100mg/kg IV q24h
			
			60mg/kg/d IV div q6h
			
			<u>< 5 years old</u>
			30mg/kg/d IV/PO div q8h
			<u>> 5 years old</u>
			20mg/kg/d IV/PO div q12h
				7 days**
				
				7 days**
				
				Minimum 14 days for confirmed MRSA
				Minimum 14 days for confirmed MRSA
					* Linezolid preferred over vancomycin if:
					  • MRSA with vancomycin MIC ≥ 1.5μg/mL
					  • concomitant nephrotoxic therapy
					  • pre-existing renal dysfunction.
					**1 week duration has been shown to be as effective as 2 weeks and associated with less antimicrobial resistance. Two weeks recommended when MRSA, Pseudomonas, Acinetobacter, and other nonfermenting Gram negative bacilli isolated.

Late onset • aspiration	See Aspiration Pneumonia, Hospital acquired				

D. Desired vancomycin trough is 15-20mg/L. Monitor renal function closely. See Vancomycin Dosing & Monitoring Guidelines.

RECOMMENDED EMPIRIC THERAPY OF SELECTED INFECTIONS IN NEONATAL/PAEDIATRIC PATIENTS[A]

Infection	Usual Pathogens	Recommended Empiric Therapy	Recommended Paediatric Dose[B]	Recommended Duration	Comments
Respiratory					
HAP (cont'd) Late onset (> 4 days hospitalization) • prior (≤ 3 months) broad spectrum antibiotics[†] • structural lung disease (bronchiectasis/cystic fibrosis) • immunosuppression	Enterobacteriaceae P. aeruginosa* Acinetobacter spp S. aureus/MRSA**	**[Piperacillin-tazobactam** or **Imipenem** or **Meropenem]** +/- **Tobramycin[‡]** If MRSA suspected add:** **Vancomycin[D]** or **Linezolid**	240-300mg/kg/d IV div q6-8h 100mg/kg/d IV div q6h 120mg/kg/d IV div q8h 7mg/kg IV q24h **or** 7.5mg/kg/d IV div q8h 60mg/kg/d IV div q6h ≤ 5 years old 30mg/kg/d IV/PO div q8h > 5 years old 20mg/kg/d IV/PO div q12h	7-14 days*** 7-14 days*** 7-14 days*** 5 days Minimum 14 days for confirmed MRSA Minimum 14 days for confirmed MRSA	† If possible, use agents from a different antibiotic class than was previously used. - Tailor antibiotics to C&S results. * If culture proven bacteremia or sepsis due to P. aeruginosa, continue two antipseudomonal agents (associated with decreased mortality [Arch Intern Med 1985;145:1621-9. Am J Med 1989;87:540-8]). ** Linezolid preferred over vancomycin if: • MRSA with vancomycin MIC ≥ 1.5µg/mL • concomitant nephrotoxic therapy • pre-existing renal dysfunction. ***1 week duration has been shown to be as effective as 2 weeks and associated with less antimicrobial resistance. Two weeks still recommended when MRSA, Pseudomonas, Acinetobacter, and other nonfermenting Gram negative bacilli isolated. ‡ Consider giving tobramycin if severely ill to cover multi-resistant Gram negative organisms until C&S results available.

D. Desired vancomycin trough is 15-20mg/L. Monitor renal function closely. See Vancomycin Dosing & Monitoring Guidelines.

RECOMMENDED EMPIRIC THERAPY OF SELECTED INFECTIONS IN NEONATAL/PAEDIATRIC PATIENTS[A]

Infection	Usual Pathogens	Recommended Empiric Therapy	Recommended Paediatric Dose[B]	Recommended Duration	Comments
Respiratory					
Ventilator-associated pneumonia (VAP)	VAP = pneumonia that develops >48-72 hours after intubation. Prevention • elevate head of bed 30°- 45° • remove NG, ET tubes ASAP • appropriate infection control measures, including hand hygiene in healthcare workers. Diagnosis NB: Start antibiotics as soon as diagnosis is considered likely. - Endotracheal (ET) aspirate with Gram stain and C&S recommended. May be significant if increased purulence (3-4+ WBC), intracellular organisms present , and/or predominant organism. - Bronchoscopically obtained specimens may be considered in immunocompromised patients. Treatment - Insufficient evidence that administration of topical (nebulized or instilled via ET tube) antibiotics as an adjunct to systemic antibiotics is beneficial.				

RECOMMENDED EMPIRIC THERAPY OF SELECTED INFECTIONS IN NEONATAL/PAEDIATRIC PATIENTS[A]

Infection	Usual Pathogens	Recommended Empiric Therapy	Recommended Paediatric Dose[B]	Recommended Duration	Comments
Respiratory					
Ventilator-associated pneumonia (VAP) (cont'd) • **≤ 5 days of hospitalization** AND • **No prior (≤ 3 months) broad spectrum antibiotics**	Enterobacteriaceae P. aeruginosa[†] S. pneumoniae* H. influenzae** S. aureus**	<u>< 3 months old</u> **Cefotaxime** <u>≥ 3 months old</u> **Ceftriaxone**	200mg/kg/d IV q6h 100mg/kg IV q24h	7 days*** 7 days***	† If culture proven bacteremia or sepsis due to P. aeruginosa, recommend two antipseudomonal agents (associated with decreased mortality in bacteremia [Arch Intern Med 1985;145:1621-9, Am J Med 1989;87:540-8]). * At risk for these organisms if < 72 hours mechanical ventilation. **S. aureus coverage is suboptimal with these regimens. Tailor antibiotics to C&S results. Use vancomycin or linezolid for documented MRSA. ***1 week duration has been shown to be as effective as 2 weeks, and associated with less antimicrobial resistance. Two weeks recommended when MRSA Pseudomonas, Acinetobacter, and other non fermenting Gram negative bacilli isolated.

- 161 -

RECOMMENDED EMPIRIC THERAPY OF SELECTED INFECTIONS IN NEONATAL/PAEDIATRIC PATIENTS[A]

Infection	Usual Pathogens	Recommended Empiric Therapy	Recommended Paediatric Dose[B]	Recommended Duration	Comments
Respiratory					
VAP (cont'd) • > 5 days of hospitalization AND/OR • Prior (≤ 3 months) broad-spectrum antibiotics[Ø]	Enterobacteriaceae P. aeruginosa[†] S. aureus/MRSA Acinetobacter spp Stenotrophomonas maltophilia	[Piperacillin-tazobactam or Imipenem or Meropenem] +/- Tobramycin[‡] If MRSA suspected add:[∞] Vancomycin[D] or Linezolid	240-300mg/kg/d IV div q6-8h 100mg/kg/d IV div q6h 120mg/kg/d IV div q8h 7mg/kg IV q24h **or** 7.5mg/kg/d IV div q8h 60mg/kg/d IV div q6h < 5 years old 30mg/kg/d IV/PO div q8h > 5 years old 20mg/kg/d IV/PO div q12h	7-14 days* 7-14 days* 7-14 days* 5 days Minimum 14 days for confirmed MRSA Minimum 14 days for confirmed MRSA	Ø If possible, use agents from a different antibiotic class than was previously used. † If culture proven bacteremia or sepsis due to P. aeruginosa, continue two antipseudomonal agents (associated with decreased mortality [Arch Intern Med 1985;145:1621-9. Am J Med 1989;87:540-8]). ‡ Consider giving tobramycin if severely ill to cover multi-resistant Gram negative organisms until C&S results available. ∞ Linezolid preferred over vancomycin if: • MRSA with vancomycin MIC ≥ 1.5μg/mL • concomitant nephrotoxic therapy • pre-existing renal dysfunction. *1 week duration has been shown to be as effective as 2 weeks, and associated with less antimicrobial resistance. Two weeks recommended when MRSA Pseudomonas, Acinetobacter, and other non fermenting Gram negative bacilli isolated.

D. Desired vancomycin trough is 15-20mg/L. Monitor renal function closely. See Vancomycin Dosing & Monitoring Guidelines.

RECOMMENDED EMPIRIC THERAPY OF SELECTED INFECTIONS IN NEONATAL/PAEDIATRIC PATIENTS[A]

Infection	Usual Pathogens	Recommended Empiric Therapy	Recommended Paediatric Dose[B]	Recommended Duration	Comments
Respiratory					
Aspiration pneumonitis	- Chemical injury caused by the inhalation of gastric contents, resulting in inflammatory reaction. - Clinical: • patient with decreased level of consciousness • pulmonary infiltrate apparent on x-ray • episode of aspiration often witnessed • respiratory symptoms range from mild to severe and develop 2-5 hours after aspiration.				
	Sterile*	**No antibiotic therapy recommended.**** **Corticosteroids of no proven benefit.**			* Secondary bacterial infection not important in early stages. At higher risk of bacterial infection if: • receiving gastric acid suppression (antacids, H$_2$ receptor antagonists, proton pump inhibitors) • receiving enteral feeds • gastroparesis • small bowel obstruction. ** No role for prophylactic antibiotics. Reassess patient in 24-48 hours – If x-ray abnormality and above risk factors, consider antibiotic therapy.
Aspiration pneumonia	- Development of radiographically evident infiltrate following the aspiration of colonized oropharyngeal material. - Risk factors: • decreased level of consciousness • dysphagia • anatomic abnormality of upper GI tract • mechanical interference of GI tract (ET/NG tubes). - Clinical: • infiltrates in dependent lung segments, especially RLL • episode of aspiration often not witnessed • may progress to abscess/empyema within 1-2 weeks. - Etiology: • role of anaerobes is controversial and may have been overemphasized in the past • ceftriaxone has activity against many oral anaerobes. - For immunocompromised patients, recommend Infectious Diseases consult.				

RECOMMENDED EMPIRIC THERAPY OF SELECTED INFECTIONS IN NEONATAL/PAEDIATRIC PATIENTS[A]

Infection	Usual Pathogens	Recommended Empiric Therapy	Recommended Paediatric Dose[B]	Recommended Duration	Comments
Respiratory					
Aspiration pneumonia (cont'd) **Community acquired**	Oral anaerobes Streptococci spp Eikenella corrodens	**[Penicillin VK** or **Penicillin G]** + **Metronidazole IV/PO**[C]	40mg/kg/d PO div qid or tid 150,000-250,000 units/ kg/d IV div q6h 30mg/kg/d IV div q12h/ 15-30mg/kg/d PO div bid	7-14 days 7-14 days	
		β-lactam allergy **Clindamycin IV/PO**[C]	20-40mg/kg/d IV div q8h/ 20-40mg/kg/d PO div qid	7-14 days	
Hospital acquired	Polymicrobial: • S. aureus • Enterobacteriaceae • Pseudomonas spp • Oral anaerobes Occasionally: • H. influenzae • S. pneumoniae	≤ 4 days hospitalization **Amoxicillin-clavulanate** or **[Ceftriaxone** + **Metronidazole IV/PO**[C]] or	40mg/kg/d PO div tid 100mg/kg IV q24h 30mg/kg/d IV div q12h/ 15-30mg/kg/d PO div bid	7-14 days* 7-14 days*	*If x-ray evidence of necrotizing pneumonia or abscess, longer therapy recommended (3-6 weeks). - Anaerobes may be more significant in witnessed aspiration and/or recent abdominal surgery. **If recent ventilatory support and/or prior broad spectrum antibiotics, use this regimen.
		[Clindamycin[C] + **Gentamicin]**	20-40mg/kg/d IV div q8h 7mg/kg IV q24h **or** 7.5mg/kg/d IV div q8h	7-14 days*	
		> 4 days hospitalization** **[Piperacillin-tazobactam** or **Imipenem]** +/- **Tobramycin**	240-300mg/kg/d IV div q6-8h 100mg/kg/d IV div q6h 7mg/kg IV q24 h **or** 7.5mg/kg/d IV div q8h	7-14 days* 5 days	

RECOMMENDED EMPIRIC THERAPY OF SELECTED INFECTIONS IN NEONATAL/PAEDIATRIC PATIENTS[A]

Infection	Usual Pathogens	Recommended Empiric Therapy	Recommended Paediatric Dose[B]	Recommended Duration	Comments
Respiratory					

Pleural Space Infections		Diagnosis:
		- Chest x-ray +/- ultrasound or CT
		- Thoracentesis
		  • Pleural fluid for Gram stain/culture, AFB stain/culture, WBC
		- Sputum for C&S/AFB
		
		Management:
		- Pleural fluid drainage with chest tube recommended if:
		  • respiratory distress
		  • large parapneumonic effusions
		  • purulent effusions.
		- If incomplete drainage, consider early administration of fibrinolytic agents and surgical consult.
		- If pleural peel, surgical consult for decortication/VATS.			

Pleural effusion	S. pneumoniae S. aureus/MRSA Group A Streptococci H. influenzae Enterobacteriaceae	**Ceftriaxone** If MRSA suspected/documented, add:[†] **Vancomycin**[D] or **Linezolid**	100mg/kg IV q24h 60mg/kg/d IV div q6h ≤ 5 years old 30mg/kg/d IV/PO div q8h > 5 years old 20mg/kg/d IV/PO div q12h	2-4 weeks 2-4 weeks 2-4 weeks	† Linezolid preferred over vancomycin if: • MRSA with vancomycin MIC ≥ 1.5ug/mL • concomitant nephrotoxic therapy • pre-existing renal dysfunction.

D. Desired vancomycin trough is 15-20mg/L. Monitor renal function closely. See Vancomycin Dosing & Monitoring Guidelines.

RECOMMENDED EMPIRIC THERAPY OF SELECTED INFECTIONS IN NEONATAL/PAEDIATRIC PATIENTS[A]

Infection	Usual Pathogens	Recommended Empiric Therapy	Recommended Paediatric Dose[B]	Recommended Duration	Comments
Respiratory					
Pleural Space Infections (cont'd)					
• **Community acquired Empyema**	S. anginosus group* S. pneumoniae Anaerobes S. aureus/MRSA Enterobacteriaceae H. influenzae Rare: • Mycobacterium tuberculosis • Nocardia spp	**Ceftriaxone** If MRSA suspected/documented add:[†] **Vancomycin**[D] or **Linezolid**	100mg/kg IV q24h 60mg/kg/d IV div q6h < 5 years old 30mg/kg/d IV/PO div q8h ≥ 5 years old 20mg/kg/d IV/PO div q12h	3-6 weeks 3-6 weeks 3-6 weeks	* Includes: • S. anginosus • S. constellatus • S. intermedius. - Tailor antibiotics to C&S results but maintain anaerobic coverage. † Linezolid preferred over vancomycin if: • MRSA with vancomycin MIC ≥ 1.5ug/mL • concomitant nephrotoxic therapy • pre-existing renal dysfunction.
• **Hospital acquired**	S. aureus/MRSA Enterobacteriaceae Enterococcus spp Anaerobes P. aeruginosa S. anginosus group*	**Piperacillin-tazobactam** + **[Vancomycin**[D] or **Linezolid]**[†]	240-300mg/kg/d IV div q6-8h 60mg/kg/d IV div q6h < 5 years old 30mg/kg/d IV/PO div q8h ≥ 5 years old 20mg/kg/d IV/PO div q12h	3-6 weeks 3-6 weeks 3-6 weeks	
Lung abscess	S. aureus Oral anaerobes Enterobacteriaceae	**Clindamycin**[C] + **Ceftriaxone**	30-40mg/kg/d IV div q8h 100mg/kg IV q24h	minimum 3 weeks	- Treat until pulmonary infiltrate has cleared. - Consider echinococcal infection in appropriate clinical setting.

D. Desired vancomycin trough is 15-20mg/L. Monitor renal function closely. See Vancomycin Dosing & Monitoring Guidelines.

RECOMMENDED EMPIRIC THERAPY OF SELECTED INFECTIONS IN NEONATAL/PAEDIATRIC PATIENTS[A]

Infection	Usual Pathogens	Recommended Empiric Therapy	Recommended Paediatric Dose[B]	Recommended Duration	Comments
Gastrointestinal					

Gastroenteritis	- Stool specimens in patients hospitalized for > 3 days should not be submitted for C&S unless patient admitted with diarrhea or there is nosocomial outbreak of diarrhea. Diarrhea in hospitalized children (≥ 1 year old) warrants investigation for C. difficile.
	- Recommend blood culture if febrile and systemically unwell.
	- Causes of bloody diarrhea:
	  - Campylobacter spp
	  - Shigella spp
	  - Nontyphoidal Salmonella spp
	  - Shiga toxin-producing E. coli, including E. coli O157:H7
	  - Aeromonas spp
	  - Vibrio spp, not V. cholerae
	  - Yersinia spp
	  - E. histolytica
	- Severe bloody diarrhea in afebrile patients should increase suspicion of E. coli O157:H7. Most common in children < 5 years old.
	- Avoid antimotility agents in children < 2 years old, or in children of any age if fever present and/or if blood in stool.				

Mild-moderate	Viral
	Parasitic:
	  • Giardia
	  • Cryptosporidium
	  • Cyclospora
	Bacterial:
	  • diarrheagenic E. coli
	  • Campylobacter spp
	  • Shigella spp
	  • Salmonella spp
	Uncommonly:
	  • Aeromonas spp
	  • Plesiomonas spp
	  • Vibrio spp, non cholerae
	  • Yersinia spp
		Fluid replacement			- These organisms usually cause self-limiting diarrhea. Antibiotic therapy is generally not recommended unless symptoms are severe or prolonged, or patient is immunocompromised.
					- For treatment of enteric parasites, see Recommended Empiric Therapy of Enteric Parasitic Infections.

- 167 -

RECOMMENDED EMPIRIC THERAPY OF SELECTED INFECTIONS IN NEONATAL/PAEDIATRIC PATIENTS[A]

Infection	Usual Pathogens	Recommended Empiric Therapy	Recommended Paediatric Dose[B]	Recommended Duration	Comments
Gastrointestinal					
Gastroenteritis (cont'd)	Culture pending, **no clinical signs of hemolytic uremic syndrome (HUS)/ thrombotic thrombocytopenic purpura (TTP)***	**[TMP/SMX** (if > 1 month old)	8mg TMP/kg/d PO div bid	3-5 days	* NB: Antibiotic therapy contraindicated if clinical suspicion of HUS as it may enhance toxin release and increase risk of HUS.
Severe		or			Clinical signs of HUS/TTP:
• > 6 diarrheal episodes/day		**Cefixime]**	8mg/kg/d PO div q12-24h	3-5 days	• diarrhea that becomes bloody after 1-4 days
• bloody diarrhea		+/-			• elevated serum creatinine/ oliguria/anuria
• persistent (> 1 week) diarrhea		**Azithromycin**	10mg/kg PO daily	3 days	• thrombocytopenia (platelets <15 x 10^9/L)
• fever		or			• microangiopathic hemolytic anemia (Hgb < 100g/L)
		[Ceftriaxone	50mg/kg IV q24h	3-5 days	- Culture recommended.
		+/-			- Tailor antibiotics to C&S results.
		Azithromycin]	10mg/kg PO daily	3 days	See below for recommendations.

- 168 -

RECOMMENDED EMPIRIC THERAPY OF SELECTED INFECTIONS IN NEONATAL/PAEDIATRIC PATIENTS[A]

Infection	Usual Pathogens	Recommended Empiric Therapy	Recommended Paediatric Dose[B]	Recommended Duration	Comments
Gastrointestinal					
Gastroenteritis (cont'd)					
Severe (cont'd) • > 6 diarrheal episodes/day • bloody diarrhea • persistent (> 1 week) diarrhea	Campylobacter spp	No therapy unless <u>severe, prolonged, or immunocompromised</u> **Azithromycin** or **Erythromycin**	 10mg/kg PO daily 40mg/kg/d PO div qid	 3 days 5 days	- Symptoms occur 1-10 days after exposure and usually resolve within 2-5 days.
• fever	Shiga toxin-producing E. coli, including E. coli O157:H7	**Antibiotic therapy contraindicated.***			* NB: Antibiotic therapy may enhance toxin release and increase risk of hemolytic uremic syndrome. - Avoid antimotility agents.
Culture-directed	Salmonella typhi Salmonella paratyphi	**Azithromycin** Hospitalized/Bacteremic **Ceftriaxone**	20mg/kg PO daily 100mg/kg IV q24h	7 days 10-14 days, or at least 5 days after defervescence, whichever is longer	- Relapse rate 10% after antibiotic therapy.

RECOMMENDED EMPIRIC THERAPY OF SELECTED INFECTIONS IN NEONATAL/PAEDIATRIC PATIENTS[A]

Infection	Usual Pathogens	Recommended Empiric Therapy	Recommended Paediatric Dose[B]	Recommended Duration	Comments
Gastrointestinal					
Gastrointestinal (cont'd)					
Severe (cont'd) • > 6 diarrheal episodes/day • bloody diarrhea • persistent (> 1 week) diarrhea • fever	Salmonella spp, non typhoidal*	No therapy unless high risk			* High risk: • bacteremia (use ceftriaxone) • immunocompromised • hemodialysis • hemoglobinopathy, e.g. sickle cell disease • chronic GI tract disease • age < 12 months. **14 days if immunocompromised or relapsing. ***4-6 weeks if extraintestinal site of infection (urinary tract, respiratory tract, endovascular, musculoskeletal, CNS) or immunosuppressed.
		High risk* **TMP/SMX** (if > 1 month old) or **Azithromycin**	8mg TMP/kg/d PO div bid 20mg/kg PO daily	7-10 days** 7 days**	
Culture-directed (cont'd)		Hospitalized/bacteremic **Ceftriaxone**	100mg/kg IV q24h	14 days***	
	Shigella spp	**Azithromycin** or **Ceftriaxone** Alternative **Cefixime**	10mg/kg PO daily 50mg/kg IV q24h 8mg/kg/d PO div q12-24h	3 days* 3 days* 3 days*	* 7 days if immunocompromised.
	Aeromonas spp Plesiomonas spp Vibrio spp, not V. cholerae Yersinia spp	No therapy unless Severe, prolonged or immunocompromised **TMP/SMX** (if > 1 month old) or **Azithromycin**	8mg TMP/kg/d PO div bid 10mg/kg PO daily	3 days* 3 days*	* 7 days if immunocompromised.
	Vibrio cholerae	**Azithromycin** or **Erythromycin**	20mg/kg PO once 30mg/kg/d PO div tid	1 dose 3 days	- Fluid/rehydration essential.
	Parasitic	See Treatment of Enteric Parasitic Infections.			

RECOMMENDED EMPIRIC THERAPY OF SELECTED INFECTIONS IN NEONATAL/PAEDIATRIC PATIENTS[A]

Infection	Usual Pathogens	Recommended Empiric Therapy	Recommended Paediatric Dose[B]	Recommended Duration	Comments
Gastrointestinal					
Travellers' diarrhea	- Antibiotic prophylaxis not recommended due to the potential for adverse effects/resistance and the fact that travellers' diarrhea is usually mild and self-limiting; prompt self-treatment is effective and preferred. Counsel on handwashing and food and water precautions. - For therapy of specific organisms, see previous Gastroenteritis section. - Avoid antimotility agents in children < 2 years old, or children of any age if fever present or blood in stool. - In the event of severe travellers' diarrhea, consider providing a 3-day supply of antibiotics, especially for immunocompromised patients, and in particular for asplenic patients as they are at increased risk of Salmonella/Campylobacter bacteremia.				
Mild-moderate	Viral: • Noroviruses • Rotavirus • Enteric adenovirus	Fluid replacement +/- bismuth subsalicylate +/- antimotility agents (e.g. loperamide) if > 2 years old			- Self-limiting. Usual duration of diarrhea ≤ 5 days.
Severe • > 6 diarrheal episodes/day • bloody diarrhea • persistent (>3 days) diarrhea • fever	Bacterial: • Campylobacter spp • diarrheagenic E. coli • Shigella spp • Salmonella spp** Parasitic: • Entamoeba spp • Giardia	**Azithromycin** or **TMP/SMX** (if > 1 month old)* or **Cefixime**	10mg/kg PO daily 8mg TMP/kg/d PO div bid 8mg/kg/d PO div q12-24h	3 days 3 days 3 days	- Culture recommended. - Tailor antibiotics to C&S results. * Widespread resistance but may be an option if travel to Mexico. **See previous Gastroenteritis section. - Persistent diarrhea suggests protozoal cause: Giardia, Cryptosporidium, Cyclospora, Entamoeba histolytica, Microsporidia. See Recommended Empiric Therapy of Enteric Parasitic Infections.

RECOMMENDED EMPIRIC THERAPY OF SELECTED INFECTIONS IN NEONATAL/PAEDIATRIC PATIENTS[A]

Infection	Usual Pathogens	Recommended Empiric Therapy	Recommended Paediatric Dose[B]	Recommended Duration	Comments
Gastrointestinal					
Clostridium difficile infection (CDI)					- NB: Clostridium difficile testing is not recommended in children < 12 months old. Colonization with this organism and toxin detection found in up to 60% of healthy neonates.

- Definition: presence of diarrhea (≥ 3 unformed stools in ≤ 24 hours) and either:
  - stool test positive for toxigenic C. difficile or its toxins

  or

  - colonoscopic or histopathologic findings of pseudomembranous colitis.
- History of treatment with antibiotics, proton pump inhibitors (PPIs), or antineoplastic agents within previous 8 weeks is also present in majority of patients.
- **Discontinue antibiotics if possible, especially cephalosporins and clindamycin, as these agents have been associated with the highest risk of CDI. If not possible, consider changing to lower CDI risk group of antibiotics if appropriate (e.g. aminoglycosides, TMP/SMX (> 1 month old), tetracyclines (> 8 years old), and/or metronidazole). Prevention of CDI with metronidazole or vancomycin while on antimicrobial therapy is NOT recommended as no evidence of efficacy.**
- PPIs/H₂ blockers are associated with a 2-3 fold increased risk for CDI, and recurrent CDI. Assess need for use, or continued use, of these agents vs. benefit and discontinue if possible.
- **Do NOT use antidiarrheals, e.g. loperamide (Imodium®), diphenoxylate (Lomotil®) as they may obscure symptoms and precipitate toxic megacolon.**
- Vancomycin IV not effective. Metronidazole IV of uncertain efficacy (only use if very strict NPO or in combination for severe/toxic megacolon).
- Do not submit post treatment stool sample if asymptomatic and/or formed stools as toxin may persist for weeks post treatment.
- Infection Control:
  - Hospitalized patients with CDI should be isolated with contact precautions.
  - Strict adherence to handwashing with soap and water essential (alcohol does not kill C. difficile spores).

RECOMMENDED EMPIRIC THERAPY OF SELECTED INFECTIONS IN NEONATAL/PAEDIATRIC PATIENTS[A]

Infection	Usual Pathogens	Recommended Empiric Therapy	Recommended Paediatric Dose[B]	Recommended Duration	Comments
Gastrointestinal					
Clostridium difficile infection (CDI) (cont'd) Initial episode	Clostridium difficile	<u>Mild-moderate</u> **Metronidazole**	30mg/kg/d PO div qid (max 250mg PO qid)	10-14 days	* Severe = WBC >15x10⁹/L, serum creatinine ≥1.5x baseline, hypotension, shock, megacolon. **Do not assume therapeutic failure of metronidazole until minimum of 3-5 days of therapy completed without symptomatic improvement.
		<u>Severe*/unresponsive to metronidazole**</u> **Vancomycin**	50mg/kg/d PO div qid (max 125mg PO qid)	10-14 days	
Ileus/NPO	Clostridium difficile	<u>Mild-moderate</u> **Metronidazole**	30mg/kg/d IV div q8h (max 500mg IV q8h)*	10-14 days	* Switch to NG/PO as soon as possible; little clinical data for IV metronidazole. **Severe = WBC >15x10⁹/L, serum creatinine ≥1.5x baseline, hypotension, shock, megacolon.
		<u>Severe**</u> **Metronidazole IV** + **Vancomycin NG/PR**	30mg/kg/d IV div q8h (max 500mg IV q8h) 50mg/kg/d NG/PR div qid (max 500mg qid)		
Recurrence		- Recurrence after first episode occurs in up to 30% of patients, and as high as 65% after first recurrence. - The role of probiotics for the prevention or treatment of CDI remains controversial. Clinical data is limited. Potential for bacteremia/fungemia in immunocompromised patients. Multiple formulations exist but labeling regulations and quality control are lacking. Further research is needed to clarify the role of probiotics in CDI.			

RECOMMENDED EMPIRIC THERAPY OF SELECTED INFECTIONS IN NEONATAL/PAEDIATRIC PATIENTS[A]

Infection	Usual Pathogens	Recommended Empiric Therapy	Recommended Paediatric Dose[B]	Recommended Duration	Comments
Gastrointestinal					
Necrotizing enterocolitis (NEC)[†]	Enterobacteriaceae Streptococcus spp Coagulase negative Staph* Perforation add: Anaerobes	**Vancomycin**[D] + **Cefotaxime** Perforation add **Metronidazole**[C] Severely ill **Meropenem** + **Vancomycin**[D]	40-60mg/kg/d IV div q6h 150-200mg/kg/d IV div q8h 30mg/kg/d IV div q12h 60mg/kg/d IV div q8h 40-60mg/kg/d IV div q6h	7-14 days 7-14 days 7-14 days	* This may be a significant pathogen in some centres. May need to consider vancomycin + gentamicin. - Adjust therapy based on Gram stain and/or culture, including antifungal therapy if applicable.
Appendicitis	Enterobacteriaceae Anaerobes +/- Enterococcus spp	Uncomplicated Empiric therapy not necessary; surgical prophylaxis recommended. Complicated* See 2° Peritonitis			* Complicated: • gangrene • perforation • abscess • peritonitis.
Helicobacter pylori	See Recommended Empiric Therapy of Selected Infections in **Adult** Patients. Use pediatric doses.				

[†] Neonatal doses listed are for term infants > 7 days old. For neonates outside of this range, refer to Neofax or Lexi-Comp or Pediatric Red Book, or consult pharmacy for dosing.
D. Desired vancomycin trough is 10-20mg/L. Monitor renal function closely. See Vancomycin Dosing & Monitoring Guidelines.

RECOMMENDED EMPIRIC THERAPY OF SELECTED INFECTIONS IN NEONATAL/PAEDIATRIC PATIENTS[A]

Infection	Usual Pathogens	Recommended Empiric Therapy	Recommended Paediatric Dose[B]	Recommended Duration	Comments
Gastrointestinal					
Peritonitis					
Spontaneous bacterial peritonitis (SBP)	\- Occurs in the setting of cirrhosis or nephrotic syndrome, but can rarely occur in healthy children, especially school age girls. \- Spontaneous bacterial peritonitis is usually monomicrobial. Polymicrobial infections suggest bowel perforation. See 2° peritonitis. Diagnosis: \- Ascitic fluid positive for bacteria and PMNs ≥0.25×10^9/L. \- Blood/peritoneal fluid cultures recommended. Management: \- Urinary/intravascular catheterization may increase risk of infection in patients with ascites - avoid if possible. \- Aminoglycosides should be avoided in patients with cirrhosis. \- Increased risk of SBP (and Clostridium difficile infection) in cirrhotic patients on proton pump inhibitors (PPIs). Therefore use PPIs judiciously and only when clearly indicated in cirrhotic patients.			
	S. pneumoniae Group A. Streptococci Enterobacteriaceae Occasionally: • S. aureus • Enterococcus spp • Anaerobes	**Ceftriaxone**	100mg/kg IV q24h	5-10 days*	\- 10 days recommended if bacteremic. Five days if repeat paracentesis (at 48 hours) shows < 0.25×10^9/L PMNs and culture negative.

Infection	Usual Pathogens	Recommended Empiric Therapy	Recommended Paediatric Dose[B]	Recommended Duration	Comments
Gastrointestinal					

Peritonitis (cont'd)	- All abscess collections require drainage.
	- Cultures of perforated or gangrenous appendix offer no benefit. However, distal colonic perforations warrant aerobic/anaerobic cultures as antibiotic therapy should be tailored to C&S results.
	- Duration of therapy:
	  • Peri-operative therapy ≤ 24h
	    Bowel injuries due to penetrating, blunt, or iatrogenic trauma with surgery within 12 hours of injury; acute perforations of stomach, duodenum, and proximal jejunum in absence of antacid therapy or malignancy; or acute appendicitis without gangrene, perforation, abscess, or peritonitis.
	  • Short course (5-7 days)
	    Uncomplicated peritonitis if adequate drainage.
	    Persistent clinical evidence of infection after 5-7 days warrants diagnostic investigations (CT, US).
	  • Prolonged course**
	    Complicated intraabdominal abscesses and/or severe underlying illness.
	    **Continue therapy until:
	      ⇒ afebrile
	      ⇒ normal WBC/differential
	      ⇒ no residual fluid collections
	      ⇒ return of GI function.			

Infection	Usual Pathogens	Recommended Empiric Therapy	Recommended Paediatric Dose[B]	Recommended Duration	Comments
Gastrointestinal					
Peritonitis (cont'd)	‡ Enterococcal coverage recommended if: • health care-associated infection • distal colon surgery • hepatobiliary/pancreatic infection (increased risk for enterococcal bacteremia) • patients with chronic illness or immunosuppression • valvular heart disease or prosthetic intravascular materials • previous antibiotic therapy (excluding surgical prophylaxis) • Enterococcus is a predominant organism in culture. ***Empiric coverage of Candida spp not recommended unless yeast/Candida on Gram smear/culture **AND** at least one of below: • yeast seen intracellularly or presence of pseudohyphae • patient on immunosuppres-sive therapy • multiple previous antibiotics • postoperative intra-abdominal infection • recurrent intra-abdominal infection. Add fluconazole if C. albicans, or an echinocandin (caspofungin or micafungin) if nonalbicans Candida spp.				
Secondary peritonitis • abscess* • bowel perforation • ruptured appendix	Polymicrobial: • Enterobacteriaceae • Enterococcus spp‡ • Anaerobes • Streptococcus spp • Candida spp***	<u>Mild - moderate**</u> **Ceftriaxone** + **Metronidazole**[C] Enterococcal coverage required <u>‡</u> **Ampicillin** + **Gentamicin*** + **Metronidazole**[C] <u>Alternative**</u> **Clindamycin**[C] + **Gentamicin***	100mg/kg IV q24h 30mg/kg/d IV div q12h 150-200mg/kg/d IV div q6h 5-7mg/kg IV q24h 30mg/kg/d IV div q12h 40mg/kg/d IV div q8h 5-7mg/kg IV q24h	Duration of therapy dependent on clinical picture (see previous).	* Aminoglycosides have good peritoneal penetration but unreliable activity in purulent material. If abscess present, use alternative Gram negative coverage. **These regimens do not have enterococcal coverage. - Switch to oral agents when tolerating oral intake and clinical improvement.

RECOMMENDED EMPIRIC THERAPY OF SELECTED INFECTIONS IN NEONATAL/PAEDIATRIC PATIENTS[A]

Infection	Usual Pathogens	Recommended Empiric Therapy	Recommended Paediatric Dose[B]	Recommended Duration	Comments
Gastrointestinal					
Peritonitis (cont'd) **Secondary peritonitis** (cont'd)		* Enterococcal coverage recommended if: • health care-associated infection • distal colon surgery • hepatobiliary/pancreatic infection (increased risk for enterococcal bacteremia) • patients with chronic illness or Immunosuppression • valvular heart disease or prosthetic intravascular materials • previous antibiotic therapy (excluding surgical prophylaxis) • Enterococcus is a predominant organism in culture. **Empiric coverage of Candida spp not recommended unless yeast/Candida on Gram smear/culture **AND** at least one of below: • yeast seen intracellularly or presence of pseudohyphae • patient on immunosuppressive therapy • multiple previous antibiotics • upper GI tract perforation • postoperative intra-abdominal infection • recurrent intra-abdominal infection. Add fluconazole if C. albicans, or an echinocandin (caspofungin or micafungin) if nonalbicans Candida spp.			
• abscess • bowel perforation • ruptured appendix	Polymicrobial: • Enterobacteriaceae • Enterococcus spp* • Anaerobes • Streptococcus spp • Candida spp**	Severe **Piperacillin-tazobactam** +/- **Gentamicin***** Multiple previous antibiotics**/known <u>ESBL</u> or <u>AmpC</u> **Imipenem** or **Meropenem**	240-300mg piperacillin/kg/d IV div q6-8h 7mg/kg IV q24h 60mg/kg/d IV div q6h 60mg/kg/d IV div q6-8h	Assess need for continuation of gentamicin based on C&S results	***Add gentamicin if: • septic shock • recent antibiotic use or • suspected ESBL, Amp C, carbapenemase producing organism. - Switch to oral agents when tolerating oral intake and clinical improvement.

RECOMMENDED EMPIRIC THERAPY OF SELECTED INFECTIONS IN NEONATAL/PAEDIATRIC PATIENTS[A]

Infection	Usual Pathogens	Recommended Empiric Therapy	Recommended Paediatric Dose[B]	Recommended Duration	Comments
Gastrointestinal					
Peritonitis (cont'd) Chronic/Tertiary	P. aeruginosa Coagulase negative Staph Enterobacteriaceae Enterococcus faecium Candida spp	[Imipenem or Meropenem] + Vancomycin[D] ± Fluconazole* Tailor according to C&S results.	60mg/kg/d IV div q6h 60mg/kg/d IV div q6-8h 60mg/kg/d IV div q6h 6-12mg/kg IV/PO daily	10-14 days and until: • afebrile • normal WBC/ differential • no residual fluid collections and • return of GI function	- All abscess collections require drainage. - Ideally, treat according to culture results (prior to antibiotics), if possible. * Add fluconazole if culture evidence of C. albicans. If nonalbicans Candida spp. use an echinocandin (caspofungin or micafungin).

D. Desired vancomycin trough is 10-20mg/L. Monitor renal function closely. See Vancomycin Dosing & Monitoring Guidelines.

Infection	Usual Pathogens	Recommended Empiric Therapy	Recommended Paediatric Dose[B]	Recommended Duration	Comments
Gastrointestinal					
Peritonitis (cont'd) Peritoneal dialysis (PD) related peritonitis [Perit Dial Int 2012;32:S32-86]		Prevention of catheter infections [Perit Dial Int 2011;31:614-30] - Increased risk for S. aureus infections if: • S. aureus nasal carrier • diabetic • immunocompromised. - Topical mupirocin cream at either the catheter exit site or intranasally, or both, has been recommended to decrease S. aureus exit site infections and peritonitis. Gentamicin cream and Polysporin Triple® antibiotic ointment have also been studied but lead to increased fungal exit site infections and peritonitis, respectively, and are therefore not recommended. Diagnosis • First cloudy effluent should be submitted to laboratory for culture, cell count and differential. • Repeat culture not recommended if cell count decreasing and symptomatic improvement. • If cell count/symptoms not improving, repeat culture within 3 days. If culture negative peritonitis consider: (1) culture volume too small, (2) prior use of antibiotics, (3) unusual causes of peritonitis: mycobacteria; fungi, including lipid-dependent yeast; Legionella spp; slow-growing/fastidious bacteria (e.g. Campylobacter spp); Ureaplasma spp. Mycoplasma spp. enteroviruses. Consult microbiologist.			

RECOMMENDED EMPIRIC THERAPY OF SELECTED INFECTIONS IN NEONATAL/PAEDIATRIC PATIENTS[A]

Infection	Usual Pathogens	Recommended Empiric Therapy	Recommended Paediatric Dose[B]	Recommended Duration	Comments
Gastrointestinal					
Peritonitis (cont'd) **Peritoneal dialysis (PD) related peritonitis** (cont'd) [Perit Dial Int 2012;32:S32-86]		Treatment - Intraperitoneal (IP) administration of antibiotics superior to IV administration. - Empiric therapy should not be based on Gram stain result. Must wait for C&S results to tailor antibiotic therapy. - For severely symptomatic peritonitis, 1-3 rapid exchanges of peritoneal dialysis solution prior to longer dwell exchange with intraperitoneal (IP) antibiotics, have been shown to provide symptomatic relief. - Recommend program specific evaluation of local susceptibility patterns. - Cefazolin plus ceftazidime is NOT an optimal empiric regimen for PD peritonitis because: • the use of 2 cephalosporins may be antagonistic • cefazolin and aminoglycoside combinations may be synergistic against certain organisms such as coagulase negative Staph. • strong association between ceftazidime and selection of β-lactamase mediated resistance in Enterobacteriaceae (both extended spectrum-β-lactamase [ESBL] and inducible [AmpC] β-lactamase). - Short courses of aminoglycosides for an episode of PD peritonitis do not adversely affect residual renal function (*Am J Kid Dis 2003;41:670-5, J Am Soc Nephrol 1999;10(1):136-45*). - Cefepime monotherapy may be considered in patients with pre-existing vestibular/cochlear toxicity. Cefepime dose: • intermittent: 15mg/kg once per day • continuous: 500mg/L LD, then 125mg/L MD. - Ciprofloxacin no longer recommended empirically due to unacceptably high resistance. - If no improvement at 48 hours, reculture and evaluate for exit site/tunnel infection or catheter colonization. - For specific treatment of positive cultures, see Recommended Therapy of Culture-Directed Infections in Adult Patients Table 2. Intraperitoneal dosing applies to paediatric patients, except where noted. For systemic antimicrobial doses, see Pediatric Antimicrobial Dosing Guide or Perit Dial Int 2012;32:S50, Table 5. - Indications for catheter removal: • refractory (failure to clear effluent after 5 days of appropriate antibiotic therapy)/relapsing (within 4 weeks of previous episode with same organism) peritonitis • refractory exit site and tunnel infection • fungal peritonitis - Consider catheter removal for: • repeat (more than 4 weeks from previous episode with same organism) peritonitis • mycobacterial peritonitis • polymicrobial peritonitis (high relapse rate; evaluate for intra-abdominal abscess)			

Infection	Usual Pathogens	Recommended Empiric Therapy	Recommended Paediatric Dose[B]		Comments
Gastrointestinal					
Peritonitis (cont'd) **Peritoneal dialysis (PD) related peritonitis** (cont'd) [Perit Dial Int 2012;32:S32-86]	Coagulase negative Staph S. aureus Enterobacteriaceae Occasionally: • Streptococcus spp • Pseudomonas spp • Anaerobes • Candida spp	**Cefazolin IP** + **Gentamicin IP**[†] Severe penicillin allergy/anaphylaxis/ Cephalosporin allergy/ MRSA colonization **Vancomycin IP** + **Gentamicin IP**[†]	Intermittent dosing* Dwell time at least 6 hours 20mg/kg once per day 0.6mg/kg once per day 15-30mg/kg q 7[‡] days 0.6mg/kg once per day	Continuous dosing (per L bag)* 500mg/L LD then 125mg/L MD 8mg/L LD then 4mg/L MD 1000mg/L LD then 25mg/L MD 8mg/L LD then 4mg/L MD LD = loading dose MD = maintenance dose	- Consult Pediatric Nephrology. * Dosing recommendations for anuric (<100mL urine/24 hours) patients. Note: Patients with residual renal function may require increased doses or more frequent dosing, especially when using intermittent regimens. See treatment guidelines at www.ispd.org. ‡ For nonanuric patients, give vancomycin every 3-5 days or when serum level < 15mg/L. † To optimize concentration-dependent activity of amino-glycosides and lessen potential for toxicity, intermittent dosing is recommended over continuous dosing, especially if aminoglycoside is continued beyond empiric use/based on C&S results.

RECOMMENDED EMPIRIC THERAPY OF SELECTED INFECTIONS IN NEONATAL/PAEDIATRIC PATIENTS[A]

Infection	Usual Pathogens	Recommended Empiric Therapy	Recommended Paediatric Dose[B]	Recommended Duration	Comments
Genital					

Vulvovaginitis
Prepubertal vaginitis
	Non sexually transmitted infections:
	• Group A Streptococci
	• Shigella spp
	• Candida spp
	• Other
	Sexually transmitted infections:
	• Gonorrhea (> 1 month*)
	• Trichomoniasis (> 6 months*)
	• Chlamydia (> 6 months*)
	• HSV (> 3 months*)
	
	* Age at which nonvertical transmission becomes most likely.
		Treat according to cause.			- DDx includes: local irritation (e.g. bubblebath), foreign body, or trauma.
					- If discharge present do:
					• careful history and physical to rule out suspected abuse and
					• swabs of vagina for:
					  • Gram stain
					  • C&S
					  • Gonorrhea culture
					  • Chlamydia culture
					  • wet mount
					  • KOH/whiff test.
					- Follow-up cultures recommended for test of cure:
					• Gonorrhea - at 5 days
					• Chlamydia - at 3-4 weeks.
					- If bloody discharge, consult paediatrics or gynecology to rule out foreign body or tumor.
					- Do not do speculum exam in children.
					- In cases of suspected sexual abuse, all specimens should be submitted with chain of custody documentation.

RECOMMENDED EMPIRIC THERAPY OF SELECTED INFECTIONS IN NEONATAL/PAEDIATRIC PATIENTS[A]

Infection	Usual Pathogens	Recommended Empiric Therapy	Recommended Paediatric Dose[B]	Recommended Duration	Comments
Urinary Tract					
Asymptomatic bacteriuria	Enterobacteriaceae Enterococcus spp	Antibiotic therapy NOT recommended unless: • prior to urologic/gynecologic instrumentation/surgery, or surgery involving prosthetic material, or • prior to catheter removal in patients catheterized for > 48 hours post surgery involving prosthetic material.			

Cystitis or pyelonephritis		- 5% of children presenting with fever may have urinary tract infection (UTI); more common in girls and uncircumcised boys.
		- UTI in children <1 month most often due to hematogenous seeding rather than ascending infection. Complete septic work-up recommended.
		
		Diagnosis:
		- Blood culture recommended if:
		• febrile (NB: < 2 months old may not be febrile)
		• signs and symptoms of pyelonephritis
		• immunocompromised.
		- All children with fever and no obvious source for infection should be investigated for possible UTI.
		- Urine specimen - submit for urinalysis and urine culture:
		• Bag urine specimens are usually contaminated (false positive rate >85%) and cannot be relied upon to diagnose UTI. Only useful if negative as excludes UTI. If positive, must be confirmed with a proper specimen BEFORE antibiotics.
		• In/out catheter specimens are preferred for the diagnosis of UTI in young children. Although they have better specificity than bag specimens, contamination may also occur. Organism(s), colony count and clinical picture must all be considered when interpreting results.
		• For children < 2 years old, collect urine by suprapubic, in/out catheter, or properly collected midstream urine (MSU).
		• For children ≥ 2 years old, collect urine by in/out catheter or properly collected MSU.
		• For older children, MSU should be collected no sooner than 2 hours after last voiding.
		  ○ < 3 years old - send urine specimen for microscopic* urinalysis (WBC/bacteria) and urine culture. NB: Dipslide/macroscopic urinalysis (leukocyte esterase/nitrites) may not be as accurate in this age group. .
		  ○ > 3 years of age - send urine specimen for macroscopic +/- microscopic urinalysis and urine culture.
		NB: Pyuria alone does not confirm a diagnosis of UTI.			

RECOMMENDED EMPIRIC THERAPY OF SELECTED INFECTIONS IN NEONATAL/PAEDIATRIC PATIENTS[A]

Infection	Usual Pathogens	Recommended Empiric Therapy	Recommended Paediatric Dose[B]	Recommended Duration	Comments
Urinary Tract					

Cystitis or pyelonephritis (cont'd)	Diagnosis (cont'd):
	 - 10^5 cfu/L - significant colony count indicative of urinary tract infection WITH signs & symptoms.
	 - $\geq 10^6$ cfu/L - may be significant colony count in in/out catheter specimens and in infants/children with definite UTI symptoms and single uropathogen.
	 - 10^5 cfu/L - significant colony count with suprapubic aspirate or cystoscopy.
	 - ≥ 3 mixed organisms – probable contamination. May be significant in children with complex genitourinary abnormality.
	 - Indications for ultrasound of kidneys and bladder:
	   • septicemia
	   • children < 2 years of age after first febrile UTI
	   • UTI due to organism other than E. coli
	   • delayed (> 48h) response to appropriate therapy
	   • abdominal or bladder mass
	   • abnormal urinary stream
	   • renal function impairment
	   • recurrent febrile UTI.
	 - VCUG no longer routinely recommended after first febrile UTI, but only if US shows hydronephrosis, renal dysplasia, scarring or findings of high grade vesicoureteral reflux (VUR) or abnormal urine stream/obstructive uropathy or if there is a recurrence of a febrile UTI.
	 - DMSA scan may be used acutely to confirm pyelonephritis, or at 6-12 months to assess for renal scarring. Not optimal for diagnosing VUR.
	 Recurrent UTI:
	 - Prophylaxis with antibiotics not recommended as does not prevent recurrent UTI or new/progressive renal scarring; but does increase risk of resistant infections.
	 - Parents should be instructed to seek prompt (within 48h) medical evaluation of their child for future febrile illnesses to ensure detection and prompt treatment of recurrrent infection.
	 Treatment:
	 - Amoxicillin and cephalexin are NOT recommended empirically due to unacceptably high E. coli resistance.
	 - Cefazolin susceptibility does not predict cephalexin susceptibility of E. coli, Proteus mirabilis, and Klebsiella spp.
	 - Significant resistance to TMP/SMX, and depending on geographic location, to amoxicillin-clavulanate; knowledge of local susceptibility patterns and confirmaiton of susceptibility by culture is recommended.			

Infection	Usual Pathogens	Recommended Empiric Therapy	Recommended Paediatric Dose[B]	Recommended Duration	Comments
Urinary Tract					
Cystitis < 24 mos old or Pyelonephritis (all ages)	E. coli Other Enterobacteriaceae Enterococcus spp[†]	Infants <1 month **Ampicillin + Gentamicin**	200mg/kg/d IV div q6h 4-5mg/kg IV q24h	7-14 days	[†] Recommend empiric coverage of Enterococcus with ampicillin (200mg/kg/d IV div q6h) or amoxicillin-clavulanate (>1 month old) if: • <1 month old • urinary catheter • instrumentation of urinary tract • genitourinary abnormality. * Significant E. coli resistance - confirm susceptibility by culture. **7 days if prompt resolution of symptoms. If not, treat for 10-14 days. - Ciprofloxacin (20-30mg/kg/d PO/IV div bid) should be reserved for treatment of pyelonephritis due to P. aeruginosa or other multi-drug resistant organisms with documented susceptibility. - Nitrofurantoin should not be used for pyelonephritis or urosepsis as poor renal tissue and serum concentrations.
		Alternative **Ampicillin + Cefotaxime**	200mg/kg/d IV div q6h 100mg/kg/d IV div q8h	7-14 days	
		Children >1 month old[†] Oral: **Cefixime**	8mg/kg/d PO div q12-24h	7-14 days**	
		Alternative **TMP/SMX***	6-12mg TMP/kg/d PO div bid	7-14 days**	
		or **Amoxicillin-clavulanate***	40mg/kg/d PO div tid	7-14 days**	
		Parenteral: **Ceftriaxone**	50mg/kg IV q24h	7-14 days**	
		or **Gentamicin**	5-7mg/kg IV q24h	7-14 days**	
Cystitis > 24 mos old*	E. coli Other Enterobacteriaceae	**Nitrofurantoin** or	5-7mg/kg/d PO div q1d	3 days	* Children < 24 months, or with fever, toxicity, or CVA tenderness, should be treated as pyelonephritis. - Post-treatment urine cultures not recommended unless symptoms persist or recur. **Significant E. coli resistance - confirm susceptibility by culture.
		Cefixime	8mg/kg/d PO div q12-24h	3 days	
		Alernative **TMP/SMX*** or	6-12mg TMP/kg/d PO div bid	3 days	
		Amoxicillin-clavulanate*	40mg/kg/d PO div tid	3 days	

RECOMMENDED EMPIRIC THERAPY OF SELECTED INFECTIONS IN NEONATAL/PAEDIATRIC PATIENTS[A]

Infection	Usual Pathogens	Recommended Empiric Therapy	Recommended Paediatric Dose[B]	Recommended Duration	Comments
Urinary Tract					

Catheter-associated UTI (CA-UTI)					Definition of CA-UTI - catheter urine culture with ≥ 10⁵cfu/L of ≥ 1 organism(s) (infections may be polymicrobial) in a patient with urinary symptoms and/or signs (costovertebral tenderness, rigors) who is currently catheterized (short-term [< 30 days], long-term [≥ 30 days]‡, intermittent) or has been catheterized within previous 48 hours.
					‡ When a long-term catheterized patient has a symptomatic UTI, the catheter should be changed, and a urine specimen should be obtained through the newly placed catheter before starting antibiotics. Replacement of the catheter results in improved therapeutic outcomes, including decreased duration of fever and decreased likelihood of relapse.
					NB: Neither fever nor pyuria are diagnostic for CA-UTI. Do not treat unless evidence of urinary tract symptoms or systemic infection as:
					   • catheter often colonized with bacteria
					   • significant risk associated with inappropriate use of antibiotics including development of resistance and C. difficile infection.
					In patients with spinal cord injury, increased spasticity, autonomic dysreflexia, or sense of unease may indicate CA-UTI.
					
					Prevention:
					• Optimal hydration essential.
					• Hand hygiene before and after patient care.
					• Remove catheter as soon as not needed.
					• Screening of urine (urinalysis or culture) NOT recommended unless prior to GU surgery/instrumentation.
					NB: cloudy/foul smelling urine alone is not an indication for urine culture.
					• In catheterized patients, antibiotic prophylaxis is NOT recommended to reduce bacteriuria or UTI.
					• Prophylactic antibiotics NOT recommended at time of catheter placement, replacement or removal except prior to catheter removal in patients catheterized for > 48 hours post surgery involving prosthetic material.
					• Data inconclusive as to whether routine catheter change is effective in reducing CA-UTI.
					• NO convincing evidence for efficacy of antibiotic coated catheters.

RECOMMENDED EMPIRIC THERAPY OF SELECTED INFECTIONS IN NEONATAL/PAEDIATRIC PATIENTS[A]

Urinary Tract

Infection	Usual Pathogens	Recommended Empiric Therapy	Recommended Paediatric Dose[B]	Recommended Duration	Comments
Catheter-associated UTI (CA-UTI) (cont'd)	Enterobacteriaceae Enterococcus spp P. aeruginosa Coagulase negative Staphylococci Occasionally: • Candida spp	Asymptomatic None Symptomatic[†] Mild **Cefixime** or **Nitrofurantoin** Alternative** **Amoxicillin-clavulanate***** or **TMP/SMX** (if > 1 month old)*** Febrile, systemically unwell **Ampicillin + [Gentamicin]** or **Ceftriaxone** Septic/Hemodynamically unstable **Piperacillin-tazobactam** +/- **Gentamicin[‡]**	 8mg/kg/d PO div q12-24h 5-7mg/kg/d PO div qid 40mg/kg/d PO div tid 6-12mg TMP/kg/d PO div bid 100-200mg/kg/d IV div q6h 5-7mg/kg IV q24h 50mg/kg IV q24h 240-300mg piperacillin/kg/d IV div q6-8h 5-7mg/kg IV q24h	 7-14 days* 7-14 days* 7-14 days* 7-14 days* 7-14 days* 7-14 days*	†Tailor empiric therapy to most narrow spectrum option based on C&S results. *If prompt response (within 72 hours), treat for 7 days. If delayed response, treat for 10-14 days. **Ciprofloxacin (20-30mg/kg/d PO/IV div bid) is an alternative but should be reserved for treatment of CA-UTI due to P. aeruginosa or other multi-drug resistant organisms with documented susceptibility. ***Significant E. coli/Proteus mirabilis resistance; confirm susceptibility. ‡ Add gentamicin if: • septic shock • recent antibiotic use • suspected ESBL, Amp C, or carbapenemase producing organism.

RECOMMENDED EMPIRIC THERAPY OF SELECTED INFECTIONS IN NEONATAL/PAEDIATRIC PATIENTS[A]

Infection	Usual Pathogens	Recommended Empiric Therapy	Recommended Paediatric Dose[B]	Recommended Duration	Comments
Central Nervous System					
Meningitis		- 95% of patients with bacterial meningitis will have at least 2 of 4 of the following signs & symptoms (S&S):			

- 95% of patients with bacterial meningitis will have at least 2 of 4 of the following signs & symptoms (S&S):
  - fever
  - stiff neck
  - altered mental status
  - headache.
  NB: Absence of stiff neck does not rule out meningitis in any age group, particularly those < 2 years old.
- Blood culture recommended.
- Lumbar puncture (LP) for cell count, glucose, protein, Gram stain* and culture recommended without neuroimaging prior to antibiotic therapy **unless**:
  - S&S of increased intracranial pressure (ICP): NB: normal CT scan does NOT rule out raised ICP.
    ○ focal neurological deficit
    ○ papilledema
    ○ GCS < 11 or decrease in score of 3 or more
    ○ relative bradycardia or hypertension
  - uncorrected coagulopathy
  - hemodynamically unstable
  - extensive or spreading purpura
  - recent seizure without recovery to baseline mental status.
* Sensitivity of Gram stain is organism-specific but generally 50-90% therefore cannot be used to rule out bacterial meningitis.
  NB: Do not delay antibiotics if neuroimaging (CT/MRI) and/or LP cannot be performed expediently.
- Bacterial antigen test (latex agglutination) of CSF not recommended.
- Repeat LP should be considered if:
  - patient not responding clinically after 48h of appropriate antibiotic therapy
  - penicillin and/or cephalosporin intermediate/resistant S. pneumoniae.
- For prophylaxis of H. influenzae and N. meningitidis in close contacts, see Prophylaxis for Contacts of Communicable Diseases.
  Recommend droplet/contact precautions for 24 hours or until N. meningitidis ruled out.

RECOMMENDED EMPIRIC THERAPY OF SELECTED INFECTIONS IN NEONATAL/PAEDIATRIC PATIENTS[A]

Infection	Usual Pathogens	Recommended Empiric Therapy	Recommended Paediatric Dose[B]	Recommended Duration	Comments
Central Nervous System					
Meningitis (cont'd)					

Corticosteroid Therapy in Meningitis

- Corticosteroids are an option in bacterial meningitis in infants and children ≥ 6 weeks of age but are still controversial [Lancet Neurol 2010; 9:254-63]. **Corticosteroids are not recommended in neonatal meningitis, or if antibiotics have already been administered.**
- Dexamethasone 0.15mg/kg (maximum 10mg/dose) IV q6h x 2-4 days. Give 15-20 minutes before, or with, the first dose of antibiotics, NOT AFTER.

- Empiric vancomycin is not routinely indicated for:
  - sepsis without meningitis
  - viral meningitis
  - neonatal meningitis (unless a VLBW neonate in the NICU, particularly those with a central line where coagulase negative Staphylococcus is not an uncommon pathogen).

NB: Vancomycin has slow distribution and poor CSF penetration. It should be given as soon as possible AFTER the first dose of cefotaxime/ceftriaxone, and continued ONLY if the C&S results indicate cefotaxime/ceftriaxone resistant S. pneumoniae. Maintain trough vancomycin serum concentration of 15-20mg/L.

Typical CSF findings (beyond neonatal period)

Parameter	Bacterial	Viral
WBC count	>500 x 10⁶/L* (predominantly neutrophils)	<300 x 10⁶/L (predominantly lymphocytes, although neutrophils may be significant early in illness)
Protein	Elevated	Normal
Glucose	Reduced	Normal
CSF:serum glucose ratio	<0.4	>0.6

NB: Normal CSF findings can be found in 5% of early bacterial meningitis cases.

*Lower CSF WBC count may be seen in severe illness, septic shock.

RECOMMENDED EMPIRIC THERAPY OF SELECTED INFECTIONS IN NEONATAL/PAEDIATRIC PATIENTS[A]

Infection	Usual Pathogens	Recommended Empiric Therapy	Recommended Paediatric Dose[B]	Recommended Duration	Comments
Central Nervous System					
Meningitis (cont'd) **Neonates < 1 month[†]**	Group B Streptococci E. coli Listeria spp	**Ampicillin + [Gentamicin]** or **Cefotaxime]**	400mg/kg/d IV div q6h* 4-5mg/kg IV q24h 200mg/kg/d IV div q6h	Group B Strep, Listeria spp - 2-3 weeks E. coli - ≥ 3 weeks	- Tailor antibiotics to C&S results. - Repeat LP recommended at day 5 for Listeria and Gram negative organisms. Some experts recommend repeat LP at 48 hours for Group B Streptococci. - Consider need for acyclovir if HSV encephalitis possible. * If not Group B Streptococcal meningitis, decrease dose to 200mg/kg/d IV div q6h. - Corticosteroids are not currently recommended in neonatal meningitis due to different pathogens and lack of randomized controlled trial data.

[†] Neonatal doses listed are for term infants > 7 days old. For neonates outside of this range, refer to Neofax or Lexi-Comp or Pediatric Red Book, or consult pharmacy for dosing.

Infection	Usual Pathogens	Recommended Empiric Therapy	Recommended Paediatric Dose[B]	Recommended Duration	Comments
Central Nervous System					
Meningitis (cont'd) **Infants 1-3 months**	Group B Streptococci E. coli Listeria spp S. pneumoniae N. meningitidis H. influenzae	**Ampicillin + Cefotaxime**	300-400mg/kg/d IV div q6h 300mg/kg/d IV div q6h	S. pneumoniae - 10-14 days N. meningitidis - 5-7 days H. influenzae - 10 days Group B Strep, Listeria - 2-3 weeks Enterobacter-iaceae - ≥ 3 weeks	- Consider need for acyclovir if HSV encephalitis possible. - Tailor antibiotics to C&S results.
Children > 3 months	S. pneumoniae N. meningitidis (H. influenzae type b - if no or incomplete primary immunization)	**Ceftriaxone + Vancomycin**[D,*] Alternative only if severe/ anaphylactic β-lactam allergy** **Chloramphenicol + Vancomycin**[D]	100mg/kg/d IV div q12h 60mg/kg/d IV div q6h 75-100mg/kg/d IV div q6h 60mg/kg/d IV div q6h	S. pneumoniae - 10 days N. meningitidis - 5-7 days H. influenzae - 10 days	- Consider need for acyclovir if HSV encephalitis possible. * Vancomycin should be stopped as soon as ceftriaxone resistance excluded. **Consult Infectious Diseases.

D. Desired vancomycin trough is 15-20mg/L. Monitor renal function closely. See Vancomycin Dosing & Monitoring Guidelines.

Infection	Usual Pathogens	Recommended Empiric Therapy	Recommended Paediatric Dose[B]	Recommended Duration	Comments
Central Nervous System					
Meningitis (cont'd) **Nosocomial in neonates**[†]	Group B Streptococci Enterobacteriaceae Listeria spp If VLBW in NICU (particularly with CVL) add: • Coagulase negative Staph (CoNS) Candida spp**	**Ampicillin + [Gentamicin]** or **Cefotaxime** If high risk for CoNS **Vancomycin**[D] (pending cultures) + **Cefotaxime** Very severe **Meropenem + Vancomycin**[D] (pending cultures) **Candida spp**** **Amphotericin B +/- Flucytosine**	400mg/kg/d IV div q6h[‡] 4-5mg/kg IV q24h 200mg/kg/d IV div q6h 45mg/kg/d IV div q6h 200mg/kg/d IV div q6h 90mg/kg/d IV div q8h* 45mg/kg/d IV div q6h 0.7-1mg/kg IV daily 25mg/kg IV/PO qid	Gram positive: ≥ 14 days Gram negative: ≥ 21 days Min. 4 weeks after resolution of all signs & symptoms	[‡] If not Group B Streptococcal meningitis, decrease dose to 200mg/kg/d IV div q6h. * Use meropenem 60mg/kg/d IV div q8h if neonate < 14 days old. **Candida meningitis often a complication of candidemia in newborn infants.
Shunt or Extraventricular drain (EVD)	Coagulase negative Staph S. aureus Enterobacteriaceae Pseudomonas spp	**Vancomycin**[D] (pending cultures) + **[Ceftriaxone]** or **Meropenem***	60mg/kg/d IV div q6h 100mg/kg/d IV div q12h 120mg/kg/d IV div q8h	Gram positive: ≥ 14 days Gram negative: ≥ 21 days	- Shunt removal should be considered ASAP. * **NB:** • If Gram positive seen on smear, use vancomycin + ceftriaxone. • If Gram negative seen on smear, use meropenem. • If nothing seen on smear and recent surgery, use vancomycin + meropenem.

[†] Neonatal doses listed are for term infants > 7 days old. For neonates outside of this range, refer to Neofax or Lexi-Comp or Pediatric Red Book, or consult pharmacy for dosing.
D. Desired vancomycin trough is 15-20mg/L. Monitor renal function closely. See Vancomycin Dosing & Monitoring Guidelines.

Infection	Usual Pathogens	Recommended Empiric Therapy	Recommended Paediatric Dose[B]	Recommended Duration	Comments
Central Nervous System					
Meningitis (cont'd) **Basilar skull fracture**	S. pneumoniae H. influenzae Group A strep If prolonged hospitalization: S. aureus/MRSA Enterobacteriaceae	**Ceftriaxone** + **Vancomycin**[D] (pending cultures)	100mg/kg/d IV div q12h 60mg/kg/d IV div q6h	≥ 10 days ≥ 10 days	- Antibiotic prophylaxis in basilar skull fracture is not warranted. However antibiotics should be started if meningitis suspected or the child develops a fever.
Recurrent Meningitis	- Recurrent meningitis requires evaluation of underlying cause: • congenital anatomical defect (epidermoid/dermoid cysts, neural tube defects, asplenia) • acquired anatomical defect (head injuries, basal skull fracture, malignancy) • congenital immunodeficiencies (complement deficiency, agammaglobulinemia, IgG subclass deficiency, IRAK 4 deficiency) • acquired immunodeficiencies - HIV • chronic parameningeal infections (sinusitis, otitis media, mastoiditis) NB: - Anatomical defects most commonly cause recurrent S. pneumoniae or H. influenzae meningitis. - Complement deficiency is associated with recurrent N. meningitidis meningitis. Vaccination for S. pneumoniae, N. meningitidis, H. influenzae recommended for asplenia or complement deficiency.				
	Bacterial: S. pneumoniae N. meningitidis H. influenzae S. aureus Enterobacteriaceae	**Vancomycin**[D] + **Ceftriaxone**	60mg/kg/d IV div q6h 100mg/kg/d IV div q12h	S. pneumoniae, N. meningitidis, H. influenzae - 10 days S. aureus -14 days after last positive blood culture Enterobacteriaceae - 21 days	

D. Desired vancomycin trough is 15-20mg/L. Monitor renal function closely. See Vancomycin Dosing & Monitoring Guidelines.

RECOMMENDED EMPIRIC THERAPY OF SELECTED INFECTIONS IN NEONATAL/PAEDIATRIC PATIENTS[A]

Infection	Usual Pathogens	Recommended Empiric Therapy	Recommended Paediatric Dose[B]	Recommended Duration	Comments
Central Nervous System					
Brain Abscess	- Surgical therapy usually required with either stereotactic aspiration or open drainage. Send fluid/tissue for Gram stain and culture - Rule out: sinusitis, otitis, dental infection, endocarditis, congenital heart disease, lung abscess. - If multiple abscesses, blood cultures are recommended before antibiotics.				
	Viridans Group Streptococci Streptococcus anginosus group Anaerobes Enterobacteriaceae S. aureus	**Cloxacillin** + **Ceftriaxone*** + **Metronidazole**[C]	200mg/kg/d IV div q4h 100mg/kg/d IV div q12h 30mg/kg/d IV div q8h	6 weeks	* Use meropenem in place of ceftriaxone if increased risk of P. aeruginosa: • post neurosurgery or trauma • prolonged ventilatory support • prolonged hospitalization • previous broad spectrum antibiotics • burns.

RECOMMENDED EMPIRIC THERAPY OF SELECTED INFECTIONS IN NEONATAL/PAEDIATRIC PATIENTS[A]

Infection	Usual Pathogens	Recommended Empiric Therapy	Recommended Paediatric Dose[B]	Recommended Duration	Comments
Central Nervous System					
Epidural abcess	- Infectious complication of: • endocarditis • vertebral osteomyelitis • psoas muscle abscess. <u>Diagnosis:</u> - Classic triad of symptoms: • back pain • fever • neurologic deficit. - <u>MRI</u>				
	S. aureus/MRSA Enterobacteriaceae Streptococci CoNS P. aeruginosa Anaerobes	**Vancomycin**[D] + **Ceftriaxone*** + **Metronidazole**[C]	60mg/kg/d IV div q6h 100mg/kg/d IV div q12h 30mg/kg/d IV div q8h	6 weeks	- Surgical drainage often necessary if: • lesions > 3cm • gas present in abscess • no improvement with medical therapy. * Use meropenem in place of ceftriaxone if increased risk of P. aeruginosa: • post neurosurgery or trauma • prolonged ventilatory support • prolonged hospitalization • previous broad spectrum antibiotics • burns. - Treat according to C&S results of blood cultures or CT-guided aspirate of abscess.

D. Desired vancomycin trough is 15-20mg/L. Monitor renal function closely. See Vancomycin Dosing & Monitoring Guidelines.

RECOMMENDED EMPIRIC THERAPY OF SELECTED INFECTIONS IN NEONATAL/PAEDIATRIC PATIENTS[A]

Infection	Usual Pathogens	Recommended Empiric Therapy	Recommended Paediatric Dose[B]	Recommended Duration	Comments
Central Nervous System					
Encephalitis	Herpes simplex I virus* Enteroviruses See Recommended Empiric Therapy in Adult Patients, Encephalitis for epidemiologic clues, investigations, and other etiologies/special considerations.	Antiviral: **Acyclovir** +/- Antibacterial: (if bacterial meningitis not ruled out) **Ceftriaxone** + **Vancomycin**[D] +/- **Ampicillin**** +/- **Doxycycline*****	≤ 12 years old 60mg/kg/d IV div q8h > 12 years old 30mg/kg/d IV div q8h 100mg/kg/d IV div q12h 60mg/kg/d IV div q6h 300-400mg/kg/d IV div q6h 4mg/kg/d IV/PO div q12h	2-3 weeks if confirmed HSV encephalitis 2-3 weeks if confirmed HSV encephalitis	* Herpes simplex is the most common cause of sporadic fatal encephalitis and is one of the few treatable causes. - Infectious Diseases consult recommended. **If risk of Listeria and neutrophilis/mononuclear cells and low glucose in CSF. NB: Also consider TB/fungal pathogens if low CSF glucose +/- increased CSF protein. ***If risk of Rickettsia/Borrelia infection, and mononuclear cells, normal glucose +/- elevated protein in CSF.

D. Desired vancomycin trough is 15-20mg/L.   Monitor renal function closely.   See Vancomycin Dosing & Monitoring Guidelines.

RECOMMENDED EMPIRIC THERAPY OF SELECTED INFECTIONS IN NEONATAL/PAEDIATRIC PATIENTS[A]

Infection	Usual Pathogens	Recommended Empiric Therapy	Recommended Dose[B]	Recommended Duration	Comments
Cardiovascular					
Pericarditis	**Diagnostic criteria** • typical chest pain • pericardial friction rub • suggestive ECG charges (typically widespread ST-segment evaluation, PR depression) +/- • new or worsening pericardial effusion • increased CRP/ESR (supports diagnosis but neither sensitive nor specific for pericarditis) **Investigations** • cardiac auscultation • ECG • transthoracic echocardiogram (TTE) • ESR/CRP, CBC, creatinine, troponin, CK-MB • CXR • pericardial fluid for C&S and mycobacterial culture by Cardiology **Differential diagnosis** • infectious (viral, bacterial, mycobacterial, fungal, parasitic) • non-infectious: ○ autoimmune ○ neoplastic ○ metabolic ○ traumatic ○ drug-related				

RECOMMENDED EMPIRIC THERAPY OF SELECTED INFECTIONS IN NEONATAL/PAEDIATRIC PATIENTS[A]

Infection	Usual Pathogens	Recommended Empiric Therapy	Recommended Paediatric Dose[B]	Recommended Duration	Comments
Cardiovascular					
Pericarditis (cont'd)	Viral (~90%): • usually Enterovirus Rare: • M. tuberculosis • Ureaplasma spp • Mycoplasma spp • S. aureus/MRSA • β-haemolytic Streptococci • Enterobacteria-ceae • S. pneumoniae	Viral pericarditis Self-limited. No antiviral therapy. Purulent pericarditis*† **Vancomycin**[D] + **Ceftriaxone**	 60mg/kg/d IV div q6h 100mg/kg IV q24h	 6 weeks	* Recommend urgent surgical drainage if purulent/bacterial etiology suspected. † Tailor antibiotics to C&S results. β-lactams superior to vancomycin so preferred if susceptible.

D. Desired vancomycin trough is 15-20mg/L. Monitor renal function closely. See Vancomycin Dosing & Monitoring Guidelines.

RECOMMENDED EMPIRIC THERAPY OF SELECTED INFECTIONS IN NEONATAL/PAEDIATRIC PATIENTS[A]

Infection	Usual Pathogens	Recommended Empiric Therapy	Recommended Paediatric Dose[B]	Recommended Duration	Comments
Cardiovascular					
Endocarditis		- Diagnosis includes: • multiple positive blood cultures • new/worsening murmur • definite emboli • vegetations on echocardiogram.			

- Diagnosis includes:
  - multiple positive blood cultures
  - new/worsening murmur
  - definite emboli
  - vegetations on echocardiogram.
- For more specific diagnostic criteria, refer to Modified Duke Criteria www.circulationaha.org (*Circulation 2005;111:e394-e433*).
- Blood cultures:
  - NB: in patients who are stable (no heart failure) with subacute presentation, wait for results of blood cultures before starting antibiotic therapy.
  - draw maximum 2 sets/day
  - consult microbiology laboratory if unusual/fastidious (Bartonella, Chlamydia/Chlamydophila, Coxiella, Brucella, Legionella, Tropheryma whipplei) organism suspected
  - ensure clearance of bacteremia to guide duration of therapy.

- For specific organism recommendations or blood culture negative endocarditis, see Tables 4 & 5, respectively in Recommended Therapy of Culture-directed Infections in Adult Patients. Use pediatric doses (Table A).

Vancomycin
- Vancomycin is less rapidly bactericidal than ß-lactams, so should only be used when ß-lactams contraindicated (due to severe allergy or resistance). Longer duration of therapy may be required.
- Desired vancomycin trough is 15-20mg/L. Monitor renal function closely.

Table A. Recommended Pediatric Doses of Antibiotics Used for Treatment of Culture-proven Endocarditis

Antibiotic	Dose
Ampicillin	300mg/kg/d IV div q4h
Ceftriaxone	100mg/kg IV q24h
Cloxacillin	200mg/kg/d IV div q4h
Daptomycin	6-10mg/kg IV daily
Gentamicin synergy	3mg/kg/d IV div q8h or q24h
Gentamicin treatment	7mg/kg IV q24h
Penicillin G	200,000 units/kg/d IV div q4h
Rifampin	10mg/kg/d PO div bid
Tobramycin treatment	7mg/kg IV q24h
Vancomycin	60mg/kg/d IV div q6h

RECOMMENDED EMPIRIC THERAPY OF SELECTED INFECTIONS IN NEONATAL/PAEDIATRIC PATIENTS[A]

Infection	Usual Pathogens	Recommended Empiric Therapy	Recommended Paediatric Dose[B]	Recommended Duration	Comments
Cardiovascular					
Endocarditis (cont'd) **Native valve**	S. aureus/MRSA Viridans Group Streptococci Rare: • Enterococcus spp • HACEK organisms	**Vancomycin**[D] + **Ceftriaxone** Severe penicillin/ cephalosporin allergy **Vancomycin**[D] + **Gentamicin***	60mg/kg/d IV div q6h 100mg/kg IV daily 60mg/kg/d IV div q6h 7.5mg/kg/d IV div q8h	See Table 4 in Recommended Therapy of Culture-Directed Infections in Adult Patients. Use pediatric doses (Table A).	* For Gram positive organisms, desired gentamicin trough< 1mg/L. - Tailor antibiotic therapy to C&S results. β-lactams superior to vancomycin so preferred if susceptible.
Prosthetic valve	S. aureus/MRSA Coagulase negative Staph Viridans Group Streptococci Enterococcus spp Enterobacteriaceae Fungi	**Vancomycin**[D] + **Gentamicin*** + **Rifampin**	60mg/kg/d IV div q6h 7.5mg/kg/d IV div q8h 10mg/kg/d PO div bid	See Table 4 in Recommended Therapy of Culture-Directed Infections in Adult Patients. Use pediatric doses (Table A).	- Recommend urgent cardiovascular surgery consult if: • etiology is S. aureus, P. aeruginosa, fungi • heart failure • diabetes and/or renal failure • valve ring abscess. - Tailor antibiotic therapy to C&S results. β-lactams superior to vancomycin so preferred if susceptible. * For Gram positive organisms, desired gentamicin trough <1mg/L. See Aminoglycoside Dosing & Monitoring Guidelines.

HACEK = Haemophilus parainfluenzae, Aggregatibacter actinomycetemcomitans/aphrophilus, Cardiobacterium hominis, Eikenella corrodens, Kingella spp.
D. Desired vancomycin trough is 15-20mg/L. Monitor renal function closely. See Vancomycin Dosing & Monitoring Guidelines.

RECOMMENDED EMPIRIC THERAPY OF SELECTED INFECTIONS IN NEONATAL/PAEDIATRIC PATIENTS[A]

Infection	Usual Pathogens	Recommended Empiric Therapy	Recommended Paediatric Dose[B]	Recommended Duration	Comments
Sepsis without a focus					
Neonates	- Recommend: • blood cultures • catheter/suprapubic urine • lumbar puncture • admission for IV antibiotics. - Neonatal herpes simplex virus (HSV) infection can present like bacterial infection, testing including lumbar puncture for HSV PCR should be considered in all neonates with possible sepsis.				
< 1 month[†]	Group B Streptococci E. coli S. aureus/MRSA Coagulase negative Staph Less common: • Listeria spp • H. influenzae • Enterococcus spp • Other Enterobacteriaceae • Herpes simplex virus	**Ampicillin** + **[Gentamicin** or **Cefotaxime]** +/- **Acyclovir** If MRSA suspected, add: **Vancomycin**[D]	200mg/kg/d IV div q6h 4-5mg/kg IV q24h 200mg/kg/d IV div q6h 60mg/kg IV div q8h 45mg/kg/d IV div q8h	≥ 10 days Minimum 14 days for confirmed MRSA	- If clinical suspician or LP evidence of meningitis, see Meningitis section.

† Neonatal doses listed are for term infants > 7 days old. For neonates outside of this range, refer to Neofax or Lexi-Comp or Pediatric Red Book, or consult pharmacy for dosing.
D. Desired vancomycin trough is 15-20mg/L. Monitor renal function closely. See Vancomycin Dosing & Monitoring Guidelines.

RECOMMENDED EMPIRIC THERAPY OF SELECTED INFECTIONS IN NEONATAL/PAEDIATRIC PATIENTS[A]

Infection	Usual Pathogens	Recommended Empiric Therapy	Recommended Paediatric Dose[B]	Recommended Duration	Comments
Sepsis without a focus					
Infants 1-3 months					
Low risk [Pediatrics 2010;125:228-33]	- Low risk: watchful waiting with no empiric antibiotic therapy may be considered for low risk infants if ALL of the following criteria are met. Lumber puncture (LP) should be considered in infants with sepsis without a focus. • previously healthy – term, uncomplicated perinatal course, no chronic illness or surgery, no prior antibiotics • no focal bacterial infection on exam (including no otitis media) • non-toxic – no lethargy, good perfusion, normal respiratory rate, no cyanosis • negative laboratory screen – WBC 5-10 x 10^9/L, bands < 1.5 x 10^9/L, urinalysis < 10 WBC/hpf • parents are reliable and close follow-up is assured.				
High risk	- If not in the low risk group, recommend: • blood cultures • catheter/suprapubic urine • lumbar puncture • admission for IV antibiotics. Group B Streptococci E. coli Listeria spp S. pneumoniae N. meningitidis Occasionally: • H. influenzae	**Cefotaxime** +/- **Ampicillin**	200mg/kg/d IV div q6h 200mg/kg/d IV div q6h	≥ 10 days	
Children > 3-24 months • with fever • no focus of infection • not toxic • no shock	Viruses S. pneumoniae N. meningitidis S. aureus Occasionally: • H. influenzae	If temperature ≥ 39.5°C and WBC ≥ 15 x 10^9/L consider: **Amoxicillin**	90mg/kg/d PO div bid-tid	48 hours pending blood culture	- Follow-up in 24 hours is essential. - If treated with amoxicillin, do a blood culture first. - Recommend a urine culture in the young infant with temperature ≥ 39°C for ≥ 48 hours, and an LP if unexplained lethargy or irritability, headache or other signs/symptoms of meningeal irritation.

RECOMMENDED EMPIRIC THERAPY OF SELECTED INFECTIONS IN NEONATAL/PAEDIATRIC PATIENTS[A]

Infection	Usual Pathogens	Recommended Empiric Therapy	Recommended Paediatric Dose[B]	Recommended Duration	Comments
Sepsis					
Children > 3 months • **toxic** • **shock**	S. pneumoniae N. meningitidis S. aureus/MRSA Group A Streptococci Occasionally: • H. influenzae	**Ceftriaxone** Severe/shock/bacterial <u>meningitis suspected</u> [**Vancomycin**[D]] + **Ceftriaxone** <u>Alternative only if severe/anaphylactic β-lactam allergy</u> [**TMP/SMX**] + **Vancomycin**[D]] or [**Chloramphenicol**] + **Vancomycin**[D]]	100mg/kg/d IV div q12h 60mg/kg/d IV div q6h 100mg/kd/d IV div q12h 15-20mg TMP/kg/d IV div q6-8h 60mg/kg/d IV div q6h 75-100mg/kg/d IV div q6h 60mg/kg/d IV div q6h	<u>If no meningitis:</u> 10-14 days <u>If meningitis:</u> S. pneumoniae - 10 days N. meningitidis - 5-7 days H. influenzae - 10 days Gram negative - ≥ 3 weeks	Recommend: • blood culture • consider lumbar puncture • urine culture.

D. Desired vancomycin trough is 15-20mg/L. Monitor renal function closely. See Vancomycin Dosing & Monitoring Guidelines.

RECOMMENDED EMPIRIC THERAPY OF SELECTED INFECTIONS IN NEONATAL/PAEDIATRIC PATIENTS[A]

Infection	Usual Pathogens	Recommended Empiric Therapy	Recommended Paediatric Dose[B]	Recommended Duration	Comments
Sepsis					
Nosocomial without a focus **Neonates**[†]	Coagulase negative Staph S. aureus/MRSA Enterobacteriaceae Group B Streptococci	**Cloxacillin** + **Gentamicin** If post op heart surgery, central venous line or very low birth weight or high institutional MRSA rate **Vancomycin**[D] + **Gentamicin** Severely ill **Vancomycin**[D] + **Meropenem**	200mg/kg/d IV div q6h 4-5mg/kg IV q24h 45mg/kg/d IV div q8h 4-5mg/kg IV q24h 45mg/kg/d IV div q8h 60-90mg/kg/d IV div q8h	≥ 7 days ≥ 7 days ≥ 7 days	- Strongly consider an LP. - Tailor antibiotic therapy to C&S results.

[†] Neonatal doses listed are for term infants > 7 days old. For neonates outside of this range, refer to Neofax or Lexi-Comp or Pediatric Red Book, or consult pharmacy for dosing.
D. Desired vancomycin trough is 15-20mg/L. Monitor renal function closely. See Vancomycin Dosing & Monitoring Guidelines.

RECOMMENDED EMPIRIC THERAPY OF SELECTED INFECTIONS IN NEONATAL/PAEDIATRIC PATIENTS[A]

Infection	Usual Pathogens	Recommended Empiric Therapy	Recommended Paediatric Dose[B]	Recommended Duration	Comments
Sepsis					
Nosocomial without a focus (cont'd) > 1 month	S. aureus/MRSA Enterobacteriaceae	[Cefazolin or Cloxacillin] + Gentamicin	100mg/kg/d IV div q8h 200mg/kg/d IV div q6h 7mg/kg IV q24h or 7.5mg/kg/d IV div q8h	≥ 7 days	Recommend: • blood culture • urine culture.
		If high institutional MRSA rate Vancomycin[D] + Gentamicin	60mg/kg/d IV div q6h 7mg/kg IV q24h or 7.5mg/kg/d IV div q8h	≥ 7 days	
		Severely ill Piperacillin-tazobactam + Tobramycin	240-300mg/kg/d IV div q6h 7mg/kg IV q24h or 7.5mg/kg/d IV div q8h	≥ 7 days	
		If high institutional MRSA rate, add: Vancomycin[D]	60mg/kg/d IV div q6h		
Post op heart surgery	Coagulase negative Staph (CoNS)* S. aureus/MRSA* Enterobacteriaceae Enterococcus spp	Vancomycin[D] + Piperacillin-tazobactam +/- Gentamicin	60mg/kg/d IV div q6h 240-300mg/kg/d IV div q6h 7mg/kg IV q24h or 7.5mg/kg/d IV div q8h	≥ 7 days ≥ 7 days ≥ 7 days	* Tailor antibiotics to C&S results, including discontinuation of vancomycin if CoNS and/or MRSA not found on culture.

D. Desired vancomycin trough is 15-20mg/L. Monitor renal function closely. See Vancomycin Dosing & Monitoring Guidelines.

RECOMMENDED EMPIRIC THERAPY OF SELECTED INFECTIONS IN NEONATAL/PAEDIATRIC PATIENTS[A]

Infection	Usual Pathogens	Recommended Empiric Therapy	Recommended Paediatric Dose[B]	Recommended Duration	Comments
Sepsis					
Catheter-related bloodstream infection (CRBSI)	- See Adult Empiric Therapy, Catheter-related bloodstream infection for further information.				
	Coagulase negative Staph (CoNS) S. aureus S. lugdunensis Enterobacteriaceae	**[Cefazolin** or **Cloxacillin]*** + **[Gentamicin** or **Tobramycin]**	100mg/kg IV div q8h 200mg/kg/d IV div q6h 7mg/kg IV q24h **or** 7.5mg/kg/d IV div q8h 7mg/kg IV q24h **or** 7.5mg/kg/d IV div q8h	Duration dependent on: • ability to remove line • organism involved. Uncomplicated† BC positive with: - CoNS - 5-7 days. **Avoid treatment in response to single positive blood culture for CoNS. Repeat culture recommended.** - S. aureus & echocardio-gram negative - 14 days after first negative BC** - Gram negative organisms - 7-14 days	- Line must be removed if any of: • tunnel infection • failure to respond within 72 hours (persistent positive daily blood cultures) • fungal (with a percutaneous CVL). * Although this regimen does not cover all CoNS, it remains a reasonable empiric option. If CoNS resistant to cloxacillin isolated, suggest repeat blood cultures (BC) before switching to vancomycin. † Complicated - 4-6 weeks of therapy: • septic thrombophlebitis • endocarditis • osteomyelitis • persistent bacteremia > 72h after catheter removal despite appropriate antimicrobial therapy. **If BC negative but catheter tip ≥15 CFU of S. aureus, consider 5-7 day course of therapy after line removal.
		Definite tunnel infection **Vancomycin**[D] + **[Gentamicin** or **Tobramycin]**	60mg/kg IV div q6h 7mg/kg IV q24h **or** 7.5mg/kg/d IV div q8h 7mg/kg IV q24h **or** 7.5mg/kg/d IV div q8h		

D. Desired vancomycin trough is 15-20mg/L. Monitor renal function closely. See Vancomycin Dosing & Monitoring Guidelines.

RECOMMENDED EMPIRIC THERAPY OF SELECTED INFECTIONS IN NEONATAL/PAEDIATRIC PATIENTS[A]

Infection	Usual Pathogens	Recommended Empiric Therapy	Recommended Paediatric Dose[B]	Recommended Duration	Comments
Sepsis					
Catheter-related bloodstream infection (CRBSI) (cont'd)					
	Candida spp	**Amphotericin B** or **Fluconazole***	0.6-1mg/kg IV daily 12mg/kg/d IV/PO div q12h	14 days after first negative BC**	* Use fluconazole if no azole exposure in past 3 months and risk of C. krusei or C. glabrata low. **If BC negative but catheter tip ≥15 CFU of Candida, consider 5-7 day course of therapy after line removal.
Peripheral IV	S. aureus Streptococcus spp Coagulase negative Staph Enterobacteriaceae	Phlebitis **Cefazolin** +/- **Gentamicin**	100mg/kg/d IV div q8h 7mg/kg IV q24h or 7.5mg/kg/d IV div q8h	7-10 days	- Remove IV.

- 208 -

RECOMMENDED EMPIRIC THERAPY OF SELECTED INFECTIONS IN NEONATAL/PAEDIATRIC PATIENTS[A]

Infection	Usual Pathogens	Recommended Empiric Therapy	Recommended Paediatric Dose[B]	Recommended Duration	Comments

Febrile Neutropenia
[Clin Infect Dis 2011;52:e56-93]
		Definitions
		Febrile = oral temperature ≥ 38.3°C once or ≥ 38°C for ≥ 1 hour
		Neutropenia = absolute neutrophil count [ANC] < 0.5 x 10⁹/L
		Investigations
		• Blood and urine cultures
		• CBC with differential, electrolytes, creatinine, AST, bilirubin
		• If respiratory symptoms:
		  ○ CXR
		  ○ Nasopharyngeal swab for viral respiratory panel PCR
		  ○ Sputum/tracheal aspirate for C&S and Mycoplasma/Chlamydophila/Legionella PCR
		• Careful physical examination required including skin, oral mucosa, perianal area, respiratory system and abdomen.
		Monotherapy
		- Piperacillin-tazobactam monotherapy is recommended first-line in patients who are hemodynamically stable and no evidence of catheter-related infection, skin and soft tissue infection (SSTI), or pneumonia.
		- Ceftazidime monotherapy is not recommended as it:
		  • has no reliable Gram positive (Enterococci, Streptococci, Staphylococci) activity compared to piperacillin-tazobactam
		  • may promote antimicrobial resistance (extended-spectrum β-lactamases (ESBL) and AmpC cephalosporinases)
		  • **is not optimal in patients with profound (< 0.1 x 10⁹/L)/prolonged neutropenia.**
		- Cefepime monotherapy is an alternative to piperacillin-tazobactam:
		  • good streptococcal activity
		  • activity against methicillin-susceptible S. aureus
		  • activity against Amp C cephalosporinase-producing Gram negative organisms (but not against ESBL)
		  • lacks enterococcal coverage.
		- Carbapenem monotherapy is an alternative to piperacillin-tazobactam. In order to prevent the selection of carbapenem resistance carbapenems should not be used first-line unless:
		  • known/suspected infection with ESBL/Amp C cephalosporinase-producing organisms.
		  • penicillin allergy.
		Combination therapy (β-lactam plus an aminoglycoside and vancomycin)
		  • provides increased coverage of potential pathogens, including resistant strains.
		  • is recommended until C&S results available in patients who are hemodynamically unstable or with septic shock.			

RECOMMENDED EMPIRIC THERAPY OF SELECTED INFECTIONS IN NEONATAL/PAEDIATRIC PATIENTS[A]

Infection	Usual Pathogens	Recommended Empiric Therapy	Recommended Paediatric Dose[B]	Recommended Duration	Comments
Febrile Neutropenia (cont'd)					

		Recommendations for the Use of Vancomycin in Febrile Neutropenia
		- Empiric vancomycin should not be used routinely in febrile neutropenic patients.
		- Empiric vancomycin therapy should be considered in:
		  • clinically obvious central venous catheter-related infections (tunnel infection)
		  • skin or soft tissue infections
		  • pneumonia
		  • hemodynamic instability
		  • patients with positive blood culture for Gram-positive organisms not yet identified (NB: Leuconostoc spp. Pediococcus spp are resistant to vancomycin.)
		  • known colonization with MRSA.
		- Vancomycin therapy should be discontinued on day 2-3 if cultures negative for β-lactam resistant Gram positive organisms.			

RECOMMENDED EMPIRIC THERAPY OF SELECTED INFECTIONS IN NEONATAL/PAEDIATRIC PATIENTS[A]

Infection	Usual Pathogens	Recommended Empiric Therapy	Recommended Paediatric Dose[B]	Recommended Duration	Comments
Febrile Neutropenia (cont'd)					

No focus	**Low risk patients:**
	•clinically stable
	•no comorbidities
	•neutropenia expected to be < 7 days
	may not require such broad spectrum antibiotic therapy. Refer to local guidelines.
	
	High risk:
	• Profound neutropenia (ANC < 0.1 x 10^9/L) anticipated to be > 7 days
	• Significant comorbid conditions, including:
	  ○ hemodynamic instability
	  ○ oral or GI mucositis that impairs swallowing or causes severe diarrhea
	  ○ new onset abdominal pain, nausea or vomiting, or diarrhea
	  ○ neurologic changes/confusion
	  ○ intravascular catheter infection
	  ○ pneumonia/hypoxemia/chronic lung disease
	  ○ hepatic insufficiency (AST > 5x normal value)
	  ○ renal insufficiency (Clcr < 30mL/min).
	
	- Median time to defervescence for high risk patients treated with appropriate empiric antibiotic therapy is 5 days.
	- Antifungal therapy: using agent from a different class from that used for prophylaxis should be considered in patients who remain febrile and neutropenic at day 4-7 despite adequate antibiotic coverage.
	  • Infectious Diseases consult recommended
	  • Repeat blood cultures plus ultrasound of abdomen recommended, or
	  • If high risk for mould infections (hematologic malignancy, especially AML: repeat blood cultures including fungal blood cultures and CT chest/abdomen/sinuses.
	- Consider switch to oral therapy if:
	  • non-septic presentation (no chills, hypotension or fluid resuscitation)
	  • patient stable
	  • mucositis resolving
	  • neutrophils > 0.1x10^9/L.
	  • adequate GI absorption.				

RECOMMENDED EMPIRIC THERAPY OF SELECTED INFECTIONS IN NEONATAL/PAEDIATRIC PATIENTS[A]

Infection	Usual Pathogens	Recommended Empiric Therapy	Recommended Paediatric Dose[B]	Recommended Duration	Comments
Febrile Neutropenia (cont'd)					
High risk	**Gram positive** Coag neg Staph Enterococcus spp Viridans Grp Strep S. aureus/MRSA S. lugdunensis Corynebacterium spp Bacillus cereus Rothia spp β-haemolytic Strep S. pneumoniae Rhodococcus spp Abiotrophia spp Granulicatella spp Leuconostoc spp Pediococcus spp **Gram negative** Enterobacteriaceae Pseudomonas spp Stenotrophomonas maltophilia Achromobacter spp Acinetobacter spp Burkholderia spp Capnocytophaga spp Eikenella spp Anaerobes Polymicrobial (20-30%) Fungi (<5%)	Hemodynamically stable[*#] **Piperacillin-tazobactam** + [**Gentamicin** or **Tobramycin**] Alternative [**Cefepime** or **Imipenem** or **Meropenem**] + [**Gentamicin** or **Tobramycin**] Hemodynamically unstable **Piperacillin-tazobactam*** + **Vancomycin[D,**]** + [**Gentamicin** or **Tobramycin**] Severe β-lactam allergy/ anaphylaxis **Ciprofloxacin** + **Clindamycin** + [**Gentamicin** or **Tobramycin**]	300mg/kg/d IV div q6h 7mg/kg IV q24h x 1 dose 7mg/kg IV q24h x 1 dose 150mg/kg/d IV div q8h 80mg/kg/d IV div q6h 60mg/kg/d IV div q6-8h 7mg/kg IV q24h x 1 dose 7mg/kg IV q24h x 1 dose 300mg/kg/d IV div q6h 60mg/kg/d IV div q6h 7mg/kg IV q24h x 1 dose 7mg/kg IV q24h x 1 dose 30mg/kg/d IV/PO div q12h 40mg/kg/d IV/PO div q8h 7mg/kg IV q24h x 1 dose 7mg/kg IV q24h x 1 dose	Tailor duration of therapy to identified organism and infection. Must be afebrile for at least 48h and neutrophil count > 0.5 x 10⁹/L before discontinuing antibiotic therapy. • Bacteremia, SSTI, pneumonia - 10-14 days. No focus: • If neutrophil count ≥ 0.5×10⁹/L – 7 days minimum. • If neutrophil count < 0.5×10⁹/L - 2 weeks minimum. Longer therapy may be required if: • neutrophil count < 0.1 x 10⁹/L • severe mucositis • unstable vital signs.	* Use imipenem or meropenem if: • suspected infection with ESBL or Amp C producing organism • nonsevere penicillin allergy. # Add vancomycin (alternative linezolid) if: • suspected catheter-related infection, SSTI, pneumonia • AML patients with mucositis and persistent (> 48h) fever. • previous/current colonization or infection with MRSA. Add linezolid instead of vancomycin if: • previous/current colonization or infection with VRE. **Use linezolid instead of vancomycin if previous/current colonization or infection with VRE.

D. Desired vancomycin trough is 15-20mg/L. Monitor renal function closely. See Vancomycin Dosing & Monitoring Guidelines.

RECOMMENDED EMPIRIC THERAPY OF SELECTED INFECTIONS IN NEONATAL/PAEDIATRIC PATIENTS[A]

FOOTNOTES

A. These are empiric antibiotic recommendations based on current literature, national susceptibility patterns, and antimicrobials currently available on the Canadian market. Readers are encouraged to make antibiotic therapy choices based on usual pathogens and susceptibility patterns locally. Antibiotics listed for each condition are not all inclusive, nor are they all approved by Health Canada TPD for the listed indication. Choice of empiric antibiotic therapy should be based on the patient's age, allergies, co-morbidities, and clinical condition, as well as cost and convenience of the dosage regimen. Empiric antibiotic therapy should be modified to narrower spectrum antibiotic(s) according to culture and susceptibility (C&S) results.

B. Usual paediatric dose in patients with normal renal and hepatic function. Mg/kg/d = milligrams per kilogram per day unless otherwise specified. Neonatal doses listed are for term infants > 7 days old. For neonates ouside of this range, refer to Neofax or Lexi-Comp or the Paediatric Red Book, or consult pharmacy for dosing.

C. Oral clindamycin/metronidazole have excellent absorption. If intravenous therapy is deemed necessary, prompt switch to the oral formulation is recommended. (See IV to PO Switch Recommendations and Paediatric Dosing Guide).

D. See Vancomycin Dosing & Monitoring Guidelines.

ABBREVIATIONS
MRSA = methicillin-resistant Staphylococcus aureus

RECOMMENDED EMPIRIC THERAPY OF SELECTED INFECTIONS IN ADULT PATIENTS[A]

Infection	Usual Pathogens	Recommended Empiric Therapy	Recommended Dose[B]	Recommended Duration	Comments
Skin & Soft Tissue					

Community-associated methicillin-resistant S. aureus (CA-MRSA)

- Incidence of CA-MRSA is significant and in many locations in Canada constitutes > 20% of S. aureus isolates.

- **Screening:**

  Community - nares

  Active screening to identify MRSA carriers in the community is NOT warranted except in:
  - individuals with recurrent S. aureus skin infections (≥2 episodes in 6 months) despite enhanced hygiene measures, and in whom eradication is being considered.
  - closed community or family setting with recurrent infection despite enhanced hygiene measures.

  Institution - nares and groin

  Controversy exists as to whether to screen select high risk patient groups versus high risk settings (presurgical, ICU, hemodialysis). Regardless, the benefit of active screening and isolation is of unproven benefit without strict adherence to hand hygiene and consistent use of contact precautions.

- **Decolonization:**
  - Decolonization regimens of limited success as recolonization is frequent (up to 75% at one year post decolonization).
  - Success of decolonization is much less if extranasal colonization, presence of active skin infection, or presence of indwelling catheters/tubes.
  - Prolonged/repeated use of mupirocin has led to significant mupirocin resistance.

  Therefore decolonization should only be considered in the following circumstances:
  - recurrent CA-MRSA skin infections (≥ 2 episodes in 6 months) despite enhanced hygiene measures and with no evidence of re-exposure.
  - outbreaks in selected closed communities or family settings despite enhanced hygiene measures
  - Recommended decolonization regimen:

Mupirocin 2%	bid-tid intranasally	7 days
Chlorhexidine 2-4%	full body wash daily	7 days
2 active systemic antibiotics		
rifampin	300mg PO bid	7 days
[doxycycline or	100mg PO bid	7 days
TMP/SMX]	1 DS tab PO bid	

RECOMMENDED EMPIRIC THERAPY OF SELECTED INFECTIONS IN ADULT PATIENTS[A]

Infection	Usual Pathogens	Recommended Empiric Therapy	Recommended Dose[B]	Recommended Duration	Comments
Skin & Soft Tissue					
Impetigo*	- Superficial nonfollicular pustules				
	Bullous S. aureus Nonbullous, honey <u>crust lesions</u> Group A Streptococci	<u>Limited involvement/ disease</u> **Mupirocin 2%** or **Fusidic acid 2%** <u>Unresponsive to topical or indication for systemic antibiotic**</u> **Cloxacillin** or **Cephalexin** β-lactam allergy **Erythromycin** or **Clindamycin**	tid topically tid- qid topically 500mg PO qid 500mg PO qid 500mg PO qid 300mg PO qid	7 days 7 days 7 days 7 days 7 days 7 days	- No evidence that disinfecting solutions are of any value. * Epidemics must be reported to Public Health. **Systemic antibiotics recommended if: • multiple/extensive/recurrent lesions • fever/constitutional symptoms/ lymphadenopathy • immunocompromised • valvular heart disease.
Folliculitis/ Furunculosis	- Folliculitis – superficial inflammation/infection of hair follicle - Furunculosis – deep infection of multiple hair follicles leading to boils (furuncles)				
	S. aureus	Hot compresses + Antiseptic cleanser <u>Unresponsive to above or extensive</u> **Mupirocin 2%** or **Fusidic acid 2%**	 tid topically tid-qid topically	 7 days 7 days	- Usually self-limiting. - Recommend incision and drainage of pus, probing cavities to break up loculations, and covering with dry dressing. - Systemic antibiotics recommended if scalp folliculitis (see Carbuncles). - Unresolving furunculosis - consider mycobacterial infections.
Whirlpool/hot tub	Pseudomonas aeruginosa	Hot compresses + Antiseptic cleanser			- Self-limiting in immunocompetent individuals.

RECOMMENDED EMPIRIC THERAPY OF SELECTED INFECTIONS IN ADULT PATIENTS[A]

Infection	Usual Pathogens	Recommended Empiric Therapy	Recommended Dose[B]	Recommended Duration	Comments
Skin & Soft Tissue					
Recurrent furunculosis	S. aureus	Consider decolonization: **Mupirocin 2%**	bid-tid intranasally	5 days. Repeat monthly for 1st 5 days/mo x 6-12 mos	- If > 6 recurrences/year, some experts recommend suppressive therapy with clindamycin 150mg PO daily or azithromycin 500mg PO weekly x at least 3 months. Culture and susceptibility recommended. Benefits of this strategy must be weighed against risks of resistance.
		Alternative **Rifampin + TMP/SMX**	600mg PO daily 1 DS tab PO bid	10 days	
Carbuncles	S. aureus	Limited disease Hot compresses + Antiseptic cleanser			- Recommend incision and drainage of pus, probing cavities to break up loculations, and covering with dry dressing.
		Unresponsive to above or indication for systemic antibiotics* **Cloxacillin** or **Cephalexin**	500mg PO qid 500mg PO qid	7 days 7 days	* Systemic antibiotics recommended if: • debilitated elderly • immunosuppression/diabetes/ concurrent malignancy • surrounding cellulitis/septic phlebitis • located in area difficult to drain (face, genitalia).
		β-lactam allergy **TMP/SMX** or **Doxycycline** or **Clindamycin**	1 DS tab PO bid 100mg PO bid 300mg PO qid	7 days 7 days 7 days	• fever/constitutional symptoms **"Increased incidence of community-associated MRSA. Incision and drainage may be all that is required.
		MRSA suspected** **TMP/SMX** or **Doxycycline**	1-2 DS tabs PO bid 100mg PO bid	7 days 7 days	If antibiotic therapy is deemed necessary, cultures recommended. Check susceptibility of MRSA. Do not use clindamycin or quinolones empirically for MRSA as significant resistance.

RECOMMENDED EMPIRIC THERAPY OF SELECTED INFECTIONS IN ADULT PATIENTS[A]

Infection	Usual Pathogens	Recommended Empiric Therapy	Recommended Dose[B]	Recommended Duration	Comments
Skin & Soft Tissue					
Vesicular lesions	- Notify Public Health.				
Chickenpox	- For contact prophylaxis recommendations, see Prophylaxis for Contacts of Communicable Diseases.				
Children	Varicella zoster	See Paediatric Guidelines			
Adults Immuno-competent	Varicella zoster	**Famciclovir** or **Valacyclovir** or **Acyclovir**	500mg PO tid 1g PO tid 800mg PO qid	5 days 5 days 5 days	- Most benefit if initiate therapy within 24 hours of rash onset. - Recommend treatment, even if started later than 24 hours, in: • pneumonia or other visceral involvement (treat x 10 days) • pregnancy. Safety of acyclovir in pregnancy not fully established. Potential benefit vs. potential risk to the fetus should be discussed with the patient. Acyclovir has been used at all stages of pregnancy; no adverse effects to the fetus/newborn have been reported to date.
Adults Immunocom-promised	Varicella zoster	**Famciclovir** or **Valacyclovir** or **Acyclovir** *Severe* **Acyclovir**	500mg PO tid 1g PO tid 800mg PO qid 10mg/kg IV q8h	7-10 days 7-10 days 7-10 days 7-10 days	

RECOMMENDED EMPIRIC THERAPY OF SELECTED INFECTIONS IN ADULT PATIENTS[A]

Infection	Usual Pathogens	Recommended Empiric Therapy	Recommended Dose[B]	Recommended Duration	Comments
Skin & Soft Tissue					
Vesicular lesions (cont'd) **Zoster (Shingles)**	- Recommend HIV testing, especially in young adults. - Herpes zoster ophthalmicus - involvement of cranial nerve V_1 occurs in 10-25% of herpes zoster (HZ) cases. Blisters on tip of nose may be seen. Consult ophthalmology. - Ramsay-Hunt syndrome - severe ear pain, facial muscle weakness, and rash indicates infection of facial nerve. - Oral corticosteroid therapy may provide some benefit in acute herpes zoster (HZ) symptoms, but they have significant adverse effects and have not been shown to lower incidence or duration of postherpetic neuralgia (PHN). Therefore, the overall risk/benefit profile does not support the routine use of corticosteroids in herpes zoster. - Immunity is boosted once a person has herpes zoster, so recurrence is uncommon (≤ 5%) in immunocompetent persons. - Direct contact with the skin lesions of a person with regional/limited herpes zoster, or via airborne route in disseminated zoster, can lead to varicella (chicken pox) in persons who have not had varicella or been immunized.				
Immunocom-petent*	- Prevention - Zoster (live) vaccine (Zostavax) approved for prevention of herpes zoster and its complications in immunocompetent adults ≥ 50 years of age. NB: Antiviral medications should not be used within 24h before or 14 days after vaccination.				
	Varicella zoster	**Famciclovir**** or **Valacyclovir**** or **Acyclovir**	500mg PO tid 1g PO tid or 1.5g PO bid 800mg PO 5x/day	7 days*** 7 days*** 7 days*** 7 days***	- Topical therapy not recommended as ineffective. * Therapy recommended for all immunocompetent patients to prevent PHN; it should be started within 72 hours of rash onset, or at any time if new vesicles forming or cutaneous/motor/neurologic/ocular complications. - Early attention to pain management during acute zoster may reduce the probability and severity of PHN. **More effective than acyclovir in the treatment & resolution of PHN. ***Treat longer if: • new vesicles forming • cutaneous, motor, neurologic or ocular complications.

RECOMMENDED EMPIRIC THERAPY OF SELECTED INFECTIONS IN ADULT PATIENTS[A]

Infection	Usual Pathogens	Recommended Empiric Therapy	Recommended Dose[B]	Recommended Duration	Comments
Skin & Soft Tissue					
Vesicular lesions (cont'd)					
Zoster (Shingles) (cont'd)					
Immunocom-promised	- Prevention - Antiviral prophylaxis is recommended to prevent herpes zoster (HZ) in immunocompromised persons who cannot receive the live HZ vaccine: - Agents: **Acyclovir** 400-800mg PO daily or **Famciclovir** 500mg PO daily or **Valacyclovir** 250-500mg PO daily } until end of immunosuppressive therapy and/or at least 1 year after transplant or leukemia induction therapy				
	Varicella zoster	Mild-moderate **Famciclovir** or **Valacyclovir** or **Acyclovir**	500mg PO tid 1g PO tid 800mg PO 5x/day	7-10 days 7-10 days 7-10 days	- Therapy should be started within 72 hours of rash onset, or at any time if new vesicles forming or cutaneous/motor/neurologic/ocular complications. * Disseminated herpes zoster: bilateral involvement, spread beyond contiguous dermatomes, or organ involvement (lung, liver, brain).
		Severe/Disseminated* **Acyclovir**	10mg/kg IV q8h	7-10 days	
Mucocutaneous Immuno-competent	- For genital herpes simplex, see Genital section.				
Primary (gingivo-stomatitis)	Herpes simplex	**Famciclovir** or **Valacyclovir** or **Acyclovir**	500mg PO bid 500mg-1g PO bid 400mg PO tid	7 days 7 days 7 days	- Therapy should be started within 72 hours of symptom onset, or at any time if new lesions forming. - Topical therapy not recommended as ineffective.

RECOMMENDED EMPIRIC THERAPY OF SELECTED INFECTIONS IN ADULT PATIENTS[A]

Infection	Usual Pathogens	Recommended Empiric Therapy	Recommended Dose[B]	Recommended Duration	Comments
Skin & Soft Tissue					
Vesicular lesions (cont'd) **Mucocutaneous** (cont'd) **Immuno-competent** (cont'd) **Recurrent (fever blisters, cold sores)**	Herpes simplex	**No therapy indicated** unless recurrences are: • severe and • ≥ 6 episodes/year Suppressive therapy Valacyclovir or Acyclovir or Symptomatic therapy* Famciclovir or Valacyclovir or Acyclovir	500mg PO daily 400mg PO bid 1500mg PO daily 2g PO bid 400mg PO tid	1 day 1 day 5 days	- No role for topical acyclovir. * Initiate therapy at first sign of symptoms. No benefit if therapy started after lesions established.
Immuno-compromised	Herpes simplex	Famciclovir or Valacyclovir or Acyclovir	500mg PO bid 500mg-1g PO bid 400mg PO 5x/day	7-10 days 7-10 days 7-10 days	- HIV patients and transplant recipients may benefit from suppressive acyclovir therapy 200-400mg PO bid-tid.

RECOMMENDED EMPIRIC THERAPY OF SELECTED INFECTIONS IN ADULT PATIENTS[A]

Infection	Usual Pathogens	Recommended Empiric Therapy	Recommended Empiric Dose[B]	Recommended Duration	Comments
Skin & Soft Tissue					

Cellulitis					Cellulitis includes:
					• erysipelas – acute, superficial, nonnecrotizing infection of dermis/hypodermis typically caused by streptococci. Classically presents with well defined raised edge/erythematous plaque of sudden onset associated with pain, swelling and fever.
					• cellulitis – acute, subacute or chronic nonnecrotizing infection of dermis/ hypodermis that extends into the subcutaneous/connective tissues with/without lymphadenopathy and/or abscess formation.
					
					Investigations:
					- Superficial skin cultures not recommended.
					  Exceptions
					  • subcutaneous abscess present: incision and drainage with culture recommended.
					  • toe web intertrigo: culture of fissures may yield pathogen (β-hemolytic strep/S. aureus/MRSA) to help guide treatment. Also culture for dermatophytes and treat if positive as may be source of bacterial entry/recurrence.
					- Blood cultures recommended if septic, temp ≥ 38.5°C, immunocompromised, or diabetic.
					
					Differential Diagnosis:
					• Deep vein thrombosis/superficial thrombophlebitis
					• Venous stasis (bilateral cellulitis rare)
					• Hypersensitivity reactions/contact dermatitis
					• Drug reactions (often sulfa-based drugs)
					• Toxic epidermal necrolysis - history of drug exposure
					• Pyoderma gangrenosum (anterior shin/ulcerative) - associated with inflammatory bowel disease, rheumatologic disease, leukemia.
					• Eosinophilic cellulitis (Well's syndrome) - associated with myeloproliferative, immunological, infectious conditions
					• Acute febrile neutrophilic dermatosis (Sweet's syndrome) - associated with hematologic malignancies
					• Gouty arthritis/septic arthritis/olecranon bursitis
					• Erythema migrans - resembles erysipelas, not painful, progresses slowly, less fever
					• Erythema nodosum
					• Carcinoma erysipeloides - metastatic disease invading skin, lymphatic vessels (breast cancer)
					• Foreign body reactions - hypersensitivity to metal implants
					• Familial Mediterranean Fever
					• Myositis (viral/parasitic)
					• Relapsing polychondritis (may mimic cellulitis of ears; sparing ear lobes)
					• Polyarteritis nodosa - subcutaneous plaques due to necrotizing vasculitis (lower extremities)
					
					Management:
					• Elevate affected area if possible (essential for lower limbs)

RECOMMENDED EMPIRIC THERAPY OF SELECTED INFECTIONS IN ADULT PATIENTS[A]

Infection	Usual Pathogens	Recommended Empiric Therapy	Recommended Dose[B]	Recommended Duration	Comments
Skin & Soft Tissue					
Cellulitis (cont'd)	- If no response to initial antibiotic therapy in 5 days, consider other diagnoses (see Differential Diagnosis) and/or change the antibiotic regimen.				
Facial	Group A Streptococci S. aureus	Mild **Cloxacillin** or **Cephalexin**	500mg PO qid 500mg PO qid	7-10 days 7-10 days	* Significant Strep/Staph resistance. Monitor clinical response.
		β-lactam allergy **Clindamycin***	300mg PO qid	7-10 days	
		Moderate-severe **Cloxacillin** or **Cefazolin**	1-2g IV q6h 1-2g IV q8h	10 days 10 days	
		β-lactam allergy **Clindamycin IV/PO**[C]*	600mg IV q8h/ 300mg PO qid	10 days	
Extremities	Group A Streptococci S. aureus Group B,C,G Streptococci	Mild **Cloxacillin** or **Cephalexin**	500mg PO qid 500mg PO qid	7-10 days 7-10 days	- Check between toes for fissures ± tinea pedis → common portal of entry.
		β-lactam allergy **Clindamycin**[†]	300mg PO qid	7-10 days	* Alternative for outpatient management of uncomplicated cellulitis. Probenecid regimen is based on pharmacokinetic data and limited clinical evidence, and should only be used in patients with adequate renal function (Clcr > 50mL/min).
		Moderate-severe **Cloxacillin** or **Cefazolin** or [**Cefazolin** + **Probenecid**]* or **Ceftriaxone***	1-2g IV q6h 1-2g IV q8h 2g IV daily 2g PO daily or 1g PO bid** (give 30 min. prior to cefazolin) 1-2g IV daily	10 days*** 10 days*** 10 days*** 10 days***	**Give bid if unable to tolerate probenecid as a 2g daily dose. *** Switch to oral agent when: • resolution of systemic symptoms • no further progression of cellulitis.
		β-lactam allergy **Clindamycin IV/PO**[C][†]	600mg IV q8h/ 300mg PO qid	10 days	† Significant Strep/Staph resistance. Monitor clinical response.

- 222 -

RECOMMENDED EMPIRIC THERAPY OF SELECTED INFECTIONS IN ADULT PATIENTS[A]

Infection	Usual Pathogens	Recommended Empiric Therapy	Recommended Dose[B]	Recommended Duration	Comments
Skin & Soft Tissue					
Cellulitis (cont'd) Extremities (cont'd)	Group A Streptococci S. aureus Group B,C,G Streptococci	**MRSA suspected/ purulent** Mild I&D if abscess* +/- Cephalexin + [TMP/SMX or Doxycycline] Moderate-Severe I&D if abscess + Vancomycin[E]	500mg PO qid 1-2 DS tabs PO bid 100mg PO bid 15mg/kg IV q8-12h	7-10 days 10 days	*I&D may be all that is required for mild cellulitis. - If systemic symptoms, do blood cultures.

If severe infection or unresponsive to above suggested empiric therapy, assess for the following risk factors and modify empiric therapy to cover those specific pathogens.

Condition	Other Potential Pathogens	
Diabetes	Group B Streptococci Occasionally: Anaerobes Pseudomonas aeruginosa	Enterobacteriaceae
Neutropenia		Enterobacteriaceae
Cirrhosis	Capnocytophaga canimorsus Vibrio vulnificus (hemorrhagic bullous lessions) Campylobacter fetus	Pseudomonas aeruginosa
Intravenous drug use	MRSA	Anaerobes
Subcutaneous drug use	Eikenella corrodens Streptococcus anginosus group	
Fresh water exposure	Aeromonas hydrophila complex	
Salt water exposure	Vibrio spp	
Post trauma with soil/water exposure, cosmetic procedures, recreational water sports	Mycobacterium spp Send specimen for mycobacterial culture.	
Fish tank exposure, fisherman	Mycobacterium marinum Send specimen for mycobacterial culture.	
Reptile contact	Salmonella spp	

E. Desired vancomycin trough is 15-20 mg/L. Monitor renal function closely. See Vancomycin Dosing & Monitoring Guidelines.

RECOMMENDED EMPIRIC THERAPY OF SELECTED INFECTIONS IN ADULT PATIENTS[A]

Infection	Usual Pathogens	Recommended Empiric Therapy	Recommended Dose[B]	Recommended Duration	Comments
Skin & Soft Tissue					
Peri-rectal cellulitis/abscess	Polymicrobial: • Anaerobes • Enterobacteriaceae • S. aureus • Group A Streptococci	Mild **Amoxicillin-clavulanate**	875mg PO bid	7-10 days	- Incision/drainage necessary for abscesses.
		Moderate-severe [**Cefazolin** + **Metronidazole IV/PO**[C]]	2g IV q8h 500mg IV/PO q12h	10 days	
		or [**Clindamycin IV/PO**[C] + **Ciprofloxacin IV/PO**[D]]	600mg IV q8h/ 300mg PO qid 400mg IV q12h/ 500mg PO bid	10 days	* If ESBL or Amp C known/ suspected, use ertapenem 1g IV daily.
		or **Piperacillin-tazobactam***	3.375g IV q6h	10 days	
		MRSA suspected Mild **Amoxicillin-clavulanate** + **TMP/SMX**	875mg PO bid 1-2 DS tabs PO bid	7-10 days	
		Moderate-severe [**Vancomycin**[E] + **Ceftriaxone** + **Metronidazole IV/PO**[C]]	15mg/kg IV q8-12h 1-2g IV daily 500mg IV/PO q12h	10 days	
		or [**Vancomycin**[E] + **Piperacillin-tazobactam***]	15mg/kg IV q8-12h 3.375g IV q6h	10 days	

E. Desired vancomycin trough is 15-20 mg/L. Monitor renal function closely. See Vancomycin Dosing & Monitoring Guidelines.

RECOMMENDED EMPIRIC THERAPY OF SELECTED INFECTIONS IN ADULT PATIENTS[A]

Infection	Potential Pathogens	Potential Pathogens	Potential Pathogens	Potential Pathogens
Skin & Soft Tissue				
Lymphadenitis, infectious	Generalized: • EBV • HIV • Syphilis • Toxoplasma gondii (Toxoplasmosis) • F. tularensis (Tularemia) • Borrelia burgdorferi (Lyme disease) • Cytomegalovirus (CMV) • Brucella spp • B. henselae (Cat Scratch disease) • Mycobacterium spp • Histoplasma spp • Cryptococcus spp	Cervical: • Group A Streptococci • S. aureus • Anaerobes • Mycobacterium spp • B. henselae (Cat Scratch disease) • Toxoplasma gondii (Toxoplasmosis) • F. tularensis (Tularemia) • HIV • CMV • EBV • Mumps • Brucella spp.	Axillary: • Group A Streptococci • S. aureus • B. henselae (Cat Scratch disease) • Sporothrix schenckii (Sporotrichosis)	Inguinal: • Group A Streptococci • S. aureus • B. henselae (Cat Scratch disease) • H. ducreyi (Chancroid) • Treponema pallidum (Syphilis) • Mycobacterium spp • Herpes simplex • Lymphogranuloma venereum (Chlamydia trachomatis LGV serovars) • HIV • Yersinia pestis (Plague) • F. tularensis (Tularemia) Extremity: • Group A Streptococci • S. aureus • Mycobacterium spp • Sporothrix schenckii (Sporotrichosis) • Nocardia spp
	Treat according to etiology, after appropriate investigations.			

RECOMMENDED EMPIRIC THERAPY OF SELECTED INFECTIONS IN ADULT PATIENTS[A]

Infection	Usual Pathogens	Recommended Empiric Therapy	Recommended Dose[B]	Recommended Duration	Comments
Skin & Soft Tissue					
Breast abscess/ mastitis		- Abscess often requires incision and drainage. - Antibiotics not recommended for minimal symptoms or prophylaxis.			

Post-partum	S. aureus	- Encourage milk flow from affected breast either through breast feeding or breast pump.			- Risk factors for abscess formation:
					  • maternal age > 30 years
					  • gestational age > 41 weeks
					  • history of mastitis

		Mild **Cloxacillin** or **Cephalexin**	500mg PO qid 500mg PO qid	7-10 days 7-10 days	- Can continue breast-feeding while on therapy.
		β-lactam allergy/MRSA **Clindamycin***	300mg PO qid	7-10 days	- Consider ultrasound if no response after one course of antibiotics.
		Moderate-severe **Cloxacillin** or **Cefazolin**	1-2g IV q6h 1-2g IV q8h	7-10 days 7-10 days	*Ensure clindamycin susceptibility - increased incidence of resistance.
		β-lactam allergy/MRSA **Vancomycin**[E]	15mg/kg IV q8-12h	7-10 days	
Postsurgical	S. aureus β-haemolytic Strep-tococci (group A,B,C,G)	**Cloxacillin** or **Cephalexin**	500mg PO qid 500mg PO qid	7-10 days 7-10 days	- Post radiation it may be difficult to differentiate infection from inflammation. If no change following antibiotic therapy, consider NSAIDs or topical corticosteroids.
		β-lactam allergy **Clindamycin***	300mg PO qid	7-10 days	- If implants, other pathogens (e.g. coagulase negative Staph, MRSA, Propionibacterium spp, atypical mycobacteria) may be involved.
		Moderate-severe **Cloxacillin** or **Cefazolin**	1-2g IV q6h 1-2g IV q8h	7-10 days 7-10 days	*Ensure clindamycin susceptibility - increased incidence of resistance.
Not post-partum, not postsurgical	S. aureus Anaerobes	**Amoxicillin-clavulanate** or	875mg PO bid	7-10 days	- Strong association with smoking, and to a lesser extent, with diabetes.
		Clindamycin*	300mg PO qid	7-10 days	*Ensure clindamycin susceptibility - increased incidence of resistance.

E. Desired vancomycin trough is 15-20 mg/L. Monitor renal function closely. See Vancomycin Dosing & Monitoring Guidelines.

RECOMMENDED EMPIRIC THERAPY OF SELECTED INFECTIONS IN ADULT PATIENTS[A]

Infection	Usual Pathogens	Recommended Empiric Therapy	Recommended Dose[B]	Recommended Duration	Comments
Skin & Soft Tissue					
Animal bites		- If animal unknown or escaped, or unprovoked attack, contact local Public Health or local Medical Officer of Health re: risk/management of rabies. - Ensure tetanus status up to date. - Irrigation and debridement necessary. - Primary closure of wound(s) NOT recommended if: • puncture wounds • ≥ 12 hours post injury. - Amoxicillin-clavulanate is drug of choice. - Cloxacillin, cephalexin/cefazolin, clindamycin, and erythromycin NOT effective against Pasteurella spp or Eikenella spp. - Pus/deep wound cultures recommended in established infection. - For animal exposures below, consider also: • reptiles – Salmonella spp, Aeromonas spp • marine animals - Vibrio spp Infectious Diseases consult recommended			

RECOMMENDED EMPIRIC THERAPY OF SELECTED INFECTIONS IN ADULT PATIENTS[A]

Infection	Usual Pathogens	Recommended Empiric Therapy	Recommended Dose[B]	Recommended Duration	Comments
Skin & Soft Tissue					
Animal bites (cont'd) **Cats**	Polymicrobial: • Pasteurella spp • Streptococcus spp • Staphylococcus spp/MRSA • Anaerobes	Prophylaxis* **Amoxicillin-clavulanate**	875mg PO bid	3-5 days	* Prophylaxis within 12 hours of bite is recommended for all significant cat bites because of high rate of infection (up to 80%).
		β-lactam allergy **Doxycycline** +/- **Metronidazole**	100mg PO bid 500mg PO bid	3-5 days	
	• Neisseria spp • Moraxella spp • Corynebacterium spp • Enterococcus spp • Bacillus spp • Bergeyella spp	Treatment **Amoxicillin-clavulanate** or **[Cefuroxime axetil +/- Metronidazole]**	875mg PO bid 500mg PO bid 500mg PO bid	7-10 days* 7-10 days*	* Prolonged therapy is required if associated osteomyelitis (4-6 weeks)/septic arthritis (3-4 weeks).
	Rare: • Bartonella spp • Francisella tularensis • Yersinia pestis • Sporothrix schenckii	β-lactam allergy **[Doxycycline +/- Metronidazole]** or **[Clindamycin + Ciprofloxacin]**	100mg PO bid 500mg PO bid 300-450mg PO qid 500mg PO bid	7-10 days* 7-10 days*	
		Moderate **Ceftriaxone + Metronidazole**	1-2g IV daily 500mg PO bid	7-10 days*	
		Severe/Limb-threatening **Piperacillin-tazobactam** or **Imipenem**	3.375g IV q6h 500mg IV q6h	10-14 days* 10-14 days*	

- 228 -

RECOMMENDED EMPIRIC THERAPY OF SELECTED INFECTIONS IN ADULT PATIENTS[A]

Infection	Usual Pathogens	Recommended Empiric Therapy	Recommended Dose[B]	Recommended Duration	Comments
Skin & Soft Tissue					
Animal bites (cont'd)					
Dogs	Polymicrobial: • Pasteurella spp • Streptococcus spp • Staphylococcus spp/MRSA • Anaerobes • Capnocytophaga spp • Eikenella spp • Bergeyella spp • Neisseria spp • Moraxella spp • Corynebacterium spp • Enterococcus spp • Bacillus spp	Prophylaxis* **Amoxicillin-clavulanate** β-lactam allergy **Doxycycline** +/- **Metronidazole**	875mg PO bid 100mg PO bid 500mg PO bid	3-5 days 3-5 days	* Infection rate up to 20%. Prophylaxis within 12 hours of bite is recommended if: • moderate/severe • crush injury/edema • age > 50 years • puncture wounds • bone/joint involvement • injuries to hand, foot, face, genitalia • splenectomized patients • immunocompromised.
		Treatment **Amoxicillin-clavulanate** or [**Cefuroxime axetil** +/- **Metronidazole**] β-lactam allergy [**Doxycycline** +/- **Metronidazole**] or [**Clindamycin** + **Ciprofloxacin**] Moderate **Ceftriaxone** + **Metronidazole** Severe/Limb-threatening **Piperacillin-tazobactam** or **Imipenem**	875mg PO bid 500mg PO bid 500mg PO bid 100mg PO bid 500mg PO bid 300-450mg PO qid 500mg PO bid 1-2g IV daily 500mg PO bid 3.375g IV q6h 500mg IV q6h	7-10 days* 7-10 days* 7-10 days* 7-10 days* 7-10 days* 10-14 days* 10-14 days*	* Prolonged therapy is required if associated osteomyelitis (4-6 weeks)/septic arthritis (3-4 weeks).

RECOMMENDED EMPIRIC THERAPY OF SELECTED INFECTIONS IN ADULT PATIENTS[A]

Infection	Usual Pathogens	Recommended Empiric Therapy	Recommended Dose[B]	Recommended Duration	Comments
Skin & Soft Tissue					

Human bites	- Irrigation and debridement necessary.
	- Immobilization and wound elevation, if possible, are beneficial.
	- HIV and Hepatitis B & C have very rarely been transmitted by human bites. Assessment of risk factors and relevant management should be considered.
	- Risk factors for developing osteomyelitis:
	    • delay in initial treatment
	    • inadequate debridement
	    • primary closure of wound.
	- Amoxicillin-clavulanate is drug of choice.
	- Cloxacillin, cephalexin/cefazolin, clindamycin, and macrolides NOT effective against Eikenella spp.
	- Pus/deep wound cultures recommended in established infections.				

	Polymicrobial:
	• Streptococcus spp
	• Staphylococcus spp/
	  MRSA
	• Anaerobes
	• Eikenella spp
	• Haemophilus spp
	• Corynebacterium
	  spp
		Prophylaxis:*
		Amoxicillin-clavulanate
		
		β-lactam allergy
		Doxycycline +/-
		Metronidazole
			875mg PO bid
			
			100mg PO bid
			500mg PO bid
				3-5 days
				
				3-5 days
					* Infection rate up to 50%.
					Prophylaxis within 12 hours of bite is recommended if:
					  • moderate/severe
					  • crush injury/edema
					  • bone/joint involvement
					  • hand injuries.

RECOMMENDED EMPIRIC THERAPY OF SELECTED INFECTIONS IN ADULT PATIENTS[A]

Infection	Usual Pathogens	Recommended Empiric Therapy	Recommended Dose[B]	Recommended Duration	Comments
Skin & Soft Tissue					
Human bites (cont'd)	Polymicrobial: • Streptococcus spp • Staphylococcus spp/ MRSA • Anaerobes • Eikenella spp • Haemophilus spp • Corynebacterium spp	Treatment **Amoxicillin-clavulanate** or **[Cefuroxime axetil** +/- **Metronidazole]**	875mg PO bid 500mg PO bid 500mg PO bid	7-10 days* 7-10 days*	* Prolonged therapy is required associated osteomyelitis (4-6 weeks)/septic arthritis (3-4 weeks).
		β-lactam allergy **[Doxycycline** +/- **Metronidazole]** or **[Clindamycin** + **Ciprofloxacin]**	100mg PO bid 500mg PO bid 300-450mg PO qid 500mg PO bid	7-10 days* 7-10 days*	
		Moderate **Ceftriaxone** + **Metronidazole**	1-2g IV daily 500mg PO bid	7-10 days*	
		Severe/Limb-threatening **Piperacillin-tazobactam** or **Imipenem**	3.375g IV q6h 500mg IV q6h	10-14 days* 10-14 days*	

Infection	Usual Pathogens	Recommended Empiric Therapy	Recommended Dose[B]	Recommended Duration	Comments
Skin & Soft Tissue					

Diabetic foot infection (DFI)
 	
[Clin Infect Dis 2012;54:e132-173.]
	General Management
	- Prevention is key - proper foot care & glycemic control are essential.
	- Pressure relief on ulcers (off-loading) very important, e.g. non-weight bearing on affected foot, contact casting.
	- Debridement of devitalized tissue is essential.
	- Recommend timely referral to multidisciplinary diabetic foot team, where available.
	
	Diagnosis
	- Not all diabetic foot wounds are infected. No evidence to support using antibiotics to decrease bioburden of wounds in order to enhance healing or to prevent infection of wound.
	- Diagnosis of infection based on:
	  1. • presence of purulent secretions, or
	     • at least two signs or symptoms of inflammation:
	       ○ erythema
	       ○ warmth
	       ○ pain
	       ○ tenderness
	       ○ induration and/or swelling
	   or
	     • systemic signs and symptoms of infection (fever. increased WBC).
	  2. Wound cultures - post debridement deep tissue specimens (biopsy or curettage) or aspiration of purulent secretions recommended as correlation of superficial wound swabs/cultures to pathogens poor. Repeat cultures are not recommended unless obvious clinical deterioration.
	  3. Imaging:
	    - All patients with DFI should have plain x-ray. NB: X-ray abnormalities lag clinical infection by up to one month. Repeat x-rays indicated if deep and/or unresolving ulcer.
	    - MRI best study to diagnose and assess extent of soft tissue and bone involvement. WBC scan +/- bone scan best alternative if MRI not available.
	      • Mild - skin and subcutaneous tissues involved
	      • Moderate-severe - deeper infection, systemic signs of infection or metabolic instability
	- Osteomyelitis is more likely if ulcer > 2 cm^2, exposed bone or ulcer overlies bony prominence, positive probe to bone, ESR > 60, or abnormal plain x-ray.			

RECOMMENDED EMPIRIC THERAPY OF SELECTED INFECTIONS IN ADULT PATIENTS[A]

Infection	Usual Pathogens	Recommended Empiric Therapy	Recommended Dose[B]	Recommended Duration	Comments
Skin & Soft Tissue					

Diabetic foot infection (DFI) (cont'd)
 	
[Clin Infect Dis 2012;54:e132-173.]
	Antibiotic Therapy
	- Pseudomonas coverage not always necessary as P. aeruginosa is often a non pathogenic colonizer of diabetic wounds. Empiric coverage of P. aeruginosa should be considered if:
	   • tropical/warm climates
	   • soaking of feet
	   • failed nonpseudomonal therapy
	   • limb-threatening infection.
	- MRSA coverage recommended if:
	   • previous (prior 12 months)/current colonization/infection with MRSA
	   • recent antibiotic use
	   • recent hospitalization.				

Simple cellulitis	See Cellulitis				
Ulcer, drainage, fistula	Polymicrobial: • S. aureus/MRSA[‡] • S. epidermidis • β-haemolytic Streptococci (group A,B,C,G) • Enterococcus spp • Enterobacteriaceae • Pseudomonas spp • Anaerobes (recovered in up to 95% of diabetic wounds)	Debridement & glycemic control Mild [**Cephalexin** + **Metronidazole**] or **Amoxicillin-clavulanate** or [**Doxycycline** + **Metronidazole**] or [**Cefazolin** + **Metronidazole**] MRSA suspected[‡] [**Doxycycline** + **Metronidazole**] or add **TMP/SMX**[†] to other regimens listed under Mild	500mg PO qid 500mg PO bid 875mg PO bid 100mg PO bid 500mg PO bid 2g IV q8h 500mg PO bid 100mg PO bid 500mg PO bid 2 DS tabs PO bid	7-14 days* 7-14 days* 7-14 days* 7-14 days* 7-14 days*	- Monitor renal function and adjust dosing of antibiotics according to renal function. - Switch to oral therapy should be guided by clinical improvement and deep tissue culture & susceptibility results. * Duration dependent on clinical response. If osteomyelitis (See Osteomyelitis), 6 weeks if adequate debridement. ‡ Consider MRSA if: • previous (prior 12 months)/current MRSA colonization or infection • recent antibiotic use • recent hospitalization. † Monitor potassium.

RECOMMENDED EMPIRIC THERAPY OF SELECTED INFECTIONS IN ADULT PATIENTS[A]

Infection	Usual Pathogens	Recommended Empiric Therapy	Recommended Dose[B]	Recommended Duration	Comments
Skin & Soft Tissue					
Diabetic foot infection (cont'd) Ulcer, drainage, fistula (cont'd) [Clin Infect Dis 2012;54:e132-173.]	Polymicrobial: • S. aureus/MRSA[‡] • S. epidermidis • β-haemolytic Streptococci (group A,B,C,G) • Enterococcus spp • Enterobacteriaceae • Pseudomonas spp • Anaerobes (recovered in up to 95% of diabetic wounds)	Debridement & glycemic control Moderate-severe [Clindamycin IV/PO][C] + Ciprofloxacin]	600mg IV q6h/ 300-450mg PO qid 750mg PO bid		- Monitor renal function and adjust dosing of antibiotics according to renal function. - Switch to oral therapy should be guided by clinical improvement and deep tissue culture and susceptibility results. * Duration dependent on clinical response. If osteomyelitis (See Osteomyelitis), 6 weeks if adequate debridement. # Ertapenem does not cover P. aeruginosa or Enterococcus spp. ‡ Consider MRSA if: • previous (prior 12 months)/ current MRSA colonization or infection • recent antibiotic use • recent hospitalization. Δ If known/suspected P. aeruginosa, use ciprofloxacin or ceftazidime instead of ceftriaxone. ** If P. aeruginosa cultured, use 4.5g IV q6h if renal function allows. ***Use imipenem if known/ suspected ESBL/AmpC-producing organisms.
		Outpatient and failure of oral therapy or known/ suspected ESBL/Amp C-producing organisms Ertapenem#	1g IV daily	2-3 weeks*	
		MRSA suspected[‡] Moderate-Severe Vancomycin[E] + Ceftriaxone[Δ] + Metronidazole IV/PO[C]	15mg/kg IV q8-12h 1-2g IV daily 500mg IV/PO q12h	2-3 weeks*	
		Limb-threatening [Piperacillin-tazobactam] or Imipenem***] + Vancomycin[E]	3.375g IV q6h** 500mg IV q6h 15mg/kg IV q8-12h	2-3 weeks*	

E: Desired vancomycin trough is 15-20mg/L. Monitor renal function closely. See Vancomycin Dosing & Monitoring Guidelines.

RECOMMENDED EMPIRIC THERAPY OF SELECTED INFECTIONS IN ADULT PATIENTS[A]

Infection	Usual Pathogens	Recommended Empiric Therapy	Recommended Dose[B]	Recommended Duration	Comments
Skin & Soft Tissue					
Pressure/ decubitus ulcers/ ulcers 2° to PVD	- Topical antibiotics of no proven efficacy in colonization or infection. - Prevention is most important element in management.				
No evidence of clinical infection	Often colonized with polymicrobic flora	Local wound management: • cleansing • debridement • dressing.			- Deep cultures from cleaned ulcer base recommended. - 25% of decubitus ulcers have underlying osteomyelitis.
Evidence of clinical infection • cellulitis • regional adenopathy • extensive ulceration • fever If osteomyelitis suspected/ documented see Osteomyelitis.	Polymicrobial: • S. aureus/MRSA* • β-haemolytic Streptococci (group A,B,C,G) • Enterococcus spp • Enterobacteriaceae • Pseudomonas spp • Anaerobes	Mild [Cephalexin + Metronidazole] or Amoxicillin-clavulanate or [Doxycycline + Metronidazole] If MRSA suspected* [Doxycycline + Metronidazole] or add TMP/SMX to other regimens listed under Mild Moderate-severe Clindamycin + Ciprofloxacin For parenteral regimens see Diabetic foot infection.	500mg-1g PO qid 500mg PO bid 875mg PO bid 100mg PO bid 500mg PO bid 100mg PO bid 500mg PO bid 1-2 DS tabs PO bid 300-450mg PO qid 750mg PO bid	7-14 days** 7-14 days** 7-14 days** 7-14 days** 2-3 weeks**	* Consider MRSA if: • previous (prior 12 months)/ current MRSA colonization or infection • recent antibiotic use • recent hospitalization. **Duration dependent on clinical response. If osteomyelitis, (See Osteomyelitis). 6 weeks if adequate debridement.

- 235 -

RECOMMENDED EMPIRIC THERAPY OF SELECTED INFECTIONS IN ADULT PATIENTS[A]

Infection	Usual Pathogens	Recommended Empiric Therapy	Recommended Dose[B]	Recommended Duration	Comments
Skin & Soft Tissue					
Post-operative wounds	- Fever in first 48 hours post-op unlikely to represent wound infection. - Most important therapy for surgical site infections (SSIs) is to open the incision, drain pus and continue dressing changes until wound heals by secondary intention. - There is little evidence to support the use of antibiotics in mild SSIs.				
Involving trunk, neck, head, extremity	S. aureus/MRSA* Group A Streptococci	Mild (< 5cm erythema/ induration): - Temp < 38.5 °C and pulse < 100/min: **Local management** **No antibiotics required.**			* If previous (prior 12 months)/current MRSA colonization or infection, or high endemic rate of MRSA, add TMP/SMX or doxycycline.
		- Temp > 38.5°C or pulse > 100/min: **Cephalexin***	500mg PO qid	24-48 hours	
		β-lactam allergy **Clindamycin***	300mg PO qid	24-48 hours	
		Moderate-severe **Cefazolin***	1-2g IV q8h	7-10 days**	**Switch to oral therapy after 48-72h if clinical improvement.
		β-lactam allergy/ MRSA suspected **Vancomycin**[E]	15mg/kg IV q8-12h	7-10 days**	

E. Desired vancomycin trough is 15-20mg/L. Monitor renal function closely. See Vancomycin Dosing & Monitoring Guidelines.

RECOMMENDED EMPIRIC THERAPY OF SELECTED INFECTIONS IN ADULT PATIENTS[A]

Infection	Usual Pathogens	Recommended Empiric Therapy	Recommended Dose[B]	Recommended Duration	Comments
Skin & Soft Tissue					
Post-operative wounds (cont'd) **Involving perineum, GI tract, female genital tract, axilla**	Polymicrobial: • S. aureus/MRSA* • β-haemolytic Streptococci (group A,B,C,G) • Enterococcus spp • Enterobacteriaceae • Anaerobes	<u>Mild</u> **Amoxicillin-clavulanate*** β-lactam allergy [**Clindamycin PO** + **Ciprofloxacin PO**]* <u>β-lactam allergy and MRSA suspected</u> **Clindamycin** + **TMP/SMX** <u>Moderate</u> [**Cefazolin** + **Metronidazole**]* <u>Severe</u> **Piperacillin-tazobactam*** <u>Severe and MRSA suspected</u> **Piperacillin-tazobactam** + **Vancomycin**[E]	875mg PO bid 300mg PO qid 500-750mg PO bid 300mg PO qid 1-2DS tabs PO bid 2g IV q8h 500mg PO bid 3.375g IV q6h 3.375g IV q6h 15mg/kg IV q8-12h	All regimens: 5-10 days or until patient afebrile and wound granulating	- Anaerobic coverage is recommended. - Cephalosporins and clindamycin have no activity against Enterococcus spp. * If MRSA colonization or infection in prior 12 months) or high endemic rate of MRSA, add TMP/SMX or doxycycline. - Switch to oral therapy after 48-72h if clinical improvement.

E. Desired vancomycin trough is 15-20mg/L. Monitor renal function closely. See Vancomycin Dosing & Monitoring Guidelines.

RECOMMENDED EMPIRIC THERAPY OF SELECTED INFECTIONS IN ADULT PATIENTS[A]

Infection	Usual Pathogens	Recommended Empiric Therapy	Recommended Dose[B]	Recommended Duration	Comments
Skin & Soft Tissue					
Rapidly progressive skin & soft tissue infections	Predisposing factors • trauma/surgery • immunosuppression/malignancy • diabetes • chronic renal/hepatic disease • chicken pox • IVDU Clinical Findings Early: • pain out of proportion to appearance • swelling • cellulitis • fever • tachycardia • induration • areas of anaesthesia in affected skin Late: • severe pain • skin discoloration (purple or black) • blistering • hemorrhagic bullae • crepitus • "dishwater" gray drainage • systemic inflammatory response syndrome (SIRS)/sepsis • multi-organ failure/shock Management - Surgical debridement and irrigation are essential. Send specimens for culture. - Infectious Diseases consult strongly recommended. - Duration of therapy (IV/PO) dependent on clinical picture.				

RECOMMENDED EMPIRIC THERAPY OF SELECTED INFECTIONS IN ADULT PATIENTS[A]

Infection	Usual Pathogens	Recommended Empiric Therapy	Recommended Dose[B]	Recommended Duration	Comments
Skin & Soft Tissue					
Rapidly progressive skin & soft tissue infections (cont'd)	S. pyogenes (Group A Strep)	**Clindamycin*** + **Ceftriaxone**	600-900mg IV q8h	10-14 days	- On initial presentation it may be difficult to determine etiologic agent(s).
	Rare:		2g IV daily		* Inhibits toxin production of Streptococcal spp, Staphylococcal spp, and Clostridium spp.
	• S. agalactiae (Group B Strep)	MRSA suspected add **Vancomycin** to above or use	15mg/kg IV q8-12h	10-14 days	**If Vibrio suspected, add doxycycline.
	• Group C,G Strep				***If P. aeruginosa suspected, use regimen containing piperacillin-tazobactam, or imipenem.
	• S. pneumoniae	**Linezolid*** + **Ceftriaxone**	600mg IV/PO q12h	10-14 days	
	• S. aureus/MRSA		2g IV daily		
	• Clostridium spp				
	• Mixed aerobic/ anaerobic organisms	**Polymicrobial** **Piperacillin-tazobactam** +	4.5g IV q6h	10-14 days	
	• Vibrio vulnificus (salt water exposure)**				
	• Aeromonas hydrophila (fresh water exposure)	**[Linezolid***	600mg IV/PO q12h		
	• Enterobacteriaceae (chronic hepatic/renal disease)	or **Vancomycin[E]]**	15mg/kg IV q8-12h		
	• P. aeruginosa (neutropenia, burns, IVDU)***				

E. Desired vancomycin trough is 15-20mg/L. Monitor renal function closely. See Vancomycin Dosing & Monitoring Guidelines.

RECOMMENDED EMPIRIC THERAPY OF SELECTED INFECTIONS IN ADULT PATIENTS[A]

Infection	Usual Pathogens	Recommended Empiric Therapy	Recommended Dose[B]	Recommended Duration	Comments
Skin & Soft Tissue					
Rapidly progressive skin & soft tissue infections (cont'd) **Necrotizing fasciitis/ myositis**		- Use of IV immune globulin (1-2g/kg/day x 2 days) could be considered if streptococcal toxic shock also present.			
Culture proven	S. pyogenes (Group A Strep)	Clindamycin* + Penicillin	600-900mg IV q8h 4MU IV q4h	10-14 days	- Invasive Group A Streptococci is reportable to Public Health. - Prophylaxis of contacts of invasive Group A Streptococci is recommended by most Public Health experts. See Prophylaxis for Contacts of Communicable Diseases. *Inhibits toxin production of Streptococcal spp.
	S. agalactiae (Group B Strep) Group C, G strep S. pneumoniae	Clindamycin* + Ceftriaxone**	600-900mg IV q8h 2g IV daily	10-14 days	*Inhibits toxin production of Streptococcal spp. **If penicillin MIC ≤ 0.12 µg/mL, switch ceftriaxone to penicillin.
	Methicillin-susceptible S. aureus (MSSA)	Clindamycin* + Cloxacillin	600mg IV q8h 2g IV q4h	10-14 days	*Inhibits toxin production of Staphylococcal spp.
	MRSA	Vancomycin[E]	15mg/kg IV q8-12h	10-14 days	†Clindamycin and linezolid inhibit toxin production of Staphylococcal spp.
		Alternative Linezolid† or	600mg IV/PO q12h	10-14 days	* Ensure MRSA is susceptible to clindamycin.
		Clindamycin*†	600mg IV q8h	10-14 days	

E. Desired vancomycin trough is 15-20mg/L. Monitor renal function closely. See Vancomycin Dosing & Monitoring Guidelines.

RECOMMENDED EMPIRIC THERAPY OF SELECTED INFECTIONS IN ADULT PATIENTS[A]

Infection	Usual Pathogens	Recommended Empiric Therapy	Recommended Dose[B]	Recommended Duration	Comments
Skin & Soft Tissue					
Rapidly progressive skin & soft tissue infections (cont'd) **Synergistic necrotizing cellulitis Fournier's gangrene***	Polymicrobial: • Anaerobes • S. aureus/MRSA** • Group A Streptococci • Enterobacteriaceae	**Imipenem** +/- **Vancomycin**[E**]	1g IV q6h 15mg/kg IV q8-12h	10-14 days 10-14 days	* Fournier's gangrene: necrotizing fasciitis of abdominal wall, buttocks, and genitalia, often following trauma, perianal abscess, or diverticulitis. **Add vancomycin if MRSA suspected: • previous (prior 12 months)/current MRSA colonization or infection • recent antibiotic use • recent hospitalization.
Gas gangrene	Clostridium spp	**[Clindamycin + Penicillin]** or **Imipenem**	600-900mg IV q8h 4MU IV q4h 1g IV q6h	10-14 days 10-14 days	- Adjunctive hyperbaric oxygen therapy is controversial.

E. Desired vancomycin trough is 15-20mg/L. Monitor renal function closely. See Vancomycin Dosing & Monitoring Guidelines.

RECOMMENDED EMPIRIC THERAPY OF SELECTED INFECTIONS IN ADULT PATIENTS[A]

Infection	Usual Pathogens	Recommended Empiric Therapy	Recommended Dose[B]	Recommended Duration	Comments
Bone & Joint					

Osteomyelitis
 	
Vertebral (spinal osteomyelitis, spondylodisc-itis, septic discitis, disc space infection)
 	
[NEJM 2010;362: 1022-9]
	Investigations:
	• Blood cultures recommended. If positive, repeat blood cultures to ensure clearance of bacteremia.
	• Bone cultures recommended. CT-guided or open biopsy for culture in vertebral osteomyelitis – higher yield than blood cultures.
	• CBC and differential, serum creatinine.
	• ESR, CRP - low sensitivity for diagnosis but if initially elevated, may be useful to monitor response.
	• Plain x-ray +/- MRI, or bone scan +/- WBC scan.
	   ○ MRI superior to x-ray and bone scan for early diagnosis of bone/joint infections, and superior to CT scan for vertebral osteomyelitis and identification of epidural abscess.
	   ○ bone scan may be falsely positive if recent trauma/aspiration of joint/superficial infection, WBC or gallium scan may improve specificity.
	
	Therapy:
	- Clindamycin achieves excellent bone penetration and is a good agent for osteomyelitis if organism susceptible. However due to high resistance rates, not recommended empirically.
	- In adults, vertebral osteomyelitis most common, occurring in lumbar, thoracic, cervical sites.
	- May present acutely (evolving over days/weeks) or subacutely/chronic (weeks/months).
	- Caused by:
	   • hematogenous seeding
	   • direct inoculation at time of surgery
	   • contiguous spread from adjacent soft tissue
	- May result in paravertebral, epidural, or psoas abscess. Increased risk of neurologic sequelae. Urgent neurosurgical consult required.
	- Clinical features: back pain most common symptom (severe, sharp pain/point tenderness on physical exam suggests epidural abscess); fever not always present.
	- Endocarditis diagnosed in one-third of cases of vertebral osteomyelitis.			

RECOMMENDED EMPIRIC THERAPY OF SELECTED INFECTIONS IN ADULT PATIENTS[A]

Infection	Usual Pathogens	Recommended Empiric Therapy	Recommended Dose[B]	Recommended Duration	Comments
Bone & Joint					
Osteomyelitis (cont'd) **Vertebral (spinal osteomyelitis, spondylodisc-itis, septic discitis, disc space infection)** (cont'd) [NEJM 2010;362: 1022-9]	S. aureus/MRSA* Rare: • Streptococcus spp • Enterococcus spp • Enterobacteriaceae • P. aeruginosa • M. tuberculosis • Dimorphic fungi If spinal implant also: • Coagulase negative staphylococci • P. acnes	Cloxacillin β-lactam allergy **Vancomycin**[E] Alternative **Linezolid** or **TMP/SMX** If MRSA suspected* [**Vancomycin**[E] or **Linezolid** or **TMP/SMX**] +/- **Rifampin**[‡]	2g IV q4h 25-30mg/kg IV once then 15mg/kg IV q8-12h 600mg IV/PO q12h 15-20mg TMP/kg/day IV/PO div q6-8h 25-30mg/kg IV once then 15mg/kg IV q8-12h 600mg PO q12h 15-20mg TMP/kg/day div q6-8h 600mg PO daily or 300-450mg PO bid	6 weeks[†] 6 weeks[†] 6 weeks[†] 6 weeks[†] minimum 8 weeks[†] minimum 8 weeks[†] minimum 8 weeks[†]	* Consider MRSA especially if: • preceding trauma • multifocal lesions • disease in adjacent muscle. - If staphylococcal hardware infection, add rifampin. - Surgical debridement and drainage of associated soft tissue abscesses recommended. †Prolonged therapy recommended if abscesses cannot be drained or spinal implant. ‡ If no debridement, consider adding rifampin and continue therapy for minimum 12 weeks. NB: Ensure TB has been ruled out before starting rifampin.

E. Desired vancomycin trough is 15-20mg/L. Monitor renal function closely. See Vancomycin Dosing & Monitoring Guidelines.

RECOMMENDED EMPIRIC THERAPY OF SELECTED INFECTIONS IN ADULT PATIENTS[A]

Infection	Usual Pathogens	Recommended Empiric Therapy	Recommended Dose[B]	Recommended Duration	Comments
Bone & Joint					
Osteomyelitis (cont'd)					
Hematogenous Long Bones	S. aureus/MRSA* Rare: • Streptococcus spp • Enterobacteriaceae • M. tuberculosis • Dimorphic fungi	**Cloxacillin** or **Cefazolin** β-lactam allergy **Vancomycin**[E] or **Clindamycin**[C,**] If MRSA suspected* **Vancomycin**[E] +/- **Rifampin**[‡]	2g IV q4h 2g IV q8h 15mg/kg IV q8-12h 600mg IV q8h/ 450mg PO qid 15mg/kg IV q8-12h 600mg PO daily or 300-450mg PO bid	4-6 weeks 4-6 weeks 4-6 weeks 4-6 weeks minimum 8 weeks ‡ If no debridement, consider adding rifampin and continue therapy for minimum 12 weeks.	* Consider MRSA especially if: • preceding trauma • multifocal lesions • disease in adjacent muscle. - Surgical debridement and drainage of associated soft tissue abscesses recommended. **Clindamycin can be used if: • bacteremia cleared • no intravascular infection AND • documented susceptibility. - Recommend minimum 2 weeks IV antibiotics. Switch to oral agents with good bioavailability and bone penetration [Clin Pharmacokinetics 2009;48;89-124] may be considered with clinical improvement. Oral ß-lactams should not be used as low bioavailability. Ceftriaxone 2g IV daily may be an option for outpatient management [Clin Infect Dis 2012;54; 585-90] but has not been studied in a prospective, randomized controlled trial.

E. Desired vancomycin trough is 15-20mg/L. Monitor renal function closely. See Vancomycin Dosing & Monitoring Guidelines.

RECOMMENDED EMPIRIC THERAPY OF SELECTED INFECTIONS IN ADULT PATIENTS[A]

Infection	Usual Pathogens	Recommended Empiric Therapy	Recommended Dose[B]	Recommended Duration	Comments
Bone & Joint					
Osteomyelitis (cont'd) **Intravenous drug use**	S. aureus/MRSA* P. aeruginosa Occasionally: • Salmonella spp • Serratia spp • Candida spp • Anaerobes Rare: • M. tuberculosis	**Vancomycin** [E,*] + [**Ciprofloxacin** or **Tobramycin**]**	15mg/kg IV q8-12h 750mg PO bid 7mg/kg IV q24h	6 weeks	- Predilection for sternoclavicular or sacroiliac joint, ribs, vertebrae, long bones - Must rule out endocarditis. * If MSSA, drug of choice is cloxacillin or cefazolin. If MRSA, use vancomycin alone. **Reassess need for quinolone or aminoglycoside therapy as soon as C&S results available.

E. Desired vancomycin trough is 15-20mg/L. Monitor renal function closely. See Vancomycin Dosing & Monitoring Guidelines.

RECOMMENDED EMPIRIC THERAPY OF SELECTED INFECTIONS IN ADULT PATIENTS[A]

Infection	Usual Pathogens	Recommended Empiric Therapy	Recommended Dose[B]	Recommended Duration	Comments
Bone & Joint					
Osteomyelitis (cont'd) **Contiguous Vascular insufficiency, diabetic foot**	Polymicrobial: • S. aureus/MRSA[†] • Streptococcus spp • Enterococcus spp • Enterobacteriaceae • P. aeruginosa • Anaerobes • Candida spp	Mild-moderate [**Clindamycin** + **Ciprofloxacin**] or [**Cefazolin** + **Metronidazole**]** If MRSA suspected[†] Add **TMP/SMX** to regimens above Outpatient and failure of oral therapy or known/ suspected ESBL/Amp C-producing organisms **Ertapenem**** Moderate-severe and MRSA suspected[†],** **Vancomycin**[‡] + **Ceftriaxone**[‡] + **Metronidazole IV/PO**[C] Severe/Limb threatening [**Piperacillin-tazobactam***] or **Imipenem**[***] + **Vancomycin**[‡]	450mg PO qid 750mg PO bid 2g IV q8h 500mg PO bid 2DS tabs PO bid 1g IV daily 15mg/kg IV q8-12h 1-2g IV daily 500mg IV/PO q12h 3.375g IV q6h* 500mg IV q6h 15mg/kg IV q8-12h	≥ 6 weeks ≥ 6 weeks ≥ 6 weeks ≥ 6 weeks ≥ 6 weeks ≥ 6 weeks	- Tetanus prophylaxis recommended. - Bone biopsy recommended. - Anaerobic coverage recommended. - Switch to oral therapy should be guided by clinical improvement and deep tissue culture and susceptibility results. May need prolonged therapy with oral agents. - Monitor renal function and adjust dosing of antibiotics according to renal function. * If P. aeruginosa cultured, use 4.5g q6h if renal function allows. **Regimen does not cover P. aeruginosa. † Consider MRSA if: • previous (in prior 12 months)/current MRSA infection or colonization • recent antibiotic use • recent hospitalization. Surgical debridement and drainage of associated soft tissue abscesses recommended. ***Use imipenem if known/suspected ESBL/AmpC-producing organism. ‡ If known/suspected P. aeruginosa, use ciprofloxacin or ceftazidime instead of ceftriaxone.

E. Desired vancomycin trough is 15-20mg/L. Monitor renal function closely. See Vancomycin Dosing & Monitoring Guidelines.

Infection	Usual Pathogens	Recommended Empiric Therapy	Recommended Dose[B]	Recommended Duration	Comments
Bone & Joint **Osteomyelitis** (cont'd) **Contiguous** (cont'd) **Post-nail puncture of foot**	P. aeruginosa Occasionally: • S. aureus • Bacillus spp • Anaerobes	Prophylaxis* **Ciprofloxacin**	750mg PO bid	5 days	- Local debridement/tetanus prophylaxis recommended. * Osteomyelitis develops in 1-2% of plantar puncture wounds. Consider prophylaxis if within 24h of nail puncture.
		Treatment **Piperacillin-tazobactam** Oral therapy **Ciprofloxacin**	4.5g IV q6h 750mg PO bid	minimum 2 weeks (IV + PO) to complete minimum 2 weeks	- Tetanus prophylaxis recommended. - Surgical debridement always necessary. - Culture recommended prior to institution of therapy.

RECOMMENDED EMPIRIC THERAPY OF SELECTED INFECTIONS IN ADULT PATIENTS[A]

Infection	Usual Pathogens	Recommended Empiric Therapy	Recommended Dose[B]	Recommended Duration	Comments
Bone & Joint					

Osteomyelitis (cont'd)
Post-operative sternotomy/ mediastinitis
	- Sternal debridement and bone cultures recommended. Tailor antibiotics to C&S results.
	- If S. aureus confirmed, and sternal wires cannot be removed, consider follow-up prolonged (months) oral therapy with:
	    • (ciprofloxacin or levofloxacin or minocycline or TMP/SMX) + rifampin
	    NB: Moxifloxacin also has good Gram positive coverage but not recommended as no clinical data available and increased risk of C. difficile infection [CMAJ 2008; 179:767-72].
	- Tetanus prophylaxis recommended.				

	S. aureus/MRSA S. epidermidis Rare: • Enterobacteriaceae • Corynebacterium spp • Candida spp	**Vancomycin** [E,*] +/- **[Ciprofloxacin** or **Gentamicin]** **	15mg/kg IV q8-12h 500-750mg PO bid/ 400mg IV q12h 7mg/kg IV q24h	6-8 weeks	* Vancomycin has slow distribution in tissues and delayed bactericidal activity. It should only be used long term when it is the only agent to which the organism is susceptible. **Reassess need for quinolone or aminoglycoside therapy as soon as C&S results available.

E. Desired vancomycin trough is 15-20mg/L. Monitor renal function closely. See Vancomycin Dosing & Monitoring Guidelines.

RECOMMENDED EMPIRIC THERAPY OF SELECTED INFECTIONS IN ADULT PATIENTS[A]

Infection	Usual Pathogens	Recommended Empiric Therapy	Recommended Dose[B]	Recommended Duration	Comments
Bone & Joint					
Prosthetic joint infections	Diagnosis [NEJM 2009;361:787-94]:- Presence of at least one of the following: • sinus tract communicating with prosthesis • isolation of same organism from ≥ 2 cultures of joint aspirates or periprosthetic tissue • gross purulence in joint space • acute inflammation on histological exam (> 5 PMNs/hpf). - ESR, CRP - low sensitivity for diagnosis but if initially elevated, may be useful to monitor response. - Imaging - Plain x-ray not useful for diagnosis but may identify loosening of prosthesis or osteolysis. Bone scan is sensitive for detecting failed implant but nonspecific for detecting infection. May remain abnormal for more than a year after implantation. Consider combining with WBC or gallium scan to improve specificity. - Antimicrobial therapy should be discontinued ≥ 2 weeks prior to surgery and perioperative antibiotics should be deferred until after intraoperative cultures have been taken. Treatment options: 1. Debridement + replacement of liner and retention of prosthesis followed by prolonged systemic antibiotic therapy - option for patients with early postoperative (within 3 months) or acute hematogenous infection with symptoms for < 3 weeks, stable implant, bone and soft tissue in good condition, and known susceptible organism. 2. One-stage exchange: removal of infected prosthesis and implantation of new prosthesis +/- antibiotic- impregnated cement in same surgery, followed by systemic antibiotic therapy. Option for patients with satisfactory condition of soft tissue, no severe comorbidities, and absence of difficult to treat organism (MRSA, enterococci, Pseudomonas aeruginosa, fungal, mycobacterial). 3. Two-stage exchange: removal of infected prosthesis, placement of temporary antibiotic-impregnated cement spacer and administration of systemic antibiotic therapy, and reimplantation of new prosthesis 6-12 weeks later. Post re-implantation duration of antibiotic therapy: • until intraoperative cultures come back negative (as long as antibiotics were stopped ≥ 2 weeks prior to surgery), or • 6-12 weeks if positive intraoperative cultures. 4. Removal of prosthesis without replacement or arthrodesis followed by systemic antibiotic therapy in patients with serious comorbidities where repeat surgery not an option. In some cases of uncontrolled infection, amputation may be necessary. 5. Long term antibiotic suppression in patients where surgery is contraindicated.			

RECOMMENDED EMPIRIC THERAPY OF SELECTED INFECTIONS IN ADULT PATIENTS[A]

Infection	Usual Pathogens	Recommended Empiric Therapy	Recommended Dose[B]	Recommended Duration	Comments
Bone & Joint					
Prosthetic joint infections (cont'd)	Intraoperative: - Gram stain of synovial fluid has poor sensitivity (< 26%). Use of intraoperative Gram stain to rule out prosthetic joint infection is NOT recommended. - Cultures of periprosthetic tissue x 5-6 samples recommended; same organism from ≥ 2 samples considered diagnostic. NB: Cultures should be sent for aerobic and anaerobic culture and kept for 14 days. - Swab cultures have low sensitivity and should be avoided. Cultures of superficial wound or sinus tract exudate often contaminated from surrounding skin so should not be done. - Tailor therapy to C&S results. If bacterial cultures negative, but patient septic/not improving, recommend empiric therapy, and discuss value of specialized bacterial, fungal and mycobacterial cultures with microbiologist. - Polymicrobial infections may occur in up to 20% of cases.			

RECOMMENDED EMPIRIC THERAPY OF SELECTED INFECTIONS IN ADULT PATIENTS[A]

Infection	Usual Pathogens	Recommended Empiric Therapy	Recommended Dose[B]	Recommended Duration	Comments
Bone & Joint					
Prosthetic joint infections (cont'd)	**Early (<3 months) after implant:** • S. aureus • Coagulase negative Staphylococci (CoNS) • Enterobacteriaceae **Delayed (3-24 months):** • CoNS • Propionibacterium spp • Anaerobes (other) • S. aureus **Late/Hematogenous (>2 years):** • Streptococcus spp • Enterococcus spp • Abiotrophia spp • Granulicatella spp • S. aureus • CoNS • Enterobacteriaceae • P. aeruginosa Polymicrobial (20%) Culture-negative(7-11%) Fungi (1%)	**Vancomycin**[*,±] + **Rifampin** +/- **Ciprofloxacin**[**] _Alternative oral therapy_ [Ciprofloxacin[***] or Levofloxacin[***] or Minocycline or Doxycycline or TMP/SMX] + **Rifampin** _If surgery contra-indicated:_ Long-term/life-long suppressive therapy[†] Agent according to C&S result or **TMP/SMX** or **Minocycline** or **Doxycycline**	15mg/kg IV q8-12h 450mg PO bid 750mg PO bid 750mg PO bid 750mg PO daily 100mg PO bid 100mg PO bid 1DS tab PO tid 450mg PO bid 1DS tab PO tid 100mg PO bid 100mg PO bid	**Debridement and retention or One-stage exchange:** 2-4 weeks IV followed by oral therapy for total of 3 months for hip and 3-6 months for knee prostheses. **Two-stage exchange:** 4-8 weeks of antimicrobial therapy + ≥ 2 weeks antibiotic-free interval before re-implantation. Postop: continue antimicrobial therapy until intraoperative cultures come back negative (as long as antibiotics were stopped ≥ 2 weeks prior to surgery) or for 6-12 weeks if positive intraoperative cultures. Tailor to C&S results.	* Vancomycin has slow, erratic distribution in tissues and delayed bactericidal activity. It should only be used long term when it is the only agent to which the organism is susceptible. **Ciprofloxacin may be considered empirically for Gram negative coverage, especially if early (<3 months). ***Moxifloxacin also has good Gram positive coverage but not recommended as no clinical data available and increased risk of C. difficile infection [CMAJ 2008; 179:767-72]. † Rifampin is not necessary since goal is to control clinical manifestations of infection rather than eradication.

E. Desired vancomycin trough is 15-20mg/L. Monitor renal function closely. See Vancomycin Dosing & Monitoring Guidelines.

RECOMMENDED EMPIRIC THERAPY OF SELECTED INFECTIONS IN ADULT PATIENTS[A]

Infection	Usual Pathogens	Recommended Empiric Therapy	Recommended Dose[B]	Recommended Duration	Comments
Bone & Joint					
Prosthetic joint infections (cont'd)					
Shoulder arthroplasty, rotator cuff surgery	P. acnes* S. aureus Occasionally polymicrobial	**Vancomycin**[E] Documented P. acnes infection* **Penicillin** or **Ceftriaxone**	15mg/kg IV q8-12h 4MU IV q6h 2g IV daily	4-6 weeks** 4-6 weeks** 4-6 weeks**	- Debridement of all necrotic tissue and removal of all nonabsorbable sutures and implants is recommended. Consider adding rifampin 450mg PO bid if hardware cannot be removed. * P. acnes is a common pathogen after these types of surgery. Alert lab to hold culture for 14 days. **May need additional oral therapy on an individualized basis.

E. Desired vancomycin trough is 15-20mg/L. Monitor renal function closely. See Vancomycin Dosing & Monitoring Guidelines.

RECOMMENDED EMPIRIC THERAPY OF SELECTED INFECTIONS IN ADULT PATIENTS[A]

Infection	Usual Pathogens	Recommended Empiric Therapy	Recommended Dose[B]	Recommended Duration	Comments
Bone & Joint					

Septic arthritis	Investigations:
	• Blood cultures recommended (positive in 60%). If positive, repeat blood cultures to ensure clearance of bacteremia.
	• Synovial fluid for cell count, C&S, and crystal analysis.
	  ○ Typical findings of septic arthritis: purulence, variable viscosity, WBC > 50 x 10⁹/L with > 75% neutrophils. Protein and glucose levels are not diagnostically useful.
	  ○ Gram stain lacks sensitivity (only positive in 1/3); whereas culture is positive in 90%.
	  ○ Tailor antibiotics according to C&S results.
	• CBC and differential, serum creatinine.
	• ESR, CRP - low sensitivity for diagnosis but if initially elevated, may be useful to monitor response.
	• Plain x-ray +/- MRI, or bone scan +/- WBC or gallium scan.
	  ○ MRI superior to x-ray and bone scan for early diagnosis of bone/joint infections
	  ○ Bone scan may be falsely positive if recent trauma/aspiration of joint/superficial infection (WBC or gallium scan may improve specificity).
	- Drainage and/or debridement of the joint space recommended.				

Adults • Native joints • +/- non-penetrating trauma	S. aureus* Streptococcus spp Rare: • Candida spp • P. aeruginosa** • Enterobacteriaceae**	[**Cloxacillin** or **Cefazolin**] +/- [**Ciprofloxacin** or **Gentamicin**]** [β-lactam allergy/MRSA* **Vancomycin**[E] or **Clindamycin**] +/- [**Ciprofloxacin** or **Gentamicin**]**	2g IV q4h 2g IV q8h 750mg PO bid 7mg/kg IV q24h 15mg/kg IV q8-12h 600mg IV q8h/ 450mg PO qid 750mg PO bid 7mg/kg IV q24h	2-4 weeks 2-4 weeks	* Consider MRSA especially if: • preceding trauma • multifocal lesion • disease in adjacent muscle. **Consider adding ciprofloxacin or gentamicin if IVDU (sternoclavicular/ sacroiliac joints), immuno-compromised, or elderly, as increased risk of Gram negative infection. - For chronic monoarticular arthritis consider mycobacterial infection.

E. Desired vancomycin trough is 15-20mg/L. Monitor renal function closely. See Vancomycin Dosing & Monitoring Guidelines.

RECOMMENDED EMPIRIC THERAPY OF SELECTED INFECTIONS IN ADULT PATIENTS[A]

Infection	Usual Pathogens	Recommended Empiric Therapy	Recommended Dose[B]	Recommended Duration	Comments
Bone & Joint					
Septic arthritis (cont'd)					
Gonococcal	http://www.phac-aspc.gc.ca/std-mts/sti-its/pdf/506gonococcal-eng.pdf and http://www.phac-aspc.gc.ca/std-mts/sti-its/alert/2011/alert-gono-eng.php				
• **Tenosynovitis /dermatitis/ polyarthralgia syndrome**	Neisseria gonorrhoeae†	**Ceftriaxone**	2g IV daily	3-7 days* *Continue IV for 24 hours after improvement of symptoms, then follow-up with oral therapy to complete 7 days total IV/PO:	† All patients: • empiric treatment for concomitant Chlamydia trachomatis infection with: azithromycin 1g PO single dose or doxycycline 100mg PO bid x 7 days. • test for HIV, syphilis, hepatitis B • culture urine (males), vagina/cervix (females), rectum, throat, blood, and joint fluid (and treat accordingly). - Test, and treat regardless of clinical signs/symptoms, all recent (60 days) sexual contacts.
		Oral therapy* **Cefixime**	400mg PO bid	to complete 7 days	
		Alternative oral therapy** **Ciprofloxacin****	500mg PO bid	to complete 7 days	**High quinolone resistance; only use if susceptibility documented.
• **Purulent arthritis**		Joint drainage plus **Ceftriaxone**	2g IV daily	7-14 days	- Recurrent gonococcal septic arthritis warrants investigation for complement deficiency.
Rheumatoid arthritis-associated infection	S. aureus Streptococcus spp Enterobacteriaceae	**Cefazolin** +/- [**Ciprofloxacin** or **Gentamicin**] β-lactam allergy **Clindamycin IV/PO**[C] + **Ciprofloxacin**	2g IV q8h 750mg PO bid 7mg/kg IV q24h 600mg IV q8h/ 450mg PO qid 500mg PO bid	4 weeks 4 weeks	- Involvement of multiple joints common. - Recommend culture of joint prior to institution of therapy. - Tailor antibiotics to C&S results. - If on TNF inhibitors, consider unusual bacterial, mycobacterial, or fungal pathogens.

RECOMMENDED EMPIRIC THERAPY OF SELECTED INFECTIONS IN ADULT PATIENTS[A]

Infection	Usual Pathogens	Recommended Empiric Therapy	Recommended Dose[B]	Recommended Duration	Comments
Bone & Joint (cont'd) **Septic arthritis Intravenous drug use**	S. aureus/MRSA P. aeruginosa Occasionally: • Candida spp	**Vancomycin**[E] + [**Ciprofloxacin** or **Tobramycin**]	15mg/kg IV q8-12h 750mg PO bid 7mg/kg IV q24h	3-4 weeks	- May have concomitant osteomyelitis with predilection for sternoclavicular/sacroiliac joint, ribs, vertebral discs, long bones. - Must rule out endocarditis. - Joint/blood cultures recommended prior to institution of therapy. Tailor antibiotics to C&S results. • If methicillin-sensitive S. aureus, use cloxacillin or cefazolin as superior to vancomycin. • Reassess need for quinolone or aminoglycoside therapy as soon as C&S results available.

E: Desired vancomycin trough is 15-20mg/L. Monitor renal function closely. See Vancomycin Dosing & Monitoring Guidelines.

RECOMMENDED EMPIRIC THERAPY OF SELECTED INFECTIONS IN ADULT PATIENTS[A]

Infection	Usual Pathogens	Recommended Empiric Therapy	Recommended Dose[B]	Recommended Duration	Comments
Bone & Joint					
Septic bursitis, olecranon, pre-patellar	\- Absence of pain with joint movement may help differentiate septic bursitis from septic arthritis. \- Recommend: • Blood cultures if systemically ill. • Baseline and follow-up x-rays to rule out bone or joint involvement. • Aspirate fluid initially for drainage and C&S, and aspirate daily until fluid sterile and no longer accumulating.				
	S. aureus/MRSA Group A Streptococci	**Mild** **Cloxacillin** or **Cephalexin**	500mg PO qid 500mg PO qid	2-3 weeks* 2-3 weeks*	\- For chronic bursitis consider mycobacterial infection; send fluid or tissue for mycobacterial culture. * 7 days of therapy may be sufficient if: • short duration of symptoms and • early aspiration/drainage, and • immunocompetent patients. Longer therapy (2-3 weeks) if: • immunocompromised or • initial symptoms >7 days. \- In patients who fail to respond to antibiotic therapy and percutaneous drainage, surgical drainage and/or bursectomy may be required.
		<u>MRSA suspected</u> **TMP/SMX** + **[Cephalexin** or **Cloxacillin]**	2 DS tabs PO bid 500mg PO qid 500mg PO qid	2-3 weeks*	
		Moderate-severe **Cloxacillin** or **Cefazolin**	2g IV q4h 2g IV q8h	2-3 weeks* 2-3 weeks*	
		<u>β-lactam allergy/</u> <u>MRSA suspected</u> **Vancomycin**[E]	15mg/kg IV q8-12h	2-3 weeks*	

E. Desired vancomycin trough is 15-20mg/L. Monitor renal function closely. See Vancomycin Dosing & Monitoring Guidelines.

RECOMMENDED EMPIRIC THERAPY OF SELECTED INFECTIONS IN ADULT PATIENTS[A]

Infection	Usual Pathogens	Recommended Empiric Therapy	Recommended Dose[B]	Recommended Duration	Comments
Respiratory					
Pharyngitis					

Etiology
- **Majority of adult cases (80-90%) of pharyngitis are of viral etiology and do not require antimicrobial therapy.**
- Group A Streptococcus (GAS) is most common bacterial cause of pharyngitis.
- Occasionally pharyngitis is caused by Group C, G Streptococci and Arcanobacterium haemolyticum. A. haemolyticum causes pharyngitis in young adults (12-30 years old). Many have scarlatiniform rash, most marked on the extremities. Notify laboratory if clinically suspected as culture requires prolonged incubation.

Clinical presentation
- The following suggests a viral etiology: conjunctivitis, cough, hoarseness, rhinorrhea, and/or diarrhea. Patients with these symptoms should not have a throat swab taken for culture or rapid antigen-detection test (RADT).
- Typical signs/symptoms of GAS pharyngitis:
   1. pharyngeal or tonsillar exudate
   2. fever
   3. tenderness/enlargement of anterior cervical lymph nodes
   4. absence of cough
   Increased risk if exposure to individual with strep throat in previous 2 weeks.
- Infectious for 2-5 days prior to symptoms.
- GAS pharyngitis is most common in children between 5-10 years old, and in fall and winter.
- Consider Lemierre's syndrome (jugular vein suppurative phlebitis) in teenagers/young adults with pharyngitis, persistent fever, and neck pain. Recommend aerobic and anaerobic blood cultures and imaging of neck veins with ultrasound or CT.

Diagnosis
- Cannot diagnose GAS pharyngitis with symptoms alone (even if all 4 signs/symptoms listed above are present). **Throat swab for culture or rapid antigen-detection test recommended.**
- Newer RADT have high specificity and much improved sensitivity therefore confirmatory throat culture is no longer recommended for negative RADT results.

Antibiotic therapy
- Awaiting throat culture results before initiating antibiotic therapy remains a reasonable strategy as:
   • Group A Strep pharyngitis is a self-limited disease (8-10 days)
   • antibiotic therapy can be delayed for up to 9 days after onset of illness and still prevent acute rheumatic fever
   • delay in antibiotic therapy may decrease reinfection rates
   • unnecessary antibiotic use can be avoided in ~50% of patients.

RECOMMENDED EMPIRIC THERAPY OF SELECTED INFECTIONS IN ADULT PATIENTS[A]

Infection	Usual Pathogens	Recommended Empiric Therapy	Recommended Dose[B]	Recommended Duration	Comments
Respiratory					

Pharyngitis (cont'd)	Antibiotic Therapy (cont'd)
	- Antibiotic therapy decreases: severity of symptoms, duration of symptoms by ~1 day, risk of transmission (after 24h of therapy), and likelihood of suppurative complications and of rheumatic fever.
	  • Group A Streptococci:
	    • No in vitro resistance to penicillin
	    • Significant macrolide and clindamycin resistance
	    • TMP/SMX – no activity against Group A Streptococcus
	- Quinolones and broad-spectrum cephalosporins NOT indicated in pharyngitis – too broad-spectrum, potential to increase resistance.
	
	- **Follow up cultures are not routinely recommended** unless:
	  • history of rheumatic fever (increased risk for recurrence)
	  • persistent symptoms
	  • recurrent symptoms.				

Acute	Group A Streptococci	Symptomatic therapy <u>Analgesic/antipyretic</u> **Penicillin VK** <u>Penicillin allergy</u> **Cephalexin**** or **Clindamycin** or **Azithromycin** or **Clarithromycin**	600mg PO bid **or** 300mg PO tid 500mg PO bid 300mg PO tid 500mg PO daily 250mg PO bid	10 days* 10 days 10 days 3 days 10 days	* Meta-analysis indicates that 5 days of penicillin therapy is inferior to 10 days of therapy. **Do not use if anaphylaxis/severe penicillin allergy.

RECOMMENDED EMPIRIC THERAPY OF SELECTED INFECTIONS IN ADULT PATIENTS[A]

Infection	Usual Pathogens	Recommended Empiric Therapy	Recommended Dose[B]	Recommended Duration	Comments
Respiratory					
Pharyngitis (cont'd)					* Consider:
Non-responders* (after 72 hours of therapy) **or** **Early relapse[†]** (2-7 days post therapy)	Group A Streptococci	<u>Non-responders*</u> Change in antibiotic therapy may not be required.			• noncompliance • concurrent viral infection in a Group A Strep carrier • suppurative complication of Group A Strep pharyngitis (e.g. peritonsillar, tonsillar, or retropharyngeal abscess).
		<u>Early relapse*[†]</u> **Clindamycin*** or	300mg PO tid	10 days	[†] Early relapse: repeat throat swab; only treat if culture positive for Group A Strep.
		Amoxicillin-clavulanate	875mg PO bid	10 days	** Group A Streptococci resistance to macrolides and clindamycin is significant.
		<u>Alternative</u> **Azithromycin**** or	500mg PO daily	3 days	
		Clarithromycin**	250mg PO bid	10 days	
Late relapse **or** **Recurrent**	Group A Streptococci	**Clindamycin** or	300mg PO tid	10 days	- Late relapse or recurrence should be confirmed by culture. - Consider:
		Amoxicillin-clavulanate	875mg PO bid	10 days	• concurrent viral infection in a Group A Strep carrier • new infections with Group A Strep.
		<u>Alternative</u> **Azithromycin** or	500mg PO daily	3 days	- **Continuous antibiotic prophylaxis is not recommended.**
		Clarithromycin or	250mg PO bid	10 days	* Although pen VK should be effective, there is some evidence that antibiotics with activity against β-lactamase producing organisms (e.g. anaerobes) may be superior.
		Penicillin VK*	600mg PO bid or 300mg PO tid	10 days	

RECOMMENDED EMPIRIC THERAPY OF SELECTED INFECTIONS IN ADULT PATIENTS[A]

Infection	Usual Pathogens	Recommended Empiric Therapy	Recommended Dose[B]	Recommended Duration	Comments
Respiratory					
Pharyngitis (cont'd)					
Asymptomatic carrier	- Up to 20% of the paediatric population may carry Group A Strep asymptomatically. Carriage rate is much lower in older adolescents and adults (2.4-3.7%). - Chronic carriers are not significant in the spread of Group A Strep and are at little risk of rheumatic fever. These individuals do not need to be identified or treated.				
Gonococcal	Neisseria gonorrhoeae*	**Ceftriaxone** + **[Azithromycin** or **Doxycycline]****	250mg IM 1g PO 100mg PO bid	single dose single dose 7 days	* Throat swabs not rountinely cultured for N. gonorrhoeae; notify lab if clinically suspected. **All regimens should be followed by empiric treatment for chlamydial infection; azithromycin preferred. - Test of cure recommended after completion of therapy.

- 260 -

RECOMMENDED EMPIRIC THERAPY OF SELECTED INFECTIONS IN ADULT PATIENTS[A]

Infection	Usual Pathogens	Recommended Empiric Therapy	Recommended Dose[B]	Recommended Duration	Comments
Respiratory					
Ulcerative gingivitis (Vincent's Angina)	Anaerobes Spirochetes	**Penicillin + Metronidazole IV/PO**[C] β-lactam allergy **Clindamycin IV/PO**[C]	4MU IV q4h 500mg IV/PO q12h 600mg IV q8h or 300mg PO qid	10 days 10 days	- Associated with vitamin deficiency.
Jugular Vein Septic Phlebitis (Lemierre's Syndrome)	Fusobacterium necrophorum* or Polymicrobial (1/3) • Oral anaerobes • Streptococcus spp	Surgical drainage as appropriate + **Penicillin + Metronidazole** β-lactam allergy **Clindamycin + Metronidazole******	3-4MU IV q4h 500mg IV q8h** 600mg IV q8h** 500mg IV q8h**	6-12 weeks 6-12 weeks	- Suspect in teenagers/young adults with pharyngitis/fever and neck pain/swelling. - May occur as a rare complication of otitis media, tonsillitis, or dental infections. * Organism difficult to grow; notify lab if suspected. **May switch to oral therapy when clinically stable. ***Combination recommended due to increasing clindamycin resistance in oral anaerobes but need for aerobic Strep coverage with clindamycin.
Parapharyngeal space infections*	Polymicrobial: • Anaerobes • Streptococcus spp • Eikenella corrodens	Surgical drainage + **Penicillin + Metronidazole** β-lactam allergy **Clindamycin**	3-4MU IV q4h 500mg IV q12h** 600mg IV q8h**	10-14 days 10-14 days	* Includes sublingual, submandibular (Ludwig's angina), lateral pharyngeal, retropharyngeal, pretracheal infections. - Consult ENT. **May switch to oral therapy when clinically stable.
Odontogenic	See Recommended Empiric Therapy of Dental Infections				

RECOMMENDED EMPIRIC THERAPY OF SELECTED INFECTIONS IN ADULT PATIENTS[A]

Infection	Usual Pathogens	Recommended Empiric Therapy	Recommended Dose[B]	Recommended Duration	Comments
Respiratory					
Epiglottitis	Group A, B, C Streptococci S. pneumoniae S. aureus H. influenzae H. parainfluenzae N. meningitidis	**Ceftriaxone** β-lactam allergy **Levofloxacin**	1-2g IV q24h 750mg IV daily	7-10 days 7-10 days	- If suspected, admit to hospital immediately, call ICU, anaesthesia, and ENT without distressing the patient. - Keep in position of comfort (usually sitting).
Laryngitis	Viruses	**No antibiotic therapy recommended**			
Rhinitis	- Adults get an average of 3-4 colds per year. (Children 6-10 colds per year) - Counsel on importance of handwashing in preventing spread of viruses. - Yellow/green nasal discharge is NOT an indicator of bacterial infection.				
	Viruses (up to 200 different viruses) or Allergic	**No antibiotic therapy recommended.** Saline nasal irrigation* + Steam inhalation + Decongestant**			* Saline solutions are available commercially or can be made at home. Saline solution recipe: 250mL (3 oz or 1 cup) warm distilled or previously boiled/filtered water ½ tsp noniodinated salt ½ tsp baking soda • Place solution in neti pot or bulb syringe • Gently squeeze water into upper nostril; water will drain from other nostril. • Repeat on other side. **May alleviate symptoms but will not shorten duration of symptoms.

RECOMMENDED EMPIRIC THERAPY OF SELECTED INFECTIONS IN ADULT PATIENTS[A]

Infection	Usual Pathogens	Recommended Empiric Therapy	Recommended Dose[B]	Recommended Duration	Comments
Respiratory					
Otitis Media					
Acute	S. pneumoniae H. influenzae M. catarrhalis Group A Streptococci S. aureus	**Amoxicillin** Alternative **Doxycycline**	1g PO tid 200mg PO once, then 100mg PO bid	5 days 5 days	- Acute otitis media is uncommon in adults.
Failure of first line agents: • persistent • prolonged • recurrent*	S. pneumoniae H. influenzae M. catarrhalis Group A Streptococci S. aureus	**Amoxicillin-clavulanate** Penicillin allergy **Cefuroxime axetil** Severe penicillin allergy or cephalosporin allergy **Levofloxacin**	875mg PO bid 500mg-1g PO bid 750mg PO daily	10 days 10 days 10 days	- For pen (I) S. pneumoniae, amoxicillin is most active of all oral β-lactam agents. * For recurrences > 6 weeks apart, see Acute otitis media.
Chronic	S. aureus Enterobacteriaceae P. aeruginosa Anaerobes	Treat according to C&S results.			- Recommend ENT consult.
Hospital acquired otitis	See Sinusitis - Hospital acquired				

RECOMMENDED EMPIRIC THERAPY OF SELECTED INFECTIONS IN ADULT PATIENTS[A]

Infection	Usual Pathogens	Recommended Empiric Therapy	Recommended Dose[B]	Recommended Duration	Comments
Respiratory					
Otitis externa					

Swimmer's ear		Prevention
		- Consider wearing earplugs during swimming.
		- After swimming, remove as much water from ears as possible by:
		  • tilting head to allow water to drain from ears
		  • using hair dryer set on low
		  • **if intact eardrum and no ear tubes**, dry ears with a few drops of vinegar +/- rubbing alcohol in each ear after swimming
					* If condition persists after 7 days, then re-assess. May require debridement. Consider referral to ENT specialist.

	P. aeruginosa Enterobacteriaceae S. aureus†	**Aluminum acetate/ benzethonium** (Buro-Sol)	2-3 drops tid-qid	max. 7 days*	**Corticosteroid-containing preparations are useful when there is underlying dermatitis.
		Alternative** **Gentamicin/betameth- asone** (Garasone)*** or	3-4 drops tid	max. 7 days*	***Risk of ototoxicity (hearing loss, tinnitus, vertigo, imbalance) if perforated eardrum, ear tubes, or > 7 days therapy.
		Framycetin/gramicidin/ dexamethasone (Sofracort)*** or	2-3 drops tid-qid	max. 7 days*	† If severe/acute onset, consider adding cloxacillin 500mg PO qid to cover methicillin-susceptible
		Ciprofloxacin/dexa- methasone (Ciprodex) or	4 drops bid	max. 7 days*	S. aureus, or TMP/SMX 1 tab PO bid or doxycycline 100mg PO bid to cover methicillin-resistant S. aureus.
		Clioquinol/flumethasone (Locacorten Vioform)	2-3 drops bid	max 7 days*	
Invasive otitis externa	P. aeruginosa	Surgical debridement + **Piperacillin +** **Tobramycin** <u>Stepdown</u> **Ciprofloxacin**	4g IV q6h 7mg/kg IV q24h 750mg PO bid	6-8 weeks (IV+PO)	- Most cases occur in diabetics. - CT or MRI scan recommended.
Mastoiditis					
Acute	See Otitis media				

RECOMMENDED EMPIRIC THERAPY OF SELECTED INFECTIONS IN ADULT PATIENTS[A]

Infection	Usual Pathogens	Recommended Empiric Therapy	Recommended Dose[B]	Recommended Duration	Comments
Respiratory					
Mastoiditis (cont'd) **Chronic**	Polymicrobial: • Anaerobes • S. aureus • Enterobacteriaceae • Pseudomonas spp	Surgical drainage Treat according to C&S of surgical cultures.		minimum 2 weeks*	* Need to rule out concomitant osteomyelitis/brain abscess. Longer therapy may be required.
Sinusitis [Clin Infect Dis 2012;Mar:e1-41]	- Most common predisposing factor is viral upper respiratory tract infection (URTI). Bacterial sinusitis complicates only 0.5-2% of cases. Up to 10% of sinusitis may be related to dental disease. - The role of Mycoplasma pneumoniae and Chlamydophila pneumoniae in acute sinusitis has been suggested but not substantiated. Empiric therapy for these organisms is not recommended. Clinical presentation - A bacterial etiology is more likely if: • high fever (≥ 39°C) and purulent nasal discharge or facial pain for 3-4 consecutive days at beginning of illness or • URTI symptoms persist for at least 10 days or worsen after 5-7 days with both nasal congestion/purulent nasal discharge and facial pain/pressure (usually unilateral) +/- • fever • maxillary toothache • facial swelling. Diagnosis - The colour of nasal discharge/sputum should not be used to diagnose the sinusitis episode as bacterial since colour is related to presence of neutrophils, not bacteria. - Black, necrotic tissue or discharge in patients with poorly controlled diabetes/ketoacidosis, or with significant immunosuppression, may indicate mucormycosis. Recommend urgent ENT/ID consult. - Nasopharyngeal cultures are not helpful in identifying etiological sinus pathogen(s). - Sinus x-rays are not routinely recommended as they will not differentiate between viral URTI and bacterial sinusitis. - CT scan only recommended for complications of acute sinusitis, chronic sinusitis not responding to therapy, and/or severe presentation. - MRI not recommended due to poor bone definition. - Transillumination of the sinuses is of limited value in adults.				

RECOMMENDED EMPIRIC THERAPY OF SELECTED INFECTIONS IN ADULT PATIENTS[A]

Infection	Usual Pathogens	Recommended Empiric Therapy	Recommended Dose[B]	Recommended Duration	Comments
Respiratory					

Sinusitis (cont'd)		Antibiotic Therapy
		- The benefit of antibiotic therapy in sinusitis is controversial (~70% resolve spontaneously).
		- Some guidelines recommend high-dose amoxicillin-clavulanate instead of amoxicillin for first line treatemnt of sinusitis because of high rates of penicillin-resistant S. pneumoniae and β-lactamase producing H. influenzae and M. catarrhalis.
		- High-dose amoxicillin remains a reasonable first-line empiric option given:
		   • the lower resistance rates in Canada
		   • amoxicillin retains best coverage of all oral β-lactam agents against S. pneumoniae (even majority of penicillin-resistant strains)
		   • higher incidence of adverse effects of amoxicillin-clavulanate
		   • need to limit broad spectrum antibiotic use in order to minimize the development of antibiotic resistance.
		- Macrolides, TMP/SMX, and oral cephalosporins are no longer recommended for empiric therapy of sinusitis due to unpredictable/poor activity against S. pneumoniae and/or H. influenzae.
		- Levofloxacin has good coverage of the pathogens involved. However because of its broad spectrum, potential for increasing resistance, and risk of C. difficile infection, it should be reserved for β-lactam allergic patients or patients who have failed first line antibiotic therapy.
		
		Prevention
		   • limit spread of viral infections by handwashing
		   • avoid environmental tobacco smoke
		   • avoid allergen exposure.			

RECOMMENDED EMPIRIC THERAPY OF SELECTED INFECTIONS IN ADULT PATIENTS[A]

Infection	Usual Pathogens	Recommended Empiric Therapy	Recommended Dose[B]	Recommended Duration	Comments
Respiratory					
Sinusitis (cont'd) **Acute** • symptoms < 4 weeks • ≤ 3 episodes/year	S. pneumoniae H. influenzae M. catarrhalis Occasionally: • S. aureus • Group A Streptococci • Anaerobes	Mild – moderate <u>symptoms < 10 days</u> Symptomatic therapy[†] <u>Symptoms > 10 days or</u> <u>worsening after 5-7 days</u> **Amoxicillin** Alternative **Doxycycline** <u>Severe**/</u> <u>Immunocompromised</u> **Amoxicillin** + **Amoxicillin-clavulanate** <u>Nonsevere β-lactam</u> <u>allergy</u> **Ceftriaxone** <u>Severe β-lactam allergy/</u> <u>anaphylaxis</u> **Levofloxacin**	500mg-1g PO tid* 200mg PO once, then 100mg PO bid 1g PO bid 875mg PO bid 1-2g IV daily 750mg PO daily	5-7 days 5-7 days 5-7 days 5-7 days 5-7 days 5 days	[†] Adjunctive therapy with topical/systemic decongestant and/or nasal irrigation with sterile saline solution or steam inhalation may be helpful. Prolonged (> 5 days) use of topical decongestants should be avoided as it may lead to rebound symptoms. NB: Antihistamines and mucolytics have no role in the management of acute sinusitis. * Use higher dose if antibiotic use within past 3 months. **Severe = high fever (≥ 39°C) and purulent nasal discharge or facial pain for 3-4 consecutive days. - The use of topical (intranasal) corticosteroids is controversial but may offer some benefit in allergic rhinosinusitis. Recent evidence indicates they are not of benefit in established acute bacterial sinusitis characterized by thick secretions, closure of the ostium and systemic symptoms.

RECOMMENDED EMPIRIC THERAPY OF SELECTED INFECTIONS IN ADULT PATIENTS[A]

Infection	Usual Pathogens	Recommended Empiric Therapy	Recommended Dose[B]	Recommended Duration	Comments
Respiratory					
Sinusitis (cont'd) **Failure of first line agents:** • clinical deterioration after 72 h of antibiotic therapy • no improvement post therapy • recurrence within 3 months[†]	S. pneumoniae M. catarrhalis H. influenzae Occasionally: • S. aureus • Group A Streptococci • Anaerobes	Second line agents: **Amoxicillin-clavulanate** +/- **Amoxicillin*** β-lactam allergy **Levofloxacin**	875mg PO bid 1g PO bid 750mg PO daily	5-10 days 5-10 days 5-10 days	- Need to consider resistant organisms, especially penicillin-resistant S. pneumoniae, ampicillin-resistant H. influenzae, and M. catarrhalis. * If patient has failed high dose amoxicillin therapy, amoxicillin-clavulanate used alone is adequate to cover β-lactamase producing organisms. [†] Recommend refer to ENT if ≥ 4 episodes/year. Consider allergy testing. Topical (intranasal) corticosteroids may be of benefit in recurrent sinusitis but should be used in early stage before production of thick secretions, closure of the ostium, and development of systemic symptoms.
Chronic • symptoms ≥ 12 weeks	Anaerobes Occasionally: • S. aureus • S. pneumoniae • H. influenzae • M. catarrhalis • Group A Streptococci • Enterobacteriaceae	**Amoxicillin-clavulanate** β-lactam allergy **Clindamycin**	875mg PO bid 300mg PO qid	3 weeks* 3 weeks*	* A single prolonged (3 weeks) course of antibiotic may be of value in chronic sinusitis but controversial. - Repeated courses of antibiotics are not recommended. - Refer to ENT if not responding. Investigations for allergy +/- polyps, underlying immunodeficiency and/or odontogenic disease may be indicated.

RECOMMENDED EMPIRIC THERAPY OF SELECTED INFECTIONS IN ADULT PATIENTS[A]

Infection	Usual Pathogens	Recommended Empiric Therapy	Recommended Dose[B]	Recommended Duration	Comments
Respiratory					
Sinusitis (cont'd) **Hospital-acquired** **< 4 days hospitalization**	See Sinusitis - Acute				
≥ 4 days hospitalization	- Majority of cases occur in second week of hospitalization. - Risk factors: • mechanical ventilation • facial/cranial fractures • nasal packing • nasogastric/nasoendotracheal tubes • otitis media post head trauma. • corticosteroid therapy • prior antibiotic use. - Black, necrotic tissue or discharge in patients with poorly controlled diabetes/ketoacidosis, or with significant immunosuppression, may indicate mucormycosis. Recommend urgent ENT/ID consult. - **Recommend:** • **ENT consult** • **Remove nasogastric/nasoendotracheal tube** • **Semi-recumbent (30-45°) positioning** • **Sinus aspiration for C&S:** ⇒ tailor antibiotics to C&S results. - If no response to therapy in 7 days, insertion of a drainage catheter should be considered.				

RECOMMENDED EMPIRIC THERAPY OF SELECTED INFECTIONS IN ADULT PATIENTS[A]

Infection	Usual Pathogens	Recommended Empiric Therapy	Recommended DoseB	Recommended Duration	Comments
Respiratory					
Sinusitis (cont'd) **Hospital-** **acquired** (cont'd) **≥ 4 days** **hospitalization** (cont'd) (majority occur in second week of hospitalization)	Enterobacteriaceae P. aeruginosa* Acinetobacter spp* S. aureus/MRSA** Yeast***	**Clindamycin IV/PO**[C] + **Ciprofloxacin IV/PO**[D] Severe[†] **Piperacillin-tazobactam** or Facial fractures, head trauma, CNS infection/ meningitis suspected **Meropenem**	600mg IV q8h/ 300mg PO qid 400mg IV q12h/ 750mg PO bid 4.5g IV q6h 2g IV q8h	7-10 days 7-10 days 7-10 days	* If Pseudomonas/Acinetobacter cultured, recommend combination therapy with tobramycin. **Add vancomycin if patient is colonized with MRSA or Gram stain is suggestive of Staphylococci. ***Addition of fluconazole recommended if yeast seen on Gram stain or if cultured from sinus aspirate. [†] Consider empiric combination therapy with tobramycin if patient has received multiple courses of broad- spectrum antibiotic therapy.
Fungal	See Recommended Empiric Therapy of Fungal Infections				

RECOMMENDED EMPIRIC THERAPY OF SELECTED INFECTIONS IN ADULT PATIENTS[A]

Infection	Usual Pathogens	Recommended Empiric Therapy	Recommended Dose[B]	Recommended Duration	Comments
Respiratory					

Pertussis (Whooping cough)	- Notify Public Health.
	- For contact prophylaxis recommendations, see Prophylaxis for Contacts of Communicable Diseases.
	- Persistent cough (≥ 6 days) in adults and adolescents may indicate whooping cough in up to 32%.
	- Cough with vomiting in adults represents high likelihood for whooping cough.
	- Typical course of pertussis:
	  1) catarrhal phase - lasts 1-2 weeks; most contagious
	  2) paroxysmal phase - 3-6 weeks.
	  3) convalescent phase - > 6 weeks (mean duration of cough is 6 weeks).
	
	<u>Diagnosis</u>
	- cough present for up to 3 weeks - order culture and PCR of posterior nasopharynx (aspirate/swab)
	- cough present > 3 weeks - order PCR (beyond 4 weeks, PCR likely to be negative)
	
	<u>Antibiotic therapy</u>
	- Antibiotic therapy may reduce the duration or severity of symptoms (only if started in catarrhal phase) and limits transmission to susceptible contacts. Because viable organisms can be recovered from untreated patients for 3 weeks after onset of cough, a 5-7 day course of antibiotics is recommended during the first 4 weeks of illness. For individuals likely to be in contact with high risk contacts (infants, pregnant women in 3rd trimester, health care workers, child care workers who care for infants), a 5-7 day course of antibiotics is recommended during the 6-8 weeks after onset of illness.
	
	<u>Prevention</u>
	- Adults are an important reservoir for pertussis and transmission to children, and pertussis in adults is associated with considerable morbidity (otitis, sinusitis, pneumonia, urinary incontinence).
	- All adults who have not previously had a dose of acellular pertussis vaccine should receive a single dose.				

	Bordetella pertussis	**Treatment** **Azithromycin** or **Clarithromycin** or **Erythromycin base** **Alternative** **TMP/SMX****	500mg PO first day then 250mg PO daily x 4 days 500mg PO bid or XL 1g PO daily 500mg PO qid 1 DS tab PO bid	5 days* 7 days* 7 days* 10 days*	* No longer infectious after 5 days of therapy. ** Efficacy not established.

- 271 -

RECOMMENDED EMPIRIC THERAPY OF SELECTED INFECTIONS IN ADULT PATIENTS[A]

Infection	Usual Pathogens	Recommended Empiric Therapy	Recommended Dose[B]	Recommended Duration	Comments
Respiratory					

Bronchitis	- Cough in the absence of fever, tachypnea, and tachycardia suggests bronchitis rather than pneumonia.
	- Acute bronchitis in adults and children is almost exclusively viral in etiology (≥ 90%).
	- Respiratory syncytial virus is a significant pathogen in adults with acute bronchitis, especially elderly.
	- Mycoplasma pneumoniae and Chlamydophila pneumoniae have been implicated but not fully established as pathogens in acute bronchitis. Empiric therapy for these organisms is not recommended.
	- Prolonged cough (>3 weeks) is not unusual in acute viral bronchitis (45% of patients still coughing at 2 weeks and 25% after 3 weeks). NB: Pertussis may mimic acute bronchitis and is underdiagnosed. Investigate if persistent cough (≥ 6 days), especially if associated with vomiting.
	- Postnasal drip, asthma, and GERD account for > 75% of coughs lasting at least 3 weeks with negative chest x-ray.
	- Purulent (green/yellow) sputum production is indicative of inflammatory reaction and does not necessarily imply bacterial infection.
	- In most patients the respiratory exam is normal (few patients may have wheezes). Chest x-ray is indicated if there is any suspicion of pneumonia on history or physical exam.
	- Follow-up not recommended unless:
	   • symptoms worsen or new symptoms develop (dyspnea, persistent fever, vomiting)
	   • coughing >1 month
	   • symptoms recur (>3 episodes/year)				

Acute	Viruses	**No antibiotic therapy recommended.*** Management** • increased humidity • smoking cessation • antitussives – may alleviate symptoms but will not reduce duration of illness • bronchodilators – should not be used routinely but may have modest benefit for protracted cough, dyspnea, and wheezing.			* Meta-analyses have shown no benefit of antibiotics in patients with acute bronchitis. **Corticosteroids (inhaled/oral) are not recommended as there is insufficient evidence to support their use. **Expectorants are not recommended; good hydration more effective.

RECOMMENDED EMPIRIC THERAPY OF SELECTED INFECTIONS IN ADULT PATIENTS[A]

Infection	Usual Pathogens	Recommended Empiric Therapy	Recommended Dose[B]	Recommended Duration	Comments
Respiratory					
Bronchitis (cont'd) **Acute exacerbation of chronic bronchitis (AECB)**		- Chronic bronchitis - productive cough for at least 3 months/year for at least 2 consecutive years. - Criteria for acute exacerbation of chronic bronchitis: • ↑ sputum volume • ↑ sputum purulence • ↑ dyspnea. - Antibiotic therapy is only recommended if two or more of above criteria are present. - Approximately 50% of acute exacerbations of chronic bronchitis are viral in etiology. - No class of antibiotic has been shown to be superior to amoxicillin in the management of AECB. - Adjunctive therapy is essential to management: • smoking cessation • bronchodilators: ⇒ Ipratropium (Atrovent®) and short acting B-agonists (fenoterol, salbutamol, terbutaline) are effective in combination. ⇒ Long acting B-agonists (formoterol, salmeterol) or anticholinergics (tiotropium) are not currently indicated in the management of AECB but may be useful in chronic COPD. • corticosteroids: ⇒ Systemic corticosteroids are indicated in most cases (prednisone 0.5-1mg/kg/d for 3-14 days). ⇒ Inhaled corticosteroids are not indicated in the management of AECB but may be useful in chronic COPD. • O₂ therapy. - COPD patients should be given annual influenza vaccine, and pneumococcal vaccine where indicated. - The role of Mycoplasma pneumoniae and Chlamydophila pneumoniae in AECB has not been fully established. Empiric therapy for these organisms is not recommended.			
< 4 exacerbations/ year and at least 2 of following criteria: • ↑ sputum volume • ↑ sputum purulence • ↑ dyspnea	Haemophilus spp S. pneumoniae Moraxella catarrhalis	First line agents **Amoxicillin** or **Doxycycline** or **TMP/SMX** <u>Failure of first line agents</u> See below	1g PO tid 200mg PO once, then 100mg PO bid 1 DS tab PO bid	5-7 days* 5-7 days* 5-7 days*	* Evidence indicates that 5 days of therapy may be as effective as 7-10 days.

- 273 -

RECOMMENDED EMPIRIC THERAPY OF SELECTED INFECTIONS IN ADULT PATIENTS[A]

Infection	Usual Pathogens	Recommended Empiric Therapy	Recommended Dose[B]	Recommended Duration	Comments
Respiratory					
Bronchitis (cont'd) **AECB** (cont'd)	Role of quinolones: * Ciprofloxacin has poor/no coverage of S. pneumoniae and should not be used routinely in AECB. Because it retains the best activity against Pseudomonas aeruginosa, ciprofloxacin may have a role in end stage disease with/without bronchiectasis, when there has been documentation of colonization/infection with this organism. Empiric S. pneumoniae coverage still recommended. **Levofloxacin has good coverage of the pathogens involved. However because of its broad spectrum, potential for increasing resistance, and risk of C. difficile infection, it should be reserved for β-lactam allergic patients or patients who have failed first line antibiotic therapy. Role of macrolides: ***These agents have poor Haemophilus coverage and significant S. pneumoniae resistance. The benefit of macrolides may be due more to their anti-inflammatory activity than their antibacterial activity. - Long term macrolide therapy cannot be recommended at this time given its marginal benefit in only select groups of COPD patients, unacceptably high potential for drug interactions & adverse effects, and proven significant risk of development of antibiotic resistance.				
≥ 4 exacerbations /year and at least 2 of following criteria: • ↑ sputum volume • ↑ sputum purulence • ↑ dyspnea **or** • **Failure of first line agents**† **or** • **Antibiotics in last 3 months**‡	Haemophilus spp S. pneumoniae Moraxella catarrhalis Enterobacteriaceae Pseudomonas spp*	**Amoxicillin-clavulanate** or **Cefuroxime axetil** or **Levofloxacin**** Alternative **Azithromycin***** or **Clarithromycin*****	875mg PO bid 500mg-1g PO bid 750mg PO daily 500mg PO daily 500mg PO bid **or** XL 1g PO daily	5-10 days 5-10 days 5 days 3 days 5-10 days	† Failure of first line agents: • no improvement in symptoms after completion of antibiotic therapy or • clinical deterioration after 72 h of antibiotic therapy. Risk factors for treatment failure: - suboptimal adjunctive nonantimicrobial therapy - FEV₁ < 50% predicted - chronic oral corticosteroid use - home oxygen therapy - significant comorbidities, e.g. cardiac disease, debilitation, malnutrition. ‡ Use an antibiotic from a different class than was used previously.

RECOMMENDED EMPIRIC THERAPY OF SELECTED INFECTIONS IN ADULT PATIENTS[A]

Infection	Usual Pathogens	Recommended Empiric Therapy	Recommended Dose[B]	Recommended Duration	Comments
Respiratory					

Bronchitis (cont'd)/ Bronchiectasis/ end stage lung disease	- Permanent abnormal dilatation of bronchi and bronchioles due to repeated cycles of airway infection and inflammation, leading to chronic cough, sputum hypersecretion, wheeze and dyspnea.
	- Diagnosis: high resolution CT showing dilated and thickened airways - investigate and treat possible causes; 50-80% of cases may be idiopathic.
	- Antibiotics with good lung penetration:
	  • macrolides
	  • quinolones.				

Acute exacerbation	H. influenzae P. aeruginosa Other non-fermenting Gram negative bacilli S. aureus/MRSA S. pneumoniae Nontuberculous mycobacteria Aspergillus spp	Tailor antibiotic to sputum C&S results.		Optimal duration of therapy unknown - anywhere from 7-21 days has been recommended depending on pathogen and previous response to therapy.	- Sputum for bacterial and mycobacterial culture recommended. *Prolonged courses of oral or inhaled antibiotics have been advocated/ studied for prevention of exacerbations in patients with frequent exacerbations but good quality evidence of benefit lacking.

RECOMMENDED EMPIRIC THERAPY OF SELECTED INFECTIONS IN ADULT PATIENTS[A]

Infection	Usual Pathogens	Recommended Empiric Therapy	Recommended Dose[B]	Recommended Duration	Comments

Respiratory
 	
Community acquired pneumonia (CAP)
 	
[Clin Infect Dis 2007;44(suppl 2): S27-72]
	Pathogens
	- S. pneumoniae most common bacterial pathogen causing CAP and must be covered with initial empiric antibiotic therapy.
	- Atypical pathogens 15% of CAP:
	  • Signs and symptoms are often prolonged with C. pneumoniae/M. pneumoniae/Legionella spp despite appropriate therapy
	  • C. pneumoniae recognized as a pathogen in elderly/nursing home acquired pneumonia.
	
	Antibiotic therapy
	- Amoxicillin:
	  • provides the best coverage of all oral β-lactams against S. pneumoniae, even majority of penicillin-resistant strains.
	  • no activity against S. aureus, β-lactamase (+) H. influenzae, M. catarrhalis, M. pneumoniae, C. pneumoniae, or Legionella spp.
	- Doxycycline:
	  • excellent activity against most CAP pathogens, including S. pneumoniae (increasing resistance), H. influenzae, M. catarrhalis, S. aureus, including MRSA, M. pneumoniae, C. pneumoniae, and Legionella spp.
	  • less resistance than macrolides in S. pneumoniae
	  • not associated with promoting penicillin resistance in S. pneumoniae (macrolides have)
	  • excellent pharmacokinetics/dynamics (high serum and lung levels, concentration-dependent killing).
	- Macrolides:
	  • significant macrolide resistance in S. pneumoniae.
	  • poor Haemophilus coverage.
	  • recent (within previous 3 months) macrolide use may predispose to infection with multi-drug resistant S. pneumoniae.
	  • monotherapy with macrolides not recommended for pneumococcal bacteremia (clinical history of rigors/positive blood cultures).
	- Quinolones:
	  • recent (within previous 3 months) quinolone use may predispose to infection with quinolone resistant S. pneumoniae.
	  • therapy in patients with undiagnosed tuberculosis may result in false negative Mycobacterium tuberculosis cultures.
	  • Moxifloxacin not listed as:
	    ○ anaerobic coverage not required for CAP
	    ○ increased risk of C. difficile infection compared to levofloxacin [CMAJ 2008; 179:767-72]
	    ○ no studies on short-course therapy in CAP.				

RECOMMENDED EMPIRIC THERAPY OF SELECTED INFECTIONS IN ADULT PATIENTS[A]

Infection	Usual Pathogens	Recommended Empiric Therapy	Recommended Dose[B]	Recommended Duration	Comments
Respiratory					

Community acquired pneumonia (CAP) (cont'd)
 	
[Clin Infect Dis 2007;44(suppl 2): S27-72]
	- The following antibiotics are not recommended empirically in adult community-acquired pneumonia:
	  • cephalexin/cefazolin - no activity against Pen I/R S. pneumoniae, Haemophilus spp, M. pneumoniae, C. pneumoniae, or Legionella spp.
	  • cefixime - no activity against pen I/R S. pneumoniae, M. pneumoniae, C. pneumoniae, or Legionella spp.
	  • ciprofloxacin – poor/no activity against S. pneumoniae
	  • TMP/SMX - increased S. pneumoniae resistance; no activity against M. pneumoniae, C. pneumoniae, or Legionella spp.
	- Other considerations:
	  • Gastric acid suppressants and inhaled corticosteroids are associated with an increased risk of CAP.
	  • The following measures are recommended:
	    ○ smoking cessation
	    ○ annual influenza vaccine
	    ○ pneumococcal vaccine where indicated
	  • Follow-up chest x-ray recommended at 6 weeks.				

Outpatient No comorbid factors[†]	S. pneumoniae Mycoplasma pneumoniae Chlamydophila pneumoniae	**Doxycycline** +/- **Amoxicillin*** Alternative **Amoxicillin** + [**Azithromycin** or **Clarithromycin**]	200mg PO once, then 100mg PO bid 1g PO tid 1g PO tid 500mg PO daily 500mg PO bid or XL 1g PO daily	5-7 days** 5-7 days** 5-7 days** 3 days 5-7 days**	*Add amoxicillin if: • lobar pneumonia with fever or rigors • recent antibiotic therapy • local S. pneumoniae tetracycline resistance > 15% Antibiotic therapy within previous 3 months is a risk factor for resistant S. pneumoniae. Amoxicillin provides the best coverage of all oral β-lactams against S. pneumoniae, even majority of penicillin-resistant strains. **Treat for a minimum of 5 days (azithromycin 3 days) and until afebrile for 48-72h.

[†] Comorbid factors: smoking, malignancy, diabetes, alcoholism, chronic heart, lung, renal or liver failure, chronic corticosteroid use/immunosuppressive therapy, malnutrition or acute weight loss (>5%), hospitalization in past 3 months, HIV/immunosuppression.

RECOMMENDED EMPIRIC THERAPY OF SELECTED INFECTIONS IN ADULT PATIENTS[A]

Infection	Usual Pathogens	Recommended Empiric Therapy	Recommended Dose[B]	Recommended Duration	Comments
Respiratory					
Community acquired pneumonia					
Outpatient (cont'd) Comorbid factors[†]	S. pneumoniae H. influenzae S. aureus[‡] Moraxella catarrhalis Enterobacteriaceae Mycoplasma pneumoniae Legionella spp Chlamydophila pneumoniae Consider influenza during epidemic season (see Influenza section).	[Amoxicillin**] or Amoxicillin-clavulanate***] + [Doxycycline or Azithromycin or Clarithromycin][‡]	1g PO tid 875mg PO bid 200mg PO once, then 100mg PO bid 500mg PO daily 500mg PO bid or XL 1g PO daily	5-7 days* 5-7 days* 5-7 days* 3 days 5-7 days*	* Treat for a minimum of 5 days (azithromycin 3 days) and until afebrile for 48-72h. ** Amoxicillin provides the best coverage of all oral β-lactams against S. pneumoniae, even majority of penicillin-resistant strains. ***Preferred regimen if Gram negative predominant on Gram stain. • alcoholism and/or recent hospitalization are risk factors for Gram negative organisms. ‡ Add doxycycline or TMP/SMX (instead of macrolide) if: • S. aureus predominant on Gram stain • diabetes • recent influenza

† Comorbid factors: smoking, malignancy, diabetes, alcoholism, chronic heart, lung, renal or liver failure, chronic corticosteroid use/immunosuppressive therapy, malnutrition or acute weight loss (>5%), hospitalization in past 3 months, HIV/immunosuppression.

RECOMMENDED EMPIRIC THERAPY OF SELECTED INFECTIONS IN ADULT PATIENTS[A]

Infection	Usual Pathogens	Recommended Empiric Therapy	Recommended Dose[B]	Recommended Duration	Comments
Respiratory					
Community acquired pneumonia (cont'd) Outpatient Failure of 1st line agents	- Failure of first line agents: • hemodynamic compromise (see CAP, Hospitalized) • no improvement in symptoms after completion of antibiotic therapy (warrants further investigation) • clinical deterioration after 72 hours of antibiotic therapy. - If deterioration or persistent respiratory/systemic symptoms, consider non-infectious etiologies as well as the following infectious etiologies (depending on epidemiologic setting/risk factors): • Methicillin-resistant S. aureus (MRSA)* • Viral pneumonia, including influenza • Mycobacterium tuberculosis • Nocardia spp • Chlamydophila psittaci • Coxiella burnetti (Q fever) • Francisella tularensis (tularemia) • Bordetella pertussis (whooping cough) • Endemic fungi (Histoplasma capsulatum, Coccidioides immitis, Cryptococcus neoformans, Blastomyces spp) • Pneumocystis jirovecii				
	S. pneumoniae H. influenzae S. aureus* Moraxella catarrhalis Enterobacteriaceae** Legionella spp Chlamydophila pneumoniae Mycoplasma pneumoniae Nocardia spp	Choose a regimen not previously used: **Amoxicillin-clavulanate** + [**Azithromycin** or **Clarithromycin**]* Alternative **Levofloxacin**	875mg PO bid 500mg PO daily 500mg PO bid or XL 1g PO daily 750mg PO daily	7 days* 3 days 7 days 5 days*	* If MRSA suspected, use doxycycline or TMP/SMX instead of macrolide. ** Pneumonia due to Klebsiella may require combination therapy for a prolonged course (minimum of 14 days).

RECOMMENDED EMPIRIC THERAPY OF SELECTED INFECTIONS IN ADULT PATIENTS[A]

Infection	Usual Pathogens	Recommended Empiric Therapy	Recommended Dose[B]	Recommended Duration	Comments
Respiratory					
Community acquired pneumonia (cont'd) Hospitalized					

- For patients in whom admission to hospital is considered, calculation of CURB-65 score is recommended (Table A). Consider hospitalization if score > 1.
- Investigations: • CBC with differential, random glucose, electrolytes, creatinine, ALT
  - Chest x-ray, PA and lateral
  - Sputum Gram stain and C&S for patients with productive cough. For organism - specific recommendations, see Recommended Therapy of Culture-Directed Infections Table 1.
  - Blood cultures
  - If interstitial pattern on chest x-ray:
    - Nasopharyngeal (NP) swab/aspirate for respiratory virus PCR
    - Sputum/NP sample for M. pneumoniae, C. pneumoniae, Legionella PCR.
    - Mycoplasma IgM - take at ≥ 7 days after symptom onset (high false negative rate if taken earlier)
    - Legionella pneumophila urine antigen
    - Consider mycobacterial/fungal culture if relevant history/travel, and PCP (P. jirovecii) in immunocompromised.
  - Arterial blood gas on room air, or on baseline O$_2$ if patient receiving chronic oxygen
- Antibiotic therapy should be administered as soon as possible after the diagnosis is considered likely. This is especially important in the elderly.
- Poor outcome risk factors:
  - respiratory rate ≥ 30/minute
  - diastolic blood pressure ≤ 60 mmHg, systolic blood pressure ≤ 90 mmHg
  - acute renal dysfunction
  - malnourishment or > 5% weight loss in past month (dietitian consult recommended)
  - functional impairment (occupational therapy and/or physiotherapy consult recommended)
  - leukopenia (< 4 x 10^9/L)
  - thrombocytopenia (< 100 x 10^9/L)
  - hypothermia (core temp < 36°C)
  - NB: age and comorbid factors are also contributors to outcome.

RECOMMENDED EMPIRIC THERAPY OF SELECTED INFECTIONS IN ADULT PATIENTS[A]

Table A. CURB-65 - Pneumonia Severity of Illness Scoring System

Patient Characteristic	Points assigned
C - confusion	1
U – blood urea nitrogen > 7 mmol/L	1
R - respiratory rate > 30/minute	1
B – systolic blood pressure < 90 mmHg or diastolic < 60 mmHg	1
Age ≥ 65 years	1

Score	30-day Mortality Risk (%)	Recommendations for Site of Care
0-1	0.7-2.1	Outpatient
2	9.2	Inpatient
3	14.5	Often ICU
4	40	Often ICU
5	57	Often ICU

Lim WS, vander Eerden MM, Laing R, et al. Defining community acquired pneumonia severity on presentation to hospital: an international derivation and validation study. Thorax 2003; 58:377-82.

RECOMMENDED EMPIRIC THERAPY OF SELECTED INFECTIONS IN ADULT PATIENTS[A]

Infection	Usual Pathogens	Recommended Empiric Therapy	Recommended Dose[B]	Recommended Duration	Comments
Respiratory					
Community acquired pneumonia (cont'd) Hospitalized (cont'd) Moderate	S. pneumoniae H. influenzae S. aureus Group A Streptococci Enterobacteriaceae Legionella spp Chlamydophila pneumoniae	**Ceftriaxone** + [**Doxycycline** or **Azithromycin**** or **Clarithromycin****]	1-2g IV daily 200mg PO once, then 100mg PO bid 500mg IV/PO daily 500mg PO bid or XL 1g PO daily	5-10 days* 5-10 days* 3 days 5-10 days*	*Treat for a minimum of 5 days (azithromycin 3 days) and until afebrile for 48-72 hours. **Avoid macrolides and quinolones if used within previous 3 months.
		Alternative **Levofloxacin IV/PO**[D]***	750mg PO/IV daily	5 days*	

- 282 -

RECOMMENDED EMPIRIC THERAPY OF SELECTED INFECTIONS IN ADULT PATIENTS[A]

Infection	Usual Pathogens	Recommended Empiric Therapy	Recommended Dose[B]	Recommended Duration	Comments
Respiratory					
Community acquired pneumonia (cont'd)					
Hospitalized (cont'd) **Severe/ICU** • respiratory rate ≥ 30/minute • PaO_2 < 60mmHg • multilobar infiltrates • confusion/ disorientation • urea > 7mmol/L • leukopenia (< 4 × 10^9/L) • thromboytopenia (< 100 x 10^9/L) • hypothermia (< 36°C) • hypotension requiring aggressive fluid resuscitation	- If deterioration or persistent respiratory/systemic symptoms, consider the following etiologies (depending on epidemiologic setting/ risk factors): • Viral pneumonia, including influenza and Hantavirus • Mycobacterium tuberculosis • Chlamydophila psittaci • Coxiella burnetti (Q fever) • Francisella tularensis (tularemia) • Endemic fungi (Histoplasma capsulatum, Coccidioides immitis, Cryptococcus neoformans, Blastomyces spp) • Pneumocytis jirovecii Corticosteroid therapy - Use of corticosteroids in CAP is controversial. Some evidence for decreased length of stay however no difference in mortality, admission to ICU, complications, 30-day pulmonary function, or readmission. Corticosteroid therapy associated with increased adverse events (hyperglycemia/GI perforation/superinfections). At time of publication, routine corticosteroid use cannot be recommended.			

RECOMMENDED EMPIRIC THERAPY OF SELECTED INFECTIONS IN ADULT PATIENTS[A]

Infection	Usual Pathogens	Recommended Empiric Therapy	Recommended Dose[B]	Recommended Duration	Comments
Respiratory					
Community acquired pneumonia (cont'd)					
Hospitalized (cont'd)					- The standard of care is with a β-lactam + macrolide. Combination therapy is associated with decreased mortality. Monotherapy (including with a quinolone) is not adequate in severe pneumonia.
Severe/ICU	S. pneumoniae	**Ceftriaxone**	1-2g IV daily	5-10 days*	
• respiratory rate ≥ 30/minute	H. influenzae	+			† Consider MRSA if:
• PaO₂ < 60mmHg	S. aureus/MRSA[†]	**Azithromycin****	500mg IV daily	3-5 days	• rapid onset
• multilobar infiltrates	Enterobacteriaceae				• necrotizing process on CXR
• confusion/disorientation	Legionella spp	If MRSA suspected[†] add:			• post-influenza
• urea > 7mmol/L	Chlamydophila pneumoniae	**Vancomycin**[E]	25-30mg/kg IV once then 15mg/kg IV q8-12h	Minimum 14 days for confirmed MRSA	• IVDU
• leukopenia (< 4 x 10⁹/L)					• colonization/recent infection with MRSA
• thrombocytopenia (< 100 x 10⁹/L)		or			• Gram positive cocci in clusters on Gram stain.
• hypothermia (< 36°C)		**Linezolid**	600mg IV/PO q12h	Minimum 14 days for confirmed MRSA	Linezolid preferred over vancomycin if:
• hypotension requiring aggressive fluid resuscitation					○ MRSA with vancomycin MIC ≥ 1.5µg/mL
		Cephalosporin allergy			○ concomitant nephrotoxic therapy
		Levofloxacin	750mg IV daily	5-10 days*	○ pre-existing renal dysfunction.
		+			* Treat until afebrile x 48-72h, hemodynamically stable, and improved O₂ saturation.
		[Vancomycin][E]	25-30mg/kg IV once then 15mg/kg IV q8-12h		**If intolerant to azithromycin, levofloxacin can be used, but does not have same immunomodulating effects.
		or			
		Clindamycin IV/PO[C]	600mg IV q8h/ 300mg PO qid		

E. Desired vancomycin trough is 15-20 mg/L. Monitor renal function closely. See Vancomycin Dosing & Monitoring Guidelines.

RECOMMENDED EMPIRIC THERAPY OF SELECTED INFECTIONS IN ADULT PATIENTS[A]

Infection	Usual Pathogens	Recommended Empiric Therapy	Recommended Dose[B]	Recommended Duration	Comments
Respiratory					
Nursing home acquired pneumonia (NHAP)	- Consider influenza during appropriate season. Recommend annual influenza vaccine, and pneumococcal vaccine where indicated. - Respiratory syncytial virus (RSV) and human metapneumovirus may cause pneumonia outbreaks in the elderly. - Chlamydophila pneumoniae also a pathogen in elderly/nursing home acquired pneumonia. Signs and symptoms may be prolonged. - Consider TB as there is a 10-30 times increased incidence of TB in long term care.				
Treated in NH	Viral	No antibiotic therapy recommended. See influenza section.			* Amoxicillin provides best coverage of all oral β-lactams against S. pneumoniae, even majority of penicillin-resistant strains.
	Bacterial S. pneumoniae H. influenzae S. aureus Enterobacteriaceae Chlamydophila pneumoniae	Amoxicillin* +/- [Doxycycline or Azithromycin or Clarithromycin]**	1g PO tid 200mg PO once, then 100mg PO bid 500mg PO daily 500mg PO bid or XL 1g PO daily	7 days 7 days 3 days 7 days	**Consider adding doxycycline, azithromycin, or clarithromycin if underlying pulmonary disease. ***Amoxicillin-clavulanate provides better coverage of H. influenzae and M. catarrhalis in patients with COPD, and is preferred post-influenza for its S. aureus coverage.
	If aspiration: See Aspiration pneumonia	Alternative Amoxicillin-clavulanate*** +/- [Doxycycline or Azithromycin or Clarithromycin]** or Levofloxacin† monotherapy	875mg PO bid 200mg PO once, then 100mg PO bid 500mg PO daily 500mg PO bid or XL 1g PO daily 750mg PO daily	7 days 7 days 3 days 7 days 7 days	† Use a different agent if any quinolone used within last 3 months Moxifloxacin not listed as: • anaerobic coverage not required for NHAP • increased risk of C. difficile infection compared to levofloxacin [CMAJ 2008; 179:767-72] • no studies on short-course therapy in pneumonia.
Transferred to Acute Care	See CAP, hospitalized, moderate or severe.				

RECOMMENDED EMPIRIC THERAPY OF SELECTED INFECTIONS IN ADULT PATIENTS[A]

Infection	Usual Pathogens	Recommended Empiric Therapy	Recommended Dose[B]	Recommended Duration	Comments
Respiratory					
Influenza	- **NB: It is essential to check resistance patterns of the current season's influenza strains.** - Vaccination is first line of defense.				
Post-exposure prophylaxis*	Influenza A Influenza B	**Oseltamivir** or **Zanamivir** or **Amantadine** for susceptible influenza A only	75mg PO daily 10mg inhaled by mouth daily ≤ 64 years old 100mg PO bid ≥ 64 years old 100mg PO daily	10 days** 10 days** 10 days** 10 days**	* Early therapy is preferred over post-exposure prophylaxis (PEP). PEP may be considered for: • exposures in closed institutional settings, e.g. long term care facilities • selectively in family settings if individuals cannot be (reliably) protected by immunization, e.g. < 6 mos old, immunocompromised, or vaccine contraindicated. **Give for 10 days, or duration of outbreak, whichever is longer.
TreatmentΦ	Influenza A Influenza B	**Oseltamivir** or **Zanamivir** or **Amantadine** for susceptible influenza A only	75mg PO bid 10mg inhaled by mouth bid ≤ 64 years old 100mg PO bid ≥ 64 years old 100mg PO daily	5 days 5 days 5 days 5 days	ΦBest efficacy of these agents if started within 48h of symptom onset. Consider even if after 48h of symptom onset if: • hospitalized patients • immunocompromised patients • progressive, severe, or complicated illness.

RECOMMENDED EMPIRIC THERAPY OF SELECTED INFECTIONS IN ADULT PATIENTS[A]

Infection	Usual Pathogens	Recommended Empiric Therapy	Recommended Dose[B]	Recommended Duration	Comments
Respiratory					
Hospital acquired pneumonia (HAP)	[Can J Infect Dis Med Microbiol 2008;19:19-53] - HAP = pneumonia that develops ≥ 48 hours after admission. - Blood cultures recommended. - For immunocompromised patients, recommend Infectious Diseases consult.				
Early onset - • ≤ 4 days hospitalization	See Community Acquired Pneumonia, Hospitalized.	Start antibiotics as soon as diagnosis is considered likely.			

Late onset -
• > 4 days hospitalization
• non-ICU
• no mechanical ventilation
• no broad-spectrum antibiotics
• no other risk factors
 	
(For associated risk factors/high endemic MRSA, see below)
	Enterobacteriaceae	**[Ceftriaxone***
		or
		Levofloxacin IV/PO[D]*]†
		+/-
		Gentamicin*
			1-2g IV daily
			
			750mg IV/PO daily
			
			7mg/kg IV daily
				7 days***
				
				7 days***
				
				Reassess once C&S results available
					* S. aureus coverage is suboptimal with these regimens. Tailor antibiotics to Gram stain/C&S results. Use vancomycin or linezolid for documented MRSA.
					† Moxifloxacin is not listed as:
					  • anaerobic coverage not required for HAP
					  • increased risk of C. difficile infection compared to levofloxacin [CMAJ 2008; 179:767-72].
					**Consider giving gentamicin to cover multi-resistant Gram negative organisms until C&S results available.
					***1 week duration has been shown to be as effective as 2 weeks and associated with less antimicrobial resistance. Two weeks is recommended when MRSA, Pseudomonas, Acinetobacter, and other nonfermenting Gram negative bacilli isolated.

RECOMMENDED EMPIRIC THERAPY OF SELECTED INFECTIONS IN ADULT PATIENTS[A]

Infection	Usual Pathogens	Recommended Empiric Therapy	Recommended Dose[B]	Recommended Duration	Comments
Respiratory					
Hospital acquired pneumonia (HAP) (cont'd)					
Late onset - (cont'd)					
• **aspiration**	See Aspiration pneumonia, Hospital acquired.				
• **coma** • **diabetes** • **head injury** • **recent influenza** • **IVDU**	Enterobacteriaceae S. aureus/MRSA*	[Ceftriaxone or Levofloxacin] +/- Gentamicin*** + [Vancomycin]E or Linezolid]*	1-2g IV daily 750mg IV/PO daily 7mg/kg IV daily 25-30mg/kg IV once then 15mg/kg IV q8-12h 600mg IV/PO q12h	7 days** 7 days** Reassess once C&S results available 14 days** 14 days**	* Rule out S. aureus bacteremia. Linezolid preferred over vancomycin if: • MRSA with vancomycin MIC ≥ 1.5µg/mL • concomitant nephrotoxic therapy • pre-existing renal dysfunction If culture proven MSSA, switch to cloxacillin or cefazolin. **1 week duration has been shown to be as effective as 2 weeks and associated with less antimicrobial resistance. Two weeks is recommended when MRSA, Pseudomonas, Acinetobacter, and other nonfermenting Gram negative bacilli isolated. ***Consider giving gentamicin to cover multi-resistant Gram negative organisms until C&S results available.

E. Desired vancomycin trough is 15-20 mg/L. Monitor renal function closely. See Vancomycin Dosing & Monitoring Guidelines.

RECOMMENDED EMPIRIC THERAPY OF SELECTED INFECTIONS IN ADULT PATIENTS[A]

Infection	Usual Pathogens	Recommended Empiric Therapy	Recommended Dose[B]	Recommended Duration	Comments
Respiratory					
Hospital acquired pneumonia (HAP) Late onset (cont'd)	Enterobacteriaceae P. aeruginosa[†] Acinetobacter spp S. aureus/MRSA**	[**Piperacillin-tazobactam**] or **Imipenem** or **Meropenem**] + **Tobramycin**	4.5g IV q6h 500mg IV q6h 500mg IV q6h or 1g IV q8h 7mg/kg IV q24h	7-14 days‡ 5 days	* If possible, use agents from a different antibiotic class than previously used. - Tailor antibiotics to C&S results. † If culture proven bacteremia or sepsis due to P. aeruginosa, continue two antipseudomonal agents for 14 days (associated with decreased mortality [Arch Intern Med 1985;145:1621-9, Am J Med 1989;87:540-8]). ** Rule out S. aureus bacteremia. Linezolid preferred over vancomycin if:
• prior (≤ 3 months) broad spectrum antibiotics* • structural lung disease (bronchiectasis /cystic fibrosis) • immunosuppression		If MRSA suspected add:** **Vancomycin**[E] or **Linezolid**	25-30mg/kg IV once then 15mg/kg IV q8-12h 600mg IV/PO q12h	Minimum 14 days for confirmed MRSA	• MRSA with vancomycin MIC ≥ 1.5μg/mL • concomitant nephrotoxic therapy • pre-existing renal dysfunction. ***Consider giving tobramycin to cover multi-resistant Gram negative organisms until C&S results available.
Mechanical ventilation (see VAP)		Severe β-lactam allergy [**Vancomycin**]** or **Linezolid**** + **Ciprofloxacin IV/PO**[D] + **Tobramycin**[†]***	25-30mg/kg IV once then 15mg/kg IV q8-12h 600mg IV/PO q12h 400mg IV q8-12h/ 750mg PO bid 7mg/kg IV q24h	Miniumum 14 days for confirmed MRSA Miniumum 14 days for confirmed MRSA 7-14 days‡ Reassess once C&S results available	‡ 1 week duration has been shown to be as effective as 2 weeks and associated with less antimicrobial resistance. Two weeks is recommended when MRSA, Pseudomonas, Acinetobacter, and other nonfermenting Gram negative bacilli isolated.

E. Desired vancomycin trough is 15-20 mg/L. Monitor renal function closely. See Vancomycin Dosing & Monitoring Guidelines.

RECOMMENDED EMPIRIC THERAPY OF SELECTED INFECTIONS IN ADULT PATIENTS[A]

Infection	Usual Pathogens	Recommended Empiric Therapy	Recommended Dose[B]	Recommended Duration	Comments
Respiratory					
Ventilator associated pneumonia (VAP) [Can J Infect Dis Med Microbiol 2008;19:19-53]	VAP = pneumonia that develops > 48-72h after intubation. Prevention • elevate head of bed 30°- 45° • oral care with chlorhexidine • oral endotracheal intubation preferred to nasotracheal - avoid re-intubation if possible • remove NG, ET tubes ASAP • continuous sub-glottic suctioning • limit stress ulcer prophylaxis • appropriate infection control measures, including hand hygiene in healthcare workers. Diagnosis NB: Start antibiotics as soon as diagnosis is considered likely. - Endotracheal (ET) aspirate with Gram stain and C&S recommended. Significant if increased purulence (3-4+ WBC), intracellular organisms present, and/or predominant organism. - Bronchoscopically obtained specimens may be considered in immunocompromised patients. Treatment - Insufficient evidence that administration of topical (nebulized or instilled via ET tube) antibiotics as an adjunct to systemic antibiotics is beneficial.			

RECOMMENDED EMPIRIC THERAPY OF SELECTED INFECTIONS IN ADULT PATIENTS[A]

Infection	Usual Pathogens	Recommended Empiric Therapy	Recommended Dose[B]	Recommended Duration	Comments
Respiratory					
Ventilator associated pneumonia (VAP) (cont'd) [Can J Infect Dis Med Microbiol 2008;19:19-53] • **≤ 5 days of hospitalization** AND • **No prior (≤ 3 months) broad spectrum antibiotics**	Enterobacteriaceae* S. pneumoniae* H. influenzae** S. aureus**	**Ceftriaxone** or **Levofloxacin IV/PO**[†]	1-2g IV daily 750mg IV/PO daily	7 days*** 7 days***	* At risk for these organisms if < 72 hours of hospitalization. **S. aureus coverage is suboptimal with these regimens. Tailor antibiotics to C&S results. Use vancomycin or linezolid for documented MRSA. Rule out bacteremia if S. aureus infection. ***1 week duration has been shown to be as effective as 2 weeks and associated with less antimicrobial resistance. Two weeks recommended when MRSA, Pseudomonas, Acinetobacter, and other nonfermenting Gram negative bacilli isolated. † Moxifloxacin not listed as: • anaerobic coverage not required for VAP • increased risk of C. difficile infection compared to levofloxacin [CMAJ 2008; 179:767-72].

RECOMMENDED EMPIRIC THERAPY OF SELECTED INFECTIONS IN ADULT PATIENTS[A]

Infection	Usual Pathogens	Recommended Empiric Therapy	Recommended Dose[B]	Recommended Duration	Comments
Respiratory					
Ventilator associated pneumonia (VAP) (cont'd) • > 5 days of hospitalization AND/OR • Prior (≤ 3 months) broad-spectrum antibiotics[Ø]	Enterobacteriaceae P. aeruginosa* S. aureus/MRSA** Stenotrophomonas maltophilia Acinetobacter spp	[Piperacillin-tazobactam or Imipenem or Meropenem] + [Tobramycin or Ciprofloxacin IV/PO[D]] If MRSA suspected add:** Vancomycin[E] or Linezolid Severe β-lactam allergy [Vancomycin[E] or Linezolid]** + [Ciprofloxacin IV/PO[‡] + Tobramycin[‡]]	4.5g IV q6h 500mg IV q6h 500mg IV q6h or 1g IV q8h 7mg/kg IV q24h 400mg IV q8-12h/ 750mg PO bid 25-30mg/kg IV once then 15mg/kg IV q8-12h 600mg IV/PO q12h 25-30mg/kg IV once then 15mg/kg IV q8-12h 600mg IV/PO q12h 400mg IV q8-12h/ 750mg PO bid 7mg/kg IV q24h	7-14 days*** 5 days* Miniumum 14 days for confirmed MRSA Miniumum 14 days for confirmed MRSA 7-14 days*** 5 days*	Ø If possible, use agents from a different antibiotic class than was previously used. * If culture proven bacteremia or sepsis due to P. aeruginosa, continue two antipseudomonal agents for 14 days (associated with decreased mortality [Arch Intern Med 1985;145:1621-9, Am J Med 1989;87:540-8]). **Rule out S. aureus bacteremia. Linezolid preferred over vancomycin if: • MRSA with vancomycin MIC ≥ 1.5µg/mL • concomitant nephrotoxic therapy • pre-existing renal dysfunction. ***1 week duration has been shown to be as effective as 2 weeks and associated with less antimicrobial resistance. Two weeks recommended when MRSA, Pseudomonas, Acinetobacter, and other nonfermenting Gram negative bacilli isolated. ‡ Consider giving tobramycin to cover multi-resistant Gram negative organisms until C&S results available.

E. Desired vancomycin trough is 15-20 mg/L. Monitor renal function closely. See Vancomycin Dosing & Monitoring Guidelines.

RECOMMENDED EMPIRIC THERAPY OF SELECTED INFECTIONS IN ADULT PATIENTS[A]

Infection	Usual Pathogens	Recommended Empiric Therapy	Recommended Dose[B]	Recommended Duration	Comments
Respiratory					
Aspiration pneumonitis	- Chemical injury caused by the inhalation of gastric contents, resulting in inflammatory reaction. - Clinical: • patient with decreased level of consciousness • pulmonary infiltrate apparent on x-ray • episode of aspiration often witnessed • respiratory symptoms range from mild to severe and develop 2-5 hours after aspiration.				
	Sterile*	**No antibiotic therapy recommended.**** **Corticosteroids of no proven benefit.**			* Secondary bacterial infection not important in early stages. At higher risk of bacterial infection if: • receiving gastric acid suppression (antacids, H_2 receptor antagonists, proton pump inhibitors) • receiving enteral feeds • gastroparesis • small bowel obstruction. ** No role for prophylactic antibiotics. Reassess patient in 24-48 hours – if x-ray abnormality and above risk factors, consider antibiotic therapy. See Aspiration Pneumonia.

RECOMMENDED EMPIRIC THERAPY OF SELECTED INFECTIONS IN ADULT PATIENTS[A]

Infection	Usual Pathogens	Recommended Empiric Therapy	Recommended Dose[B]	Recommended Duration	Comments
Respiratory					

Aspiration pneumonia	- Development of radiographically evident infiltrate following the aspiration of colonized oropharyngeal material.
	- Risk factors: • descreased level of consciousness
	  • dysphagia
	  • anatomic abnormality of upper GI tract
	  • mechanical interference of GI tract (ET/NG tubes)
	- Clinical: • usually older patient with above risk factors
	  • infiltrates in dependent lung segments, especially RLL
	  • episode of aspiration often not witnessed
	  • may progress to abscess/empyema within 1-2 weeks.
	- Etiology: • role of anaerobes is controversial and may have been overemphasized in the past
	  • Gram stain may be helpful in diagnosis and decision to use antianaerobic therapy
	  • choice of antibiotic dependent on clinical situation
	  • ceftriaxone has activity against many oral anaerobes.
	- For immunocompromised patients, recommend Infectious Diseases consult.				

Community or **Nursing home acquired**	S. pneumoniae H. influenzae S. aureus Enterobacteriaceae*	**Ceftriaxone** or **Levofloxacin**	1-2g IV daily 750mg PO daily	7-10 days 5 days	* Alcoholism and enteral feeding may be risk factors for colonization with these organisms.
Community or **Nursing home acquired with:** • poor oral hygiene • severe periodontal disease • putrid sputum	S. pneumoniae H. influenzae S. aureus Enterobacteriaceae Oral anaerobes Streptococcus spp Eikenella corrodens	**Amoxicillin-clavulanate** or [**Ceftriaxone** + **Metronidazole IV/PO**[C]] Alternative **Levofloxacin**** + **Metronidazole IV/PO**[C]	875mg PO bid 1-2g IV daily 500mg IV/PO q12h 750mg PO daily 500mg IV/PO q12h	7-14 days* 7-14 days* 7-14 days*	* If x-ray evidence of necrotizing pneumonia or abscess, treat for 3-6 weeks. **Moxifloxacin not listed as: • anaerobic coverage may not be optimal • increased risk of C. difficile infection compared to levofloxacin [CMAJ 2008; 179:767-72].

RECOMMENDED EMPIRIC THERAPY OF SELECTED INFECTIONS IN ADULT PATIENTS[A]

Infection	Usual Pathogens	Recommended Empiric Therapy	Recommended Dose[B]	Recommended Duration	Comments
Respiratory					
Aspiration pneumonia (cont'd) **Hospital acquired**	Polymicrobial: • Enterobacteriaceae • P. aeruginosa* • S. aureus • S. pneumoniae • H. influenzae • Moraxella catarrhalis • Oral anaerobes**	Mild-moderate **Amoxicillin-clavulanate** or [**Ceftriaxone** + **Metronidazole IV/PO**[C]] Severe/ICU **Piperacillin-tazobactam** or **Meropenem** β-lactam allergy **Clindamycin IV/PO**[C] + **Ciprofloxacin IV/PO**[D]	875mg PO bid 1-2g IV daily 500mg IV/PO q12h 4.5g IV q6h 500mg IV q6h or 1g IV q8h 600mg IV q8h/ 300mg PO qid 400mg IV q8-12h/ 750mg PO bid	7-14 days*** 7-14 days*** 7-14 days*** 7-14 days*** 7-14 days***	* If recent ventilatory support and/or prior multiple antibiotics, recommend anti-pseudomonal coverage. If culture proven bacteremia or sepsis due to P. aeruginosa, continue two antipseudomonal agents for 14 days (associated with decreased mortality [Arch Intern Med 1985;145:1621-9. Am J Med 1989;87:540-8]). **Anaerobes may be more significant in witnessed aspiration and/or recent abdominal surgery. ***If x-ray evidence of necrotizing pneumonia or abscess, treat for 3-6 weeks.

RECOMMENDED EMPIRIC THERAPY OF SELECTED INFECTIONS IN ADULT PATIENTS[A]

Infection	Usual Pathogens	Recommended Empiric Therapy	Recommended Dose[B]	Recommended Duration	Comments
Respiratory					

Pleural Space Infections	- Most cases secondary to pneumonia, lung abcess or complications of bronchiectasis.
	- May also occur after thoracic surgery procedures, trauma, or esophageal rupture.
	- Primary pleural effusions are as a result of hematogenous spread of oropharyngeal flora (streptococci/anaerobes) or due to M. tuberculosis.
	
	Diagnosis
	- Chest x-ray
	- Thoracentesis
	- Pleural fluid for Gram stain/culture, AFB stain/culture, pH, WBC, LDH, glucose and cytology.
	- Sputum for C&S/AFB. If TB suspected, avoid quinolones and linezolid until cultures taken.
	
	Management
	- Pleural fluid drainage (may require repeat thoracentesis):
	  • If pH > 7.2/culture negative - typical parapneumonic effusion, treat as for pneumonia.
	  • If pH < 7.2 and/or glucose < 3.4 µmol/L and/or purulent - complicated effusion, typically requires:
	    1. additional anaerobic coverage
	    2. chest tube drainage. If incomplete drainage, consider early administration of fibrinolytic agents and Thoracic Surgery consult.
	    3. thoracic CT- if pleural peel, recommend Thoracic Surgery consult for decortication/video-assisted thorascopic surgery (VATS).				

RECOMMENDED EMPIRIC THERAPY OF SELECTED INFECTIONS IN ADULT PATIENTS[A]

Infection	Usual Pathogens	Recommended Empiric Therapy	Recommended Dose[B]	Recommended Duration	Comments
Respiratory					
Pleural Space Infections (cont'd)					
Pleural effusion	S. pneumoniae S. aureus/MRSA Group A Streptococci H. influenzae Enterobacteriaceae	**Ceftriaxone**	1-2g IV daily	2-4 weeks	† Linezolid preferred over vancomycin if: • MRSA with vancomycin MIC ≥ 1.5ug/mL • concomitant nephrotoxic therapy • pre-existing renal dysfunction.
		If MRSA suspected/documented, add:[†] **Vancomycin**[E] or **Linezolid**	15mg/kg IV q8-12h 600mg IV/PO q12h	2-4 weeks 2-4 weeks	
Empyema • **Community acquired**	S. anginosus group* S. pneumoniae Anaerobes S. aureus/MRSA Enterobacteriaceae** H. influenzae Rare: • Mycobacterium tuberculosis • Nocardia spp	**Ceftriaxone** + **Metronidazole**	1-2g IV daily 500mg IV/PO q12h	3-6 weeks 3-6 weeks	* Includes: • S. anginosus • S. constellatus • S. intermedius. ** Especially Klebsiella spp in alcoholics. - Tailor antibiotics to C&S results but maintain anaerobic coverage. † Linezolid preferred over vancomycin if: • MRSA with vancomycin MIC ≥ 1.5ug/mL • concomitant nephrotoxic therapy • pre-existing renal dysfunction.
		If MRSA suspected/documented add:[†] **Vancomycin**[E] or **Linezolid** β-lactam allergy: **Vancomycin**[E] + **Levofloxacin** + **Metronidazole**	15mg/kg IV q8-12h 600mg IV/PO q12h 15mg/kg IV q8-12h 750mg IV/PO daily 500mg IV/PO q12h	3-6 weeks 3-6 weeks 3-6 weeks	

E. Desired vancomycin trough is 15-20 mg/L. Monitor renal function closely. See Vancomycin Dosing & Monitoring Guidelines.

RECOMMENDED EMPIRIC THERAPY OF SELECTED INFECTIONS IN ADULT PATIENTS[A]

Infection	Usual Pathogens	Recommended Empiric Therapy	Recommended Dose[B]	Recommended Duration	Comments
Respiratory					
Pleural Space Infections (cont'd)					

Empyema (cont'd)
• **Hospital acquired**
	S. aureus/MRSA
	Enterobacteriaceae**
	Enterococcus spp
	Anaerobes
	P. aeruginosa
	S. anginosus group*
		Piperacillin-tazobactam
		+
		[**Vancomycin**[E]
		or
		Linezolid][†]
			4.5g IV q6h
			
			15mg/kg IV q8-12h
			
			600mg IV/PO q12h
				3-6 weeks	* Includes:
					  • S. anginosus
					  •• S. constellatus
					  •• S. intermedius
					** Especially Klebsiella spp in alcoholics.
					- Tailor antibiotics to C&S results but maintain anaerobic coverage.
					† Linezolid preferred over vancomycin if:
					  • MRSA with vancomycin MIC ≥ 1.5ug/mL
					  • concomitant nephrotoxic therapy
					  • pre-existing renal dysfunction.

		β-lactam allergy **Vancomycin**[E] + **Ciprofloxacin** + **Metronidazole**	15mg/kg IV q8-12h 400mg IV q8-12h/ 750mg PO bid 500mg IV/PO q12h	3-6 weeks	

E. Desired vancomycin trough is 15-20 mg/L. Monitor renal function closely. See Vancomycin Dosing & Monitoring Guidelines.

RECOMMENDED EMPIRIC THERAPY OF SELECTED INFECTIONS IN ADULT PATIENTS[A]

Infection	Usual Pathogens	Recommended Empiric Therapy	Recommended Dose[B]	Recommended Duration	Comments
Respiratory					
Pleural Space Infections (cont'd) **Lung abscess**	- Careful assessment of risk factors recommended: • dental/gingival disease • immunosuppression • immigration/travel history • underlying lung disease. - Consider TB/mycobacterial, fungal, parasitic etiology. - Consider noninfectious etiology: malignancy, rheumatologic diseases, pulmonary emboli.				
	Polymicrobial including: • Fusobacterium spp • Prevotella spp • S. anginosus group* S. aureus/MRSA[†] Klebsiella pneumoniae S. pneumoniae Haemophilus spp Occasionally: • Nocardia spp • Legionella spp • Actinomyces spp	[Ceftriaxone + **Metronidazole**] or **Piperacillin-tazobactam** If MRSA suspected/documented add:[†] **Vancomycin**[E] or **Linezolid**	1-2g IV daily 500mg IV/PO q12h 3.375g IV q6h or 4.5g IV q8h 15mg/kg IV q8-12h 600mg IV/PO q12h	3-6 weeks** 3-6 weeks** 3-6 weeks** 3-6 weeks**	* Includes: ○ S. anginosus ○ S. constellatus ○ S. intermedius † Rule out S. aureus bacteremia/endovascular infection. Consider MRSA if: • rapid onset • post-influenza • IVDU • colonization/recent infection with MRSA • Gram positive cocci in clusters on Gram stain Linezolid preferred over vancomycin if: ○ MRSA with vancomycin MIC ≥ 1.5µg/mL ○ concomitant nephrotoxic therapy ○ pre-existing renal dysfunction. **Treat until pulmonary infiltrate has cleared.

E. Desired vancomycin trough is 15-20 mg/L. Monitor renal function closely. See Vancomycin Dosing & Monitoring Guidelines.

RECOMMENDED EMPIRIC THERAPY OF SELECTED INFECTIONS IN ADULT PATIENTS[A]

Infection	Usual Pathogens	Recommended Empiric Therapy	Recommended Dose[B]	Recommended Duration	Comments
Respiratory					
Tuberculosis (TB)	Note: Complete management of tuberculosis is beyond the scope of this book. Refer to Canadian guidelines at http://www.phac-aspc.gc.ca/tbpc-latb/pubs/tbstand07-eng.phpf.				

- Recommend investigation for TB in adults if:
  - symptoms of:
    - ⇒ cough > 2-3 weeks
    - ⇒ hemoptysis
    - ⇒ fever/night sweats
    - ⇒ anorexia/weight loss
  - high risk:
    - ⇒ foreign-born (Asia, Africa, Latin America)
    - ⇒ First Nations
    - ⇒ elderly
    - ⇒ homeless
    - ⇒ immunocompromised/HIV
    - ⇒ epidemiologic link to active TB case

  or

  - chest x-ray with upper lobe cavity or fibronodular infiltrate.

- If suspect TB, place patient in negative pressure respiratory isolation until sputum AFB smear negative on 3 consecutive days.

Diagnosis:
- Chest x-ray
- Sputum for AFB smear and culture (collect on 3 consecutive days).

NB: Do NOT use tuberculin skin test (TST) or Interferon Gamma Release Assay (IGRA) for diagnosis of active TB. These are used to diagnose latent TB infection and cannot distinguish active from latent infection.

- If AFB smear/culture positive for M. tuberculosis complex, initiate therapy and report case to Public Health. Test for HIV infection.
- Strongly consider directly observed therapy (DOT) via Public Health, especially for HIV co-infection, MDR/XDR TB, sputum smear positive pulmonary TB, and nonadherence.

- **If history of previous TB treatment or contact with drug-resistant TB*, consult TB specialist.**

* Multi-drug resistant TB (MDR-TB) = resistance to at least isoniazid and rifampin.

Extensively drug-resistant TB (XDR-TB) = resistance to isoniazid and rifampin and fluoroquinolone plus at least one of the three second-line injectable aminoglycosides drugs (capreomycin, kanamycin, or amikacin).

RECOMMENDED EMPIRIC THERAPY OF SELECTED INFECTIONS IN ADULT PATIENTS[A]

Infection	Usual Pathogens	Recommended Empiric Therapy	Recommended Dose[B]	Recommended Duration	Comments
Respiratory					
Tuberculosis (TB) (cont'd)	- Monitor for drug toxicity: • CBC with differential, ALT, AST, bilirubin, urinalysis, serum creatinine at baseline and every 1-2 weeks • Increased monitoring recommended in patients at risk for hepatotoxicity: ⇒ pre-existing liver disease ⇒ history of alcohol abuse ⇒ ≥ 35 years of age Patients should be instructed to watch for signs of hepatitis (nausea, vomiting, stomach pain, lack of appetite, fatigue, dark urine, jaundice). • visual acuity (Snellen chart/color vision (isochromatic plates) baseline and monthly while on ethambutol.				
	M. tuberculosis[‡]	**Isoniazid** + **Rifampin** + **Pyrazinamide**** + **Ethambutol***** + **Pyridoxine†** **(vitamin B$_6$)**	5mg/kg* PO daily (max 300mg/day) 10mg/kg* PO daily (max 600mg/day) 20-25mg/kg* PO daily (max 2g/day) 15-25mg/kg* PO daily (max 1.6g/day) 25mg PO daily	For fully susceptible M. tuberculosis: 2 month initial phase and continuation phase of 4 or 7 months depending on presence or absence of cavitary disease and results of sputum cultures taken at 2 months. TB osteomyelitis - 12 months. TB meningitis - 12 months.	‡ Consider adding fifth drug pending susceptibility results if: • history of previously treated active TB • patient from a country with risk of MDR or XDR TB. * Based on ideal body weight. ** Round to nearest 500mg. ***Round to nearest 400mg. †Give with INH to decrease incidence of peripheral neuropathy.

RECOMMENDED EMPIRIC THERAPY OF SELECTED INFECTIONS IN ADULT PATIENTS[A]

Infection	Usual Pathogens	Recommended Empiric Therapy	Recommended Dose[B]	Recommended Duration	Comments
Gastrointestinal					

Gastroenteritis	- Stool specimens in patients hospitalized for > 3 days should not be submitted for C&S unless patient admitted with diarrhea or nosocomial outbreak of diarrhea. Diarrhea in hospitalized patients always warrants investigation for C. d ficile.
	- Recommend blood culture if febrile and systemically unwell.
	- Causes of bloody diarrhea:
	  - Campylobacter spp
	  - Shigella spp
	  - Nontyphoidal Salmonella spp
	  - Shiga toxin-producing E. coli, including E. coli O157:H7
	  - Aeromonas spp
	  - Vibrio spp, not V. cholerae
	  - Yersinia spp
	  - E. histolytica
	- Severe bloody diarrhea in afebrile patients should increase suspicion of E. coli O157:H7. More common in children <5 years old.
	- Do not use bismuth subsalicylate with quinolones as binding decreases quinolone absorption.
	- Avoid antimotility agents if fever present or blood in stool.				

Mild-moderate	Viral
	Parasitic:
	  • Giardia
	  • Cryptosporidium
	  • Cyclospora
	Campylobacter spp
	Shigella spp
	Salmonella spp
	diarrheagenic E. coli
	Aeromonas spp
	Plesiomonas spp
	Vibrio spp,
	noncholerae
	Yersinia spp
		Fluid replacement + bismuth subsalicylate +/- antimotility agents			- These organisms usually cause self-limiting diarrhea. Antibiotic therapy is generally not recommended unless symptoms are severe or prolonged, or patient is immunocompromised.
					- For treatment of enteric parasites, see Recommended Empiric Therapy of Enteric Parasitic Infections.

- 302 -

RECOMMENDED EMPIRIC THERAPY OF SELECTED INFECTIONS IN ADULT PATIENTS[A]

Infection	Usual Pathogens	Recommended Empiric Therapy	Recommended Dose[B]	Recommended Duration	Comments
Gastrointestinal					
Gastroenteritis (cont'd) **Severe** • > 6 diarrheal episodes/day • bloody diarrhea • persistent (> 1 week) diarrhea • +/- fever	Culture pending, **no clinical suspicion of hemolytic uremic syndrome (HUS)/ thrombotic thrombocytopenic purpura (TTP)***	**Ciprofloxacin** _Alternative_ **TMP/SMX**	500mg PO bid 1 DS tab PO bid	3-5 days 3-5 days	* NB: Antibiotic therapy contraindicated if clinical suspicion of HUS as it may enhance toxin release and increase risk of HUS. Clinical signs of HUS/TTP: • diarrhea that becomes bloody after 1-4 days • elevated serum creatinine/ oliguria/anuria • thrombocytopenia (platelets <15 x 10⁹/L) • microangiopathic hemolytic anemia (Hgb < 100g/L). - Culture recommended. - Tailor antibiotics to C&S results. See below for recommendations.
Culture-directed	Campylobacter spp	No therapy unless severe, prolonged, or immunocompromised **Azithromycin** or **Erythromycin** _Alternative_ **Ciprofloxacin***	500mg PO daily 500mg PO qid 500mg PO bid	3 days 5 days 3 days	- Symptoms occur 1-10 days after exposure and usually resolve within 2-5 days. * Resistance to quinolones is high in Campylobacter spp.
	Shiga toxin-producing E. coli, including E. coli O157:H7	**Antibiotic therapy contraindicated.***			* NB: Antibiotic therapy may enhance toxin release and increase risk of hemolytic uremic syndrome (HUS). - Avoid antimotility agents.

- 303 -

RECOMMENDED EMPIRIC THERAPY OF SELECTED INFECTIONS IN ADULT PATIENTS[A]

Infection	Usual Pathogens	Recommended Empiric Therapy	Recommended Dose[B]	Recommended Duration	Comments
Gastrointestinal					
Gastroenteritis (cont'd)					
Severe (cont'd) • > 6 diarrheal episodes/day • bloody diarrhea • persistent (> 1 week) diarrhea	Salmonella typhi Salmonella paratyphi	**Ciprofloxacin*** or **Azithromycin** Hospitalized/Bacteremic **Ceftriaxone**	500mg PO bid 500mg PO daily 2g IV/IM daily	7 days 7 days 10-14 days, or at least 5 days after defervescence, whichever is longer	- Relapse rate 10% after antibiotic therapy. - Significant ciprofloxacin resistance if acquired in Asia; use azithromycin or ceftriaxone.
	Salmonella spp, non typhoidal*	No therapy unless high risk* High risk* **Ciprofloxacin** Alternative **TMP/SMX** or **Azithromycin** Hospitalized/bacteremic **Ceftriaxone**	 500mg PO bid 1 DS tab PO bid 500mg PO daily 2g IV/IM daily	 7-10 days** 7-10 days** 7 days** 14 days***	* High risk: • bacteremia (use ceftriaxone) • immunocompromised** • hemodialysis • hemoglobinopathy, e.g. sickle cell disease • chronic GI tract disease • food handlers • patients > 65 years with severe symptoms • age < 12 months. **14 days if immunocompromised or relapsing infection. ***4-6 weeks if extraintestinal site of infection (urinary tract, respiratory tract, endovascular, musculoskeletal, CNS) or immunosuppressed.
	Shigella spp	**Ciprofloxacin** or **Azithromycin**	500mg PO bid 500mg PO daily	3 days* 3 days*	* 7 days if immunocompromised.
	Vibrio cholerae	**Doxycycline** or **Azithromycin**	300mg PO once 1g PO once	1 dose 1 dose	- Fluid/rehydration essential.

RECOMMENDED EMPIRIC THERAPY OF SELECTED INFECTIONS IN ADULT PATIENTS[A]

Infection	Usual Pathogens	Recommended Empiric Therapy	Recommended Dose[B]	Recommended Duration	Comments
Gastrointestinal (cont'd)					
Severe (cont'd) • > 6 diarrheal episodes/day • bloody diarrhea • persistent (> 1 week) diarrhea	Aeromonas spp Plesiomonas spp Vibrio spp. not V. cholerae Yersinia spp	No therapy unless <u>severe, prolonged, or immunocompromised</u> **Ciprofloxacin** <u>Alternative</u> **TMP/SMX**	500mg PO bid 1 DS tab PO bid	3 days* 3 days*	* 7 days if immunocompromised.
	Parasitic	See Treatment of Enteric Parasitic Infections.			

RECOMMENDED EMPIRIC THERAPY OF SELECTED INFECTIONS IN ADULT PATIENTS[A]

Infection	Usual Pathogens	Recommended Empiric Therapy	Recommended Dose[B]	Recommended Duration	Comments
Gastrointestinal					
Travellers' diarrhea	- Antibiotic prophylaxis not recommended due to the potential for adverse effects/resistance and the fact that travellers' diarrhea is usually mild and self-limiting; prompt self-treatment is effective and preferred. Counsel on handwashing and food and water precautions. - For therapy of specific organisms, see previous Gastroenteritis section. - Avoid antimotility agents if fever present or blood in stool. - In the event of severe travellers' diarrhea, consider providing a 3-day supply of antibiotics, especially for immunocompromised patients, and in particular for asplenic patients as they are at increased risk of Salmonella/Campylobacter bacteremia.				
Mild-moderate	diarrheagenic E. coli Campylobacter spp Shigella spp Salmonella spp	Fluid replacement + bismuth subsalicylate +/- antimotility agents (e.g. loperamide)			- Self-limiting. Usual duration of diarrhea 3-5 days. - Persistent diarrhea suggests protozoal causes: Giardia, Cryptosporidium, Cyclospora, Entamoeba histolytica, Microsporidia. See Treatment of Enteric Parasitic Infections.
Severe • > 6 diarrheal episodes/day • bloody diarrhea • persistent (> 3 days) diarrhea • fever	diarrheagenic E. coli Campylobacter spp Shigella spp Enterotoxigenic Bacteroides fragilis	**Azithromycin** or **Levofloxacin*** or **Norfloxacin*** or **Ciprofloxacin*** or **TMP/SMX***	1g PO or 500mg PO daily 500mg PO or 500mg PO daily 800mg PO or 400mg PO bid 750mg PO or 500mg PO bid 2 DS tabs PO or 1 DS tab PO bid	1 dose*** 3 days 1 dose*** 3 days 1 dose*** 3 days 1 dose*** 3 days 1 dose*** 3 days	- Culture recommended. - Tailor antibiotics to C&S results. * Resistance to quinolones is high in Campylobacter spp., especially in Asia. Do not use bismuth subsalicylate with quinolones, or doxycycline for malaria, as binding decreases antibiotic absorption. **Widespread resistance but may be an option if travel to Mexico. ***A single dose can be taken initially and response assessed. If diarrhea is not improved, continue antibiotics for up to 3 days.
	Salmonella spp	See previous Gastroenteritis section.			

RECOMMENDED EMPIRIC THERAPY OF SELECTED INFECTIONS IN ADULT PATIENTS[A]

Infection	Usual Pathogens	Recommended Empiric Therapy	Recommended Dose[B]	Recommended Duration	Comments
Gastrointestinal					
Clostridium difficile infection (CDI)					

- Definition: presence of diarrhea (≥ 3 unformed stools in ≤ 24 hours) and either:
  - stool positive for toxigenic C. difficile or its toxins
  - or
  - colonoscopic or histopathologic findings of pseudomembranous colitis.
- History of treatment with antibiotics, proton pump inhibitors (PPIs), or antineoplastic agents within previous 8 weeks is also present in majority of patients.
- **Discontinue antibiotics if possible, especially cephalosporins, quinolones** (risk: moxifloxacin>ciprofloxacin>levofloxacin [CMAJ 2008; 179:767-72]), **and clindamycin, as these agents have been associated with the highest risk of CDI. If not possible, consider changing to lower CDI risk group of antibiotics if appropriate (e.g. aminoglycosides, TMP/SMX, tetracyclines, and/or metronidazole). Prevention of CDI with metronidazole or vancomycin while on antimicrobial therapy is NOT recommended as no evidence of efficacy.**
- PPIs/H₂ blockers are associated with a 2-3 fold increased risk for CDI and recurrent CDI. Assess need for use, or continued use, of these agents vs. benefit and discontinue if possible.
- **Do NOT use antidiarrheals, e.g. loperamide (Imodium®), diphenoxylate (Lomotil®) as they may obscure symptoms and precipitate toxic megacolon.**
- Vancomycin IV not effective. Metronidazole IV of uncertain efficacy (only use if very strict NPO or in combination for severe/toxic megacolon).
- Fidaxomicin has recently been approved in Canada but its place in CDI therapy has not been established and may be cost-prohibitive.
- Do not submit post treatment stool sample if asymptomatic and/or formed stools as toxin may persist for weeks post treatment.
- Infection Control:
  - Hospitalized patients with CDI should be isolated with contact precautions.
  - Strict adherence to handwashing with soap and water essential (alcohol does not kill C. difficile spores).

RECOMMENDED EMPIRIC THERAPY OF SELECTED INFECTIONS IN ADULT PATIENTS[A]

Infection	Usual Pathogens	Recommended Empiric Therapy	Recommended Dose[B]	Recommended Duration	Comments
Gastrointestinal					
Clostridium difficile infection (CDI) (cont'd)					
Initial episode	Clostridium difficile	Mild-moderate **Metronidazole**	500mg PO tid	10-14 days	* Severe = WBC >15x10⁹/L, serum creatinine ≥1.5x baseline, hypotension, shock, megacolon. **Do not assume therapeutic failure of metronidazole until minimum of 3-5 days of therapy completed without symptomatic improvement.
		Severe*/unresponsive to metronidazole** **Vancomycin**	125mg PO qid	10-14 days	
Ileus/NPO	Clostridium difficile	Mild-moderate **Metronidazole**	500mg IV q8h*	10-14 days	* Switch to NG/PO as soon as possible; little clinical data for IV metronidazole. **Severe = WBC >15x10⁹/L, serum creatinine ≥1.5x baseline, hypotension, shock, megacolon. ***Consider intracolonic instillation of vancomycin 500mg in 100mL NS via colonic tube q6h clamped x 3 hours.
		Severe** **Metronidazole IV + Vancomycin NG/PR***	500mg IV q8h 500mg NG/PR qid	10-14 days	
Recurrence					

- Recurrence after first episode occurs in up to 30% of patients, and as high as 65% after first recurrence.
- The role of probiotics for the prevention or treatment of CDI remains controversial. Clinical data is limited. Potential for bacteremia/fungemia in immunocompromised patients. Multiple formulations exist but labeling regulations and quality control are lacking. Further research is needed to clarify the role of probiotics in CDI.

Infection	Usual Pathogens	Recommended Empiric Therapy	Recommended Dose[B]	Recommended Duration	Comments
• **Initial recurrence**	Clostridium difficile	Mild-moderate **Metronidazole**	500mg PO tid	10-14 days	* Severe = WBC >15x10⁹/L, serum creatinine ≥1.5x baseline, hypotension, shock, megacolon.
		Severe*/unresponsive to metronidazole **Vancomycin**	125mg PO qid	10-14 days	

RECOMMENDED EMPIRIC THERAPY OF SELECTED INFECTIONS IN ADULT PATIENTS[A]

Infection	Usual Pathogens	Recommended Empiric Therapy	Recommended Dose[B]	Recommended Duration	Comments
Gastrointestinal					
Clostridium difficile infection (CDI) (cont'd) • Subsequent recurrence	Clostridium difficile	**Vancomycin pulse** or **Vancomycin taper**	Pulse regimen* 125mg PO qid then 125mg PO q3days Taper regimen 125mg PO qid 125mg PO bid 125mg PO daily 125mg PO q 2 days 125mg PO q 3 days	10-14 days 3 weeks 10-14 days 1 week 1 week 1 week 1 week	* Recurrence rate may be lower with pulse regimen (14%) than taper regimen (31%). [Clin Microbiol Infect 2009;15:1067-79] - Metronidazole should not be used for more than 2 consecutive courses or in a pulse or taper regimen due to cumulative risk of neurotoxicity. - Fecal bacteriotherapy may be considered in recalcitrant CDI. Consultation with specialist recommended.

RECOMMENDED EMPIRIC THERAPY OF SELECTED INFECTIONS IN ADULT PATIENTS[A]

Infection	Usual Pathogens	Recommended Empiric Therapy	Recommended Dose[B]	Recommended Duration	Comments
Gastrointestinal					

Helicobacter pylori associated duodenal/gastric ulcer	- Indications for investigation and treatment of H. pylori:
	  • active peptic ulcer (gastric or duodenal) disease (PUD)
	  • past history of PUD (if not previously treated for H. pylori)
	  • gastric MALT lymphoma
	  • after endoscopic resection of gastric cancer
	  • uninvestigated dyspepsia.
	- Investigation and treatment of H. pylori is **controversial** for following conditions:
	  • gastroesophageal reflux disease (GERD)
	  • non-ulcer dyspepsia (test and treat if H. pylori positive)
	  • NSAID - induced gastropathy
	  • unexplained iron deficiency anemia
	  • persons at risk of gastric cancer
	- **Compliance is essential to achieve expected eradication rates of 85-90% and to decrease development of antimicrobial resistance. Resistance is increasing to metronidazole and clarithromycin.** Eradication therapy regimens that include only one antibiotic are NOT recommended (potential to induce resistance).
	- H. pylori eradication should be confirmed by urea breath test ≥ 4 weeks after treatment completed.
	- More than one course of treatment is NOT appropriate without further investigation.
	- Recurrence of H. pylori infection is infrequent (3.4%/patient year).
	- Post H. pylori therapy, acid suppression course (H$_2$-receptor antagonist or proton pump inhibitor [PPI]) NOT recommended for uncomplicated ulcers. If complicated (perforation, hemorrhage, obstruction), recommend acid suppression course x 4-6 weeks following H. pylori eradication regimen. Do not continue acid supression for longer than this without a clear indication as increased risk of adverse events, including C. difficile infection, community-acquired pneumonia, SBP in cirrhotic patients, and fractures.			

- 310 -

RECOMMENDED EMPIRIC THERAPY OF SELECTED INFECTIONS IN ADULT PATIENTS[A]

Infection	Usual Pathogens	Recommended Empiric Therapy	Recommended Dose[B]	Recommended Duration	Comments
Gastrointestinal					
Helicobacter pylori associated duodenal/gastric ulcer (cont'd) **Initial therapy**	Helicobacter pylori	Triple therapy: [**Clarithromycin** + **Amoxicillin** + PPI]	500mg PO bid 1g PO bid	7 days	
		or [**Clarithromycin** + **Metronidazole** + PPI]	500mg PO bid 500mg PO bid	7 days	
		Alternative Sequential therapy*: **Amoxicillin** + PPI then **Clarithromycin** + **Metronidazole** + PPI	1g PO bid 500mg PO bid 500mg PO bid	5 days 5 days	* Sequential administration of antibiotics may help overcome clarithromycin resistance. Preliminary evidence indicates it may be superior to standard triple therapy.
Failure of therapy*	Helicobacter pylori	[**Bismuth subsalicylate** + **Metronidazole** + **Tetracycline** + PPI]	2 tabs PO qid 250mg PO qid 500mg PO qid	10-14 days	* Confirm that H. pylori infection is still present. Recommend gastroenterology consult if second treatment course fails as resistance may have developed.
		Alternative**: **Amoxicillin** + **Levofloxacin** + PPI	1g PO bid 500mg PO bid	10 days	** Not recommended if patient has received quinolones in previous 3-6 months.

RECOMMENDED EMPIRIC THERAPY OF SELECTED INFECTIONS IN ADULT PATIENTS[A]

Infection	Usual Pathogens	Recommended Empiric Therapy	Recommended Dose[B]	Recommended Duration	Comments
Gastrointestinal					
Cholecystitis **Acute**	Enterobacteriaceae Enterococcus spp* Anaerobes*	**Ceftriaxone**** +/- **Metronidazole IV/PO**[C]	1-2g IV daily 500mg IV/PO q12h	7 days***	- Mild cases do not require **antimicrobial therapy.** * Coverage of anaerobes and Enterococcus is controversial. Recommended if: • elderly • immunocompromised/ diabetic/cirrhosis • bile duct-bowel anastomosis. **These regimens do not have enterococcal coverage. ***Short course (3-5 days, or 24 hours after cholecystectomy) may be considered if: • no perforation • no abscess • no cholangitis. † Due to significant ciprofloxacin resistance in E. coli, this regimen should only be used if severe penicillin/β-lactam allergy.
		Alternative [**Ampicillin** + **Gentamicin** +/- **Metronidazole IV/PO**[C]]	2g IV q6h 5-7mg/kg IV q24h 500mg IV/PO q12h	7 days***	
		Hemodynamic instability **Piperacillin-tazobactam**	4.5g IV q8h or 3.375g IV q6h	7 days***	
		Severe β-lactam allergy [**Ciprofloxacin IV/PO*****†** or **Gentamicin**] +/- **Metronidazole IV/PO**[C]	400mg IV q12h/ 500mg PO bid 5-7mg/kg IV daily 500mg IV/PO q12h	7 days***	

RECOMMENDED EMPIRIC THERAPY OF SELECTED INFECTIONS IN ADULT PATIENTS[A]

Infection	Usual Pathogens	Recommended Empiric Therapy	Recommended Dose[B]	Recommended Duration	Comments
Gastrointestinal					
Cholangitis **Acute**	Enterobacteriaceae Enterococcus spp Anaerobes* P. aeruginosa**	**Piperacillin-tazobactam** or **Imipenem** _Severe β-lactam allergy***_ **Vancomycin**[E] + **Ciprofloxacin IV/PO**[D] +/- **Metronidazole IV/PO**[C]	4.5g IV q8h or 3.375g IV q6h 500mg IV q6h 15mg/kg IV q12h 400mg IV q12h/ 500-750mg PO bid 500mg IV/PO q12h	10 days 10 days 10 days	- Blood cultures recommended (high risk of bacteremia). * Coverage of anaerobes is controversial but recommended if previous biliary surgery. **Pseudomonas aeruginosa potential pathogen if post-ERCP. - Drainage of obstructed biliary tree is essential for therapy of cholangitis. ***Due to significant ciprofloxacin resistance in E. coli, this regimen should only be used if severe penicillin/β-lactam allergy.
Recurrent	Enterobacteriaceae Enterococcus spp	Therapy See Acute cholangitis Prophylaxis **TMP/SMX** Alternative **Ciprofloxacin**	1 DS tab PO daily 500mg PO daily	3-4 months then re-evaluate 3-4 months then re-evaluate	- May be seen following reconstructive surgery of the biliary tract.
Perforation/ pericholecystic abscess	See 2° peritonitis				

E. Desired vancomycin trough is 10-20 mg/L. Monitor renal function closely. See Vancomycin Dosing & Monitoring Guidelines.

RECOMMENDED EMPIRIC THERAPY OF SELECTED INFECTIONS IN ADULT PATIENTS[A]

Infection	Usual Pathogens	Recommended Empiric Therapy	Recommended Dose[B]	Recommended Duration	Comments
Gastrointestinal					
Pancreatitis **Acute**	- Diagnosis: presence of at least 2 of 3 following features: 1. abdominal pain 2. increased pancreatic enzyme, amylase and/or lipase levels ≥3x upper limit of normal 3. CT scan findings of acute pancreatitis (pancreatic edema, necrosis, or pseudocyst formation). - Alcohol abuse and gallstones are the two most common causes of pancreatitis.				
	Non-infected +/- necrosis on CT scan*	No antibiotic therapy**			* CT scan contrast enhanced. ** Prophylactic antibiotics are not recommended for acute necrotizing pancreatitis.
Complicated: • **pancreatic abscess** • **infected pseudocyst** • **infected necrotic pancreas**	Enterobacteriaceae Enterococcus spp S. aureus Coagulase negative Staphylococci Anaerobes Candida spp*	**Piperacillin-tazobactam** or **Imipenem** Severe β-lactam allergy:** **Vancomycin**[E] + **Ciprofloxacin IV/PO**[D] + **Metronidazole IV/PO**[C]	4.5g IV q8h or 3.375g IV q6h 500mg IV q6h 15mg/kg IV q12h 400mg IV q12h/ 500-750mg PO bid 500mg IV/PO q12h	Based on clinical improvement. May require prolonged antibiotic therapy. Based on clinical improvement. May require prolonged antibiotic therapy.	- Surgical debridement and drainage essential for established infections. * Tailor antibiotics to C&S results. * If Candida spp isolated on culture, recommend adding fluconazole if C. albicans or echinocandin (anidulafungin, caspofungin, micafungin) if nonalbicans Candida spp. **Due to significant ciprofloxacin resistance in E. coli, this regimen should only be used if severe penicillin/β-lactam allergy.

E. Desired vancomycin trough is 10-20 mg/L. Monitor renal function closely. See Vancomycin Dosing & Monitoring Guidelines.

RECOMMENDED EMPIRIC THERAPY OF SELECTED INFECTIONS IN ADULT PATIENTS[A]

Infection	Usual Pathogens	Recommended Empiric Therapy	Recommended Empiric Therapy	Recommended Dose[B]	Recommended Duration	Comments
Gastrointestinal						

Liver abscess	- Blood cultures recommended (increased risk of bacteremia).
	- Drainage required (percutaneous where feasible).
	- Investigation of GI tract recommended.
	- Surgical drainage recommended if:
	  • fever persists > 2 weeks on appropriate therapy
	  • biliary obstruction.					

Bacterial	Polymicrobial: • Enterobacteriaceae (especially Klebsiella spp[†]) • Anaerobes • Enterococcus spp • Streptococcus anginosus group	**Ampicillin + Metronidazole IV/PO**[C] **+ Gentamicin** or **Piperacillin-tazobactam*** or **Imipenem***		2g IV q6h 500mg IV/PO q12h 5-7mg/kg IV q24h 4.5g IV q8h or 3.375g IV q6h 500mg IV q6h	Minimum 4 weeks or until CT resolution (may be up to 4 months)** Minimum 4 weeks or until CT resolution (may be up to 4 months)** Minimum 4 weeks or until CT resolution (may be up to 4 months)**	† If Klebsiella pneumoniae genotype K1, serious septic ocular or central nervous system complications can occur (even in previously healthy persons). - Enterococcal coverage indicated empirically. * If E. histolytica has not been ruled out, add metronidazole. **If clinical improvement/ defervescence consider switch to oral therapy (guided by susceptibility). e.g. amoxicillin-clavulanate or (ciprofloxacin + metronidazole).
Parasitic	Entamoeba histolytica	**Metronidazole** followed by **Iodoquinol** (to eradicate luminal cysts)		500-750mg PO tid 650mg PO tid	7-10 days 20 days	- Recommend E. histolytica serology and chest x-ray. - Check for history of diarrhea. - Often do not have high spiking fevers (unlike bacterial liver abscess)

RECOMMENDED EMPIRIC THERAPY OF SELECTED INFECTIONS IN ADULT PATIENTS[A]

Infection	Usual Pathogens	Recommended Empiric Therapy	Recommended Dose[B]	Recommended Duration	Comments
Gastrointestinal					
Diverticulitis	Polymicrobial: • Enterobacteriaceae • Anaerobes • Enterococcus spp*	<u>Mild-moderate**</u> [TMP/SMX + **Metronidazole**] or **Amoxicillin-clavulanate** or [**Ciprofloxacin** + **Metronidazole**] <u>Severe/IV therapy</u> See 2° Peritonitis	1 DS tab PO bid 500mg PO bid 875mg PO bid 750mg PO bid 500mg PO bid	5-7 days*** 5-7 days*** 5-7 days***	* Coverage of Enterococcus is controversial. Only amoxicillin-clavulanate covers Enterococcus. **The benefit of antibiotics in mild, uncomplicated diverticulitis has not been proven. Antibiotic therapy may not be necessary in mild diverticulitis. ***Duration directed by clinical response. Treat until afebrile 3-5 days.
Appendicitis Acute	Enterobacteriaceae Enterococcus spp Anaerobes	<u>Uncomplicated</u> Empiric therapy not necessary. Surgical prophylaxis recommended. <u>Complicated*</u> See 2° Peritonitis			* Complicated: • gangrene • perforation • abscess • peritonitis.

RECOMMENDED EMPIRIC THERAPY OF SELECTED INFECTIONS IN ADULT PATIENTS[A]

Infection	Usual Pathogens	Recommended Empiric Therapy	Recommended Dose[B]	Recommended Duration	Comments
Gastrointestinal					
Peritonitis	- Spontaneous bacterial peritonitis is usually monomicrobial. Polymicrobial infections suggest bowel perforation. See 2° peritonitis.				
Spontaneous bacterial peritonitis (SBP)	Diagnosis: - Ascitic fluid positive for bacteria and PMNs ≥ 0.25×10^9/L. - Blood/peritoneal fluid cultures recommended. Management: - Urinary/intravascular catheterization may increase risk of infection in patients with ascites - avoid if possible. - Aminoglycosides should be avoided in patients with cirrhosis. - Increased risk of SBP (and Clostridium difficile infection) in cirrhotic patients on proton pump inhibitors (PPIs). Therefore use PPIs judiciously and only when clearly indicated in cirrhotic patients. Prophylaxis: - SBP will occur in 10-25% of cirrhotic patients with ascites. Prophylactic antibiotics decrease incidence of initial (primary prophylaxis)/ recurrent (secondary prophylaxis) episodes of SBP but have not demonstrated reduction in hospitalization or survival rates. - **Long term prophylaxis with antibiotics increases carriage of multiresistant organisms.**			
	Enterobacteriaceae Occasionally: • S. pneumoniae • Streptococcus spp	Treatment **Ceftriaxone**	1-2g IV daily	5-10 days*	* 10 days recommended if bacteremic. Five days if repeat paracentesis (at 48 hours) shows < 0.25×10^9/L PMNs and culture negative.

RECOMMENDED EMPIRIC THERAPY OF SELECTED INFECTIONS IN ADULT PATIENTS[A]

Infection	Usual Pathogens	Recommended Empiric Therapy	Recommended Dose[B]	Recommended Duration	Comments
Gastrointestinal					
Peritonitis (cont'd) **Spontaneous bacterial peritonitis (SBP)** (cont'd)	Prophylaxis: - SBP will occur in 10-25% of cirrhotic patients with ascites. Prophylactic antibiotics decrease incidence of initial (primary prophylaxis)/ recurrent (secondary prophylaxis) episodes of SBP but have not demonstrated reduction in hospitalization or survival rates. - **Long term prophylaxis with antibiotics increases carriage of multiresistant organisms.**				
	Enterobacteriaceae Occasionally: • S. pneumoniae • Streptococcus spp	Prophylaxis Primary prophylaxis in patients with cirrhosis & GI bleed*: **Ceftriaxone** then [**TMP/SMX** or **Norfloxacin** or **Ciprofloxacin**] Secondary prophylaxis in high risk patients only**: **TMP/SMX** Alternative **Norfloxacin***** or **Ciprofloxacin*****	 1-2g IV daily 1 DS tab PO bid 400mg PO bid 500mg PO bid 1 DS tab PO daily 400mg PO daily 750mg PO daily	 while NPO to complete 7 days to complete 7 days to complete 7 days lifetime lifetime lifetime	* Primary prophylaxis decreases incidence of Gram negative infections but not overall incidence of infection. **Secondary prophylaxis may be considered in high risk patients: ascitic fluid protein <10-15g/L **plus at least one of:** • bilirubin > 30mg/L • platelets < 98 x 10⁹/L • serum creatinine >100μmol/L • sodium ≤130mmol/L • Child-Pugh score ≥ 9 points. ***Quinolones are acceptable alternatives but may select for Gram positive organisms.

RECOMMENDED EMPIRIC THERAPY OF SELECTED INFECTIONS IN ADULT PATIENTS[A]

Infection	Usual Pathogens	Recommended Empiric Therapy	Recommended Dose[B]	Recommended Duration	Comments
Gastrointestinal					

Peritonitis (cont'd)					- Drainage and debridement essential.
					
					- Cultures of perforated or gangrenous appendix offer no benefit. However, distal colonic perforations warrant aerobic/anaerobic cultures as antibiotic therapy should be tailored to C&S results.
					
					- Duration of therapy:
					   • Peri-operative therapy ≤ 24h
					     Bowel injuries due to penetrating, blunt, or iatrogenic trauma with surgery within 12 hours of injury; acute perforations of stomach, duodenum, and proximal jejunum in absence of antacid therapy or malignancy; or acute appendicitis without gangrene, perforation, abscess, or peritonitis.
					   • Short course (5-7 days)
					     Uncomplicated peritonitis if adequate drainage.
					     Persistent clinical evidence of infection after 5-7 days warrants diagnostic investigations (CT, US).
					   • Prolonged course*
					     Complicated intraabdominal abscesses and/or severe underlying illness.
					     *Continue therapy until:
					     ⇒ afebrile
					     ⇒ normal WBC/differential
					     ⇒ no residual fluid collections
					     ⇒ return of GI function.

RECOMMENDED EMPIRIC THERAPY OF SELECTED INFECTIONS IN ADULT PATIENTS[A]

Infection	Usual Pathogens	Recommended Empiric Therapy	Recommended Dose[B]	Recommended Duration	Comments
Gastrointestinal					
Peritonitis (cont'd) **Secondary peritonitis** • abscess* • bowel perforation • ruptured appendix	Polymicrobial: • Enterobacteriaceae • Enterococcus spp[‡] • Anaerobes • Streptococcus spp • Candida spp***	Mild - moderate **Ceftriaxone**** + **Metronidazole IV/PO**[C] Severe β-lactam allergy[†] **Ciprofloxacin IV/PO**[D]*** + **Metronidazole IV/PO**[C] +/- **Vancomycin**[E] Enterococcal coverage required[‡] **Ampicillin** + **Gentamicin*** + **Metronidazole IV/PO**[C]	1-2g IV daily 500mg IV/PO q12h 400mg IV q12h/ 500mg PO bid 500mg IV/PO q12h 15mg/kg IV q12h 2g IV q6h 5-7mg/kg IV q24h 500mg IV/PO q12h	Duration of therapy dependent on clinical picture. See Peritonitis.	* Aminoglycosides have good peritoneal penetration but unreliable activity in purulent material. If abscess present, use alternative Gram negative coverage. **No enterococcal coverage. ‡ Enterococcal coverage is recommended if: • healthcare-associated infection • distal colon surgery • hepatobiliary/pancreatic infection (increased risk of Enterococcal bacteremia) • valvular heart disease or prosthetic intravascular materials • patients with chronic illness or immunosuppression • previous antibiotic therapy (excluding surgical prophylaxis) • Enterococcus is a predominant organism in culture. † Due to significant ciprofloxacin resistance in E. coli, this regimen should only be used if cephalosporin or severe penicillin allergy.

E. Desired vancomycin trough is 10-20mg/L. Monitor renal function closely. See Vancomycin Dosing & Monitoring Guidelines.

RECOMMENDED EMPIRIC THERAPY OF SELECTED INFECTIONS IN ADULT PATIENTS[A]

Infection	Usual Pathogens	Recommended Empiric Therapy	Recommended Dose[B]	Recommended Duration	Comments
Gastrointestinal					
Peritonitis (cont'd) **Secondary peritonitis** (cont'd)	* Enterococcal coverage is recommended if: • healthcare-associated infection • distal colon surgery • hepatobiliary/pancreatic infection (increased risk of Enterococcal bacteremia) • valvular heart disease or prosthetic intravascular materials • patients with chronic illness or immunosuppression • previous antibiotic therapy (excluding surgical prophylaxis) • Enterococcus is a predominant organism in culture. **Empiric coverage of Candida spp not recommended unless yeast/Candida on Gram smear/culture **AND** at least one of below: • yeast seen intracellularly or presence of pseudohyphae • patient on immuno-suppressive therapy • multiple previous antibiotics • upper GI tract perforation • postoperative intra-abdominal infection • recurrent intra-abdominal infection. - Add fluconazole if C. albicans or echinocandin (anidulafungin, caspofungin, micafungin) if nonalbicans Candida spp.				
• abscess • bowel perforation • ruptured appendix	Polymicrobial: • Enterobacteriaceae • Enterococcus sp* • Anaerobes • Streptococcus spp • Candida spp**	Severe/ICU **Piperacillin-tazobactam** +/- **Gentamicin***‡ Multiple previous antibiotics**/known ESBL or AmpC **Imipenem**	4.5g IV q8h or 3.375g IV q6h 7mg/kg IV q24h 500mg IV q6h	Duration of therapy dependent on clinical picture. See Peritonitis. Assess need for continuation of gentamicin based on C&S results	‡ Add gentamicin if: • septic shock • recent antibiotic use • suspected ESBL, Amp C, carbapenemase producing organism.

RECOMMENDED EMPIRIC THERAPY OF SELECTED INFECTIONS IN ADULT PATIENTS[A]

Infection	Usual Pathogens	Recommended Empiric Therapy	Recommended Dose[B]	Recommended Duration	Comments
Gastrointestinal					
Peritonitis **Secondary peritonitis** (cont'd) • abscess • bowel perforation • ruptured appendix	Polymicrobial: • Enterobacteriaceae • Enterococcus sp • Anaerobes • Streptococcus spp • Candida spp	Oral switch therapy **Amoxicillin-clavulanate** Severe β-lactam allergy* **Ciprofloxacin** + **Metronidazole**** or **TMP/SMX** + **Metronidazole****	875mg PO bid 500mg PO bid 500mg PO bid 1 DS tab PO bid 500mg PO bid	Duration of therapy dependent on clinical picture. See Peritonitis.	- Switch to oral agents when tolerating oral intake and clinical improvement. * Due to significant resistance in E. coli, these regimens should only be used if cephalosporin or severe penicillin allergy. **No enterococcal coverage.

- 322 -

RECOMMENDED EMPIRIC THERAPY OF SELECTED INFECTIONS IN ADULT PATIENTS[A]

Infection	Usual Pathogens	Recommended Empiric Therapy	Recommended Dose[B]	Recommended Duration	Comments
Gastrointestinal					
Peritonitis (cont'd) Chronic/Tertiary peritonitis	P. aeruginosa Coagulase negative Staph Enterobacteriaceae Enterococcus faecium Candida spp	[Imipenem or Meropenem] + Vancomycin[E] +/- Fluconazole* Tailor according to C&S results	500mg IV q6h 500mg IV q6h or 1g IV q8h 15mg/kg IV q12h 400mg IV/PO daily	Continue antibiotic therapy until patient: • afebrile • normal WBC/ differential • no residual fluid collect- ions. • return of GI function	- All abscess collections require drainage. * Add fluconazole if culture evidence of C. albicans. If nonalbicans Candida, use an echinocandin (anidulafungin, caspofungin, micafungin). - **Persistent peritonitis in patients with multiple organ dysfunction or immunosuppression often does not respond to antibiotic therapy alone.**
Peritoneal dialysis-related peritonitis [Perit Dial Int 2010;30:393-423]	Prevention of catheter infections [Perit Dial Int 2011;31:614-30] - Increased risk for S. aureus infections if: • S. aureus nasal carrier • diabetic • immunocompromised. - Topical mupirocin cream at either the catheter exit site or intranasally, or both, has been recommended to decrease S. aureus exit site infections and peritonitis. Gentamicin cream and Polysporin Triple® antibiotic ointment have also been studied but lead to increased fungal exit site infections and peritonitis, respectively, and are therefore not recommended. Diagnosis • First cloudy effluent should be submitted to laboratory for culture, cell count and differential. • Repeat culture not recommended if cell count decreasing and symptomatic improvement. • If cell count/symptoms not improving, repeat culture within 3 days. If culture negative peritonitis consider: (1) culture volume too small, (2) prior use of antibiotics, (3) unusual causes of peritonitis: mycobacteria; fungi, including lipid-dependent yeast; Legionella spp; slow-growing/fastidious bacteria (e.g. Campylobacter spp, Ureaplasma spp, Mycoplasma spp); enteroviruses. Consult microbiologist.				

E. Desired vancomycin trough is 10-20 mg/L. Monitor renal function closely. See Vancomycin Dosing & Monitoring Guidelines.

RECOMMENDED EMPIRIC THERAPY OF SELECTED INFECTIONS IN ADULT PATIENTS[A]

Infection	Usual Pathogens	Recommended Empiric Therapy	Recommended Dose	Recommended Dose	Comments
Gastrointestinal					

Peritonitis (cont'd) **PD peritonitis** (cont'd) [Perit Dial Int 2010;30:393-423]		Treatment
		- Intraperitoneal (IP) administration of antibiotics superior to IV administration.
		- Empiric therapy should not be based on Gram stain result. Must wait for C&S results to tailor antibiotic therapy. For organism - specific recommendations, see Recommended Therapy of Culture-Directed Infections Table 2.
		- For severely symptomatic peritonitis, 1-3 rapid exchanges of peritoneal dialysis solution prior to longer dwell exchange with intraperitoneal (IP) antibiotics, have been shown to provide symptomatic relief.
		- Recommend program specific evaluation of local susceptibility patterns.
		- Cefazolin + ceftazidime is NOT an optimal empiric regimen for PD peritonitis because:
		  • the use of 2 cephalosporins may be antagonistic
		  • cefazolin and aminoglycoside (AG) combinations may be synergistic against organisms such as coagulase negative Staph
		  • strong association between ceftazidime and selection of β-lactamase mediated resistance in Enterobacteriaceae (both extended spectrum-β-lactamase [ESBL] and inducible (AmpC) β-lactamase).
		- Short courses of aminoglycosides for an episode of PD peritonitis do not adversely affect residual renal function (Am J Kid Dis 2003;41:670-5).
		- Cefepime monotherapy is considered in patients with pre-existing vestibular/cochlear toxicity.
		Cefepime dose (> 100mL urine/24h – increase (maintenance) dose by 25%):
		  • intermittent: 1g once per day
		  • continuous: 500mg/L LD, then 125mg/L MD.
		- Ciprofloxacin no longer recommended empirically due to unacceptably high resistance.
		- If no improvement at 48 hours, reculture and evaluate for exit site/tunnel infection or catheter colonization.
		- Indications for catheter removal:
		  • refractory (failure to clear effluent after 5 days of appropriate antibiotic therapy)/relapsing (within 4 weeks of previous episode with same organism) peritonitis
		  • refractory exit site and tunnel infection
		  • fungal peritonitis
		- Consider catheter removal for:
		  • repeat (more than 4 weeks from previous episode with same organism) peritonitis
		  • mycobacterial peritonitis
		  • polymicrobial peritonitis (high relapse rate, evaluate for intra-abdominal abscess).			

RECOMMENDED EMPIRIC THERAPY OF SELECTED INFECTIONS IN ADULT PATIENTS[A]

Infection	Usual Pathogens	Recommended Empiric Therapy	Recommended Adult Dose	Comments
Gastrointestinal				
Peritonitis (cont'd) **PD peritonitis** (cont'd) [Perit Dial Int 2010;30:393-423]	Coagulase negative Staph S aureus Enterobacteriaceae	**Cefazolin IP** + **Gentamicin IP**[†]	<u>Intermittent Dosing*</u> Dwell time at least 6 hours 15mg/kg once per day** 0.6mg/kg once per day***	- Cefazolin + AG has been shown to have equivalent efficacy as vancomycin + AG as empiric therapy of PD peritonitis. * Dosing recommendations for anuric (<100 mL urine/24 hours) patients. PD patients with residual renal function may require increased doses or more frequent dosing, especially when using intermittent regimens. See treatment guidelines at www.ispd.org/ - For nonanuric patients: ** > 100 mL urine/24 hours - use 20mg/kg cefazolin *** > 100 mL urine/24 hours - increase dose by 25% ‡ > 500 mL urine/24 hours - give every 5 days, or when serum level < 15mg/L. † To optimize concentration-dependent activity of aminoglycosides and lessen potential for toxicity, intermittent dosing is recommended over continuous dosing, especially if aminoglycoside is continued beyond empiric use/based on C&S results.
			<u>Continuous dosing (per L bag)*</u> 500mg/L LD then 125mg/L MD*** 8mg/L LD then 4mg/L MD***	
		<u>Severe penicillin allergy/anaphylaxis/ Cephalosporin allergy/ MRSA colonization</u> **Vancomycin IP** +	15-30mg/kg q 7 days‡ (max 2g/dose)	
		Gentamicin IP[†]	0.6mg/kg once per day***	
			1000mg/L LD then 25mg/L MD*** 8mg/L LD then 4mg/L MD*** LD=loading dose MD=maintenance dose	

RECOMMENDED EMPIRIC THERAPY OF SELECTED INFECTIONS IN ADULT PATIENTS[A]

Infection	Usual Pathogens	Recommended Empiric Therapy	Recommended Dose[B]	Recommended Duration	Comments
Gastrointestinal					
Peritoneal dialysis catheter infections • **exit site** • **tunnel**	- C&S recommended. Tailor antibiotics to results. - Oral antibiotics as effective as intraperitoneal antibiotics. - Catheter removal should be considered if: • unresponsive to adequate course (> 3 wks) of appropriate antibiotics • exit site infection due to P. aeruginosa • tunnel infection • peritonitis (exception: coagulase negative Staph)				
	S. aureus/MRSA* P. aeruginosa	**Cephalexin** + **Ciprofloxacin**	500mg PO bid-tid 500mg PO daily	Continue until exit site looks normal; S. aureus - minimum 2 weeks P. aeruginosa - minimum 3 weeks	* If previous (prior 12 months)/ current MRSA colonization or infection, add TMP/SMX (1 SS tab PO daily) or doxycycline (100mg PO bid).

RECOMMENDED EMPIRIC THERAPY OF SELECTED INFECTIONS IN ADULT PATIENTS[A]

Infection	Usual Pathogens	Recommended Empiric Therapy	Recommended Dose[B]	Recommended Duration	Comments
Genital					
Vulvovaginitis		http://www.phac-aspc.gc.ca/std-mts/sti-its/pdf/408vagdis-eng.pdf <u>Typical features of vulvovaginitis</u> • Candidiasis - increased white, thick, curdy vaginal discharge associated with pruritus, dysuria, and burning. • Trichomoniasis - increased yellow frothy vaginal discharge associated with increased odor, pruritus, and dysuria. • Bacterial vaginosis - increased thin whitish-grey vaginal discharge with increased odor. • Group A Streptococcus - profuse watery yellow vaginal discharge +/- moderate-severe vulvar pain +/- pruritus.			
Candidiasis **Asymptomatic**	Candida spp Occasionally non-albicans spp	Treatment not necessary if asymptomatic			
Symptomatic **Uncomplicated**		**Fluconazole** or	150mg PO	1 dose*	* May be repeated in 72 hours if symptoms remain.
		Clotrimazole **2% cream** or **10% cream** or **tablet**	5g intravag hs 5g intravag hs 200mg intravag hs **or** 500mg intravag hs	3 days 1 dose 3 days 1 dose	- Treat male partner (only if Candida balanitis present) with topical azole bid x 7 days.
		or **Miconazole** **ovule** **ovule** **4% cream**	1200mg intravag hs 400mg intravag hs 5g intravag hs	1 dose 3 days 3 days	
		or **Terconazole** **0.8% cream** or **ovule**	5g intravag hs 80mg intravag hs	3 days 3 days	
		or **Butoconazole** **2% cream**	5g intravag hs	1 dose	

RECOMMENDED EMPIRIC THERAPY OF SELECTED INFECTIONS IN ADULT PATIENTS[A]

Infection	Usual Pathogens	Recommended Empiric Therapy	Recommended Dose[B]	Recommended Duration	Comments
Genital					
Vulvovaginitis (cont'd)					
Candidiasis (cont'd)	http://www.phac-aspc.gc.ca/std-mts/sti-its/pdf/408vagdis-eng.pdf				
Symptomatic Complicated Severe**	Candida spp Occasionally non-albicans spp	**Fluconazole#** or **Intravaginal azole**	150mg PO q72h See Symptomatic-Uncomplicated	2 doses 10-14 days	****Severe:** extensive vulvar erythema, edema, excoriation or fissure formation. # Fluconazole (long term use) and boric acid contraindicated in pregnancy.
Recurrent***		<u>Induction treatment</u> **Fluconazole#** or **Intravaginal azole** or **Boric acid#†** plus <u>Maintenance treatment</u> **Fluconazole#** or **Clotrimazole tablet** or **Boric acid#†**	150mg PO q72h See Symptomatic-Uncomplicated 300-600mg intravag daily 150mg PO weekly 500mg intravag monthly 300mg intravag daily x first 5 days of menstrual cycle	3 doses 10-14 days 14 days minimum 6 months minimum 6 months minimum 6 months	*****Recurrent:** ≥ 4 episodes in 12 months. Treatment requires induction, followed by a minimum of 6 months maintenance treatment. For those patients who require a course of antibiotics, prophylactic intravaginal or oral azole can be given at start of antibiotic course and once weekly during remainder of antibiotic course. Consider investigation for: • diabetes • HIV infection and ask lab to speciate Candida and perform susceptibility testing. † Pharmacy compounded product - boric acid powder in gelatin capsules. NB: Boric acid may cause vulvovaginal irritation.

RECOMMENDED EMPIRIC THERAPY OF SELECTED INFECTIONS IN ADULT PATIENTS[A]

Infection	Usual Pathogens	Recommended Empiric Therapy	Recommended DoseB	Recommended Duration	Comments
Genital					
Vulvovaginitis (cont'd)					
Candidiasis (cont'd)					
Symptomatic (cont'd)					
Complicated (cont'd)					
Pregnancy#	Candida spp Occasionally non-albicans spp				# Fluconazole (long term use) and boric acid contraindicated in pregnancy.
		Clotrimazole 2% cream or **tablet**	5g intravag hs 200mg intravag hs	7 days 7 days	
		or **Miconazole 4% cream** or **ovule**	5g intravag hs 400mg intravag hs	7 days 7 days	
		or **Terconazole 0.8% cream** or **ovule**	5g intravag hs 80mg intravag hs	7 days 7 days	
		or **Butoconazole 2% cream**	5g intravag hs	7 days	
Non-albicans Candida	Non-albicans Candida spp	**Boric acid#‡**	600mg intravag daily	14 days	† Pharmacy compounded product - boric acid powder in gelatin capsules. NB: Boric acid may cause vulvovaginal irritation. ‡ Chronic corticosteroid use, uncontrolled diabetes.
Compromised host‡	Candida spp Occasionally non-albicans spp	**Intravaginal azole** or **Boric acid#†**	See Symptomatic-Uncomplicated 600mg intravag daily	10-14 days 14 days	

Infection	Usual Pathogens	Recommended Empiric Therapy	Recommended Dose[B]	Recommended Duration	Comments
Genital					
Vulvovaginitis (cont'd) **Trichomoniasis**	http://www.phac-aspc.gc.ca/std-mts/sti-its/pdf/408vagdis-eng.pdf - Trichomoniasis may be associated with: • premature rupture of membranes (PROM) • preterm birth • low birth weig • HIV transmission • PI.				
	T. vaginalis	**Metronidazole***	2g PO	1 dose	- Treat all cases and their sexual partners regardless of symptoms. * Intravaginal metronidazole gel is NOT effective. - For metronidazole allergy/ intolerance, see Am J Obstet Gynecol 2008;198:e1370-77 for incremental dosing protocol for metronidazole. - Some (~5%) metronidazole resistance. **For cases unresponsive to longer course metronidazole, high dose oral metronidazole and intravaginal metronidazole gel has been successful [CID 2007;44(suppl 3);S123-9] however significant toxicity, including peripheral neuropathy, neutropenia, and pancreatitis may occur. Consult Infectious Diseases/STI specialist.
		<u>Failure/recurrence**</u> **Metronidazole**	500mg PO bid or 2g PO daily	7 days 3-5 days	

RECOMMENDED EMPIRIC THERAPY OF SELECTED INFECTIONS IN ADULT PATIENTS[A]

Infection	Usual Pathogens	Recommended Empiric Therapy	Recommended Dose[B]	Recommended Duration	Comments
Genital					
Vulvovaginitis (cont'd) **Bacterial vaginosis (BV)**		http://www.phac-aspc.gc.ca/std-mts/sti-its/pdf/408vagdis-eng.pdf			
	Non-inflammatory alteration of normal vaginal flora: • ↓ Lactobacillus spp • ↑ Gardnerella vaginalis • ↑ Mycoplasma hominis • ↑ Mobiluncus spp & other anaerobes	**Asymptomatic** Treatment not required unless: • high-risk pregnancy (previous pre-term delivery) • pre-IUD insertion • pre-gynecologic surgery or upper tract instrumentation • pre-induced abortion			- Risk for BV: • new and/or multiple sex partners (male/female) • lack of condom use • douching. - Treatment of male sexual partner not recommended.
		Symptomatic **Metronidazole tablet** or **0.75% intravag gel†** or **Clindamycin 2% cream***	500mg PO bid 5g intravag hs 5g intravag hs	7 days 5 days 7 days	Pregnancy: - No need to screen and/or treat low-risk pregnant women. - Treatment of asymptomatic BV in women with previous preterm birth may reduce the risk of preterm premature rupture of membranes and stillbirth. † Nidagel® NOT Metrogel®
		Alternative **Clindamycin** or **Metronidazole**	300mg PO bid 2g PO**	7 days 1 dose	*Clindamycin cream is oil based and may weaken latex condoms. **2g single metronidazole dose is an alternative but has a higher rate of relapse (50%).
		Pregnancy***/Lactation **Metronidazole** **Alternative**** **Clindamycin**	500mg PO bid 300mg PO bid	7 days 7 days	***Intravaginal agents not recommended in pregnancy (not effective in preventing pre-term delivery).

RECOMMENDED EMPIRIC THERAPY OF SELECTED INFECTIONS IN ADULT PATIENTS[A]

Infection	Usual Pathogens	Recommended Empiric Therapy	Recommended Dose[B]	Recommended Duration	Comments
Genital					
Vulvovaginitis (cont'd)					
Group A Streptococcus (GAS) [Clin Infect Dis 2008;46:e112-5]	S. pyogenes (Group A Streptococcus)	**Penicillin VK** Alternative **Clindamycin**	600mg PO bid 300mg PO tid	10 days 10 days	- Increased risk for GAS vulvovaginitis: • prepubertal • postpartum • postmenopausal. - Often related to current/recent case or household outbreak of respiratory/dermal GAS infection.

RECOMMENDED EMPIRIC THERAPY OF SELECTED INFECTIONS IN ADULT PATIENTS[A]

Infection	Usual Pathogens	Recommended Empiric Therapy	Recommended Dose[B]	Recommended Duration	Comments
Genital					

Cervicitis
[Clin Infect Dis 2007;44(suppl 3) S102-10]
	- Two most common causes are Chlamydia trachomatis and N. gonorrhoeae. Other etiologies include:
	  • Trichomonas vaginalis
	  • Herpes simplex
	  • Cytomegalovirus
	  • bacterial vaginosis
	  • Mycoplasma genitalium
	  • S. agalactiae and S. pyogenes
	  • chemical douches/spermicides.
	- For all women with cervicitis recommend test and treat, if positive, for concomitant vaginal conditions especially BV and Trichomonas vaginalis, and consider genital herpes.
	- Diagnosis: NAAT recommended for both Chlamydia trachomatis and Neisseria gonorrhoeae.
	- Test and treat regardless of clinical signs/symptoms, all recent (60 days) sexual contacts. Patients should abstain from sexual intercourse during, and for 7 days after therapy, and until all their sexual partners are treated. Repeat treatment if re-exposed to untreated partner.			

Chlamydia*
http://www.phac-aspc.gc.ca/std-mts/sti-its/pdf/502chlamydia-eng.pdf
	Chlamydia trachomatis	**Azithromycin**
		or
		Doxycycline
		or
		Ofloxacin
		
		Pregnancy/Lactation
		Amoxicillin
		or
		Azithromycin
		or
		Erythromycin base (not estolate)**
			1g PO
			100mg PO bid
			300mg PO bid
			
			500mg PO tid
			1g PO
			500mg PO qid
				1 dose
				7 days
				7 days
				
				7 days
				1 dose
				7 days
					* **Must rule out gonorrhea or treat it empirically.**
					**Erythromycin estolate is contra-indicated in pregnancy as it may cause intrahepatic cholestasis.
					- Test of cure recommended (no sooner than 4 weeks post-treatment to avoid false positive results):
					  • where compliance is suboptimal
					  • if regimen other than azithromycin or doxycycline has been used
					  • in all prepubertal children
					  • in all pregnant women.
					- Repeat testing recommended in all cases 6 months post-treatment.

RECOMMENDED EMPIRIC THERAPY OF SELECTED INFECTIONS IN ADULT PATIENTS[A]

Infection	Usual Pathogens	Recommended Empiric Therapy	Recommended Dose[B]	Recommended Duration	Comments
Genital					
Cervicitis (cont'd) Gonococcal*	http://www.phac-aspc.gc.ca/std-mts/sti-its/pdf/506gonococcal-eng.pdf and http://www.phac-aspc.gc.ca/std-mts/sti-its/alert/2011/alert-gono-eng.php Diagnosis: - NAAT recommended for both Chlamydia trachomatis and Neisseria gonorrhoeae. - Endocervical swab for N. gonorrhoeae culture should also be submitted for: • sexual assault (see Prophylaxis, Sexual Assault) • evaluation of PID • treatment failure • infection acquired abroad by patient or sexual contact. - Test and treat, regardless of clinical signs/symptoms, all recent (60 days) sexual contacts. Patients should abstain from sexual intercourse during, and for 7 days after therapy, and until all their sexual partners are treated. Repeat treatment if re-exposed to untreated partner. Test of cure: - Test of cure *by culture* 4-5 days after completion of therapy recommended if: • regimen other than recommended has been used • antimicrobial resistant organism identified on culture • concern over false-positive NAAT result • persistent signs or symptoms post-therapy • concomitant infection at non-genital site (e.g. eye, rectum, pharynx) • PID or disseminated gonococcal infection • uncertain compliance • pregnancy.			

RECOMMENDED EMPIRIC THERAPY OF SELECTED INFECTIONS IN ADULT PATIENTS[A]

Infection	Usual Pathogens	Recommended Empiric Therapy	Recommended Dose[B]	Recommended Duration	Comments
Genital					

Cervicitis (cont'd)
Gonococcal*
http://www.phac-aspc.gc.ca/std-mts/sti-its/pdf/506gonococcal-eng.pdf
and
http://www.phac-aspc.gc.ca/std-mts/sti-its/alert/2011/alert-gono-eng.php
	Neisseria gonorrhoeae	**Cefixime**
		or
		Ceftriaxone
		
		Alternative
		Azithromycin
			800mg PO
			
			250mg IM
			
			2g PO
				1 dose
				
				1 dose
				
				1 dose
					* All patients should also be **treated for chlamydial infection unless treated with azithromycin.**
					- Quinolones no longer recommended due to significant resistance. Ciprofloxacin 500mg PO x 1 dose may be considered if:
					  • penicillin anaphylaxis or cephalosporin allergy AND
					  • contraindications/intolerance/ failure of azithromycin AND
					  • known ciprofloxacin susceptibility.
					Test of cure recommended.

Nonchlamydial/ nongonococcal	Potential etiology: • Mycoplasma genitalium • Trichomonas vaginalis • Bacterial vaginosis • Herpes simplex • Cytomegalovirus	**Azithromycin** or **Doxycycline** Alternative **Erythromycin base** If unresponsive to each of above: **Doxycycline** + **Levofloxacin** +/- **Metronidazole 0.75% intravag gel†**	1g PO 100mg PO bid 500mg PO qid 100mg PO bid 500mg PO daily 5g intravag hs	1 dose 7 days 7 days 7 days 7 days 7 days	- Evaluate history for use of spermicides, deodorants, chemical douches. † Nidagel® NOT Metrogel®

RECOMMENDED EMPIRIC THERAPY OF SELECTED INFECTIONS IN ADULT PATIENTS[A]

Infection	Usual Pathogens	Recommended Empiric Therapy	Recommended Dose[B]	Recommended Duration	Comments
Genital					
Urethritis (male) **Chlamydial*** http://www.phac-aspc.gc.ca/std-mts/sti-its/pdf/502chlamydia-eng.pdf	http://www.phac-aspc.gc.ca/std-mts/sti-its/pdf/407urethritis-eng.pdf Diagnosis: - NAAT recommended for both Chlamydia trachomatis and Neisseria gonorrhoeae. - Test and treat, regardless of clinical signs/symptoms, all recent (60 days) sexual contacts. Patients should abstain from sexual intercourse during, and for 7 days after therapy, and until all their sexual partners are treated. Repeat treatment if re-exposed to untreated partner. - Test of cure recommended (no sooner than 4 weeks post-treatment to avoid false positive results): • where compliance is suboptimal • persistent signs or symptoms post-therapy • if regimen other than azithromycin or doxycycline has been used. - Repeat testing recommended in all cases 6 months post-treatment.			
	Chlamydia trachomatis	**Azithromycin** or **Doxycycline** or **Ofloxacin**	1g PO 100mg PO bid 300mg PO bid	1 dose 7 days 7 days	* **Must rule out gonorrhea or treat it empirically.** See Urethritis, Gonococcal.
		Alternative **Erythromycin base**	500mg PO qid	7 days	

RECOMMENDED EMPIRIC THERAPY OF SELECTED INFECTIONS IN ADULT PATIENTS[A]

Infection	Usual Pathogens	Recommended Empiric Therapy	Recommended Dose[B]	Recommended Duration	Comments
Genital					
Urethritis (male) (cont'd) **Gonococcal***	http://www.phac-aspc.gc.ca/std-mts/sti-its/pdf/506gonococcal-eng.pdf and http://www.phac-aspc.gc.ca/std-mts/sti-its/alert/2011/alert-gono-eng.php Diagnosis: - NAAT recommended for both Chlamydia trachomatis and Neisseria gonorrhoeae. - Urethral swab for N. gonorrhoeae culture should also be submitted for: • men who have sex with men • sexual assault • treatment failure • Infection acquired abroad by patient or sexual contact. - Test and treat, regardless of clinical signs/symptoms, all recent (60 days) sexual contacts. Patients should abstain from sexual intercourse during, and for 7 days after therapy, and until all their sexual partners are treated. Repeat treatment if re-exposed to untreated partner. - Test of cure *by culture* 4-5 days after completion of therapy recommended if: • regimen other than recommended has been used • antimicrobial resistant organism identified on culture • concern over false-positive NAAT result • persistent signs or symptoms post-therapy • concomitant infection at non-genital site (e.g. eye, rectum, pharynx) • disseminated gonococcal infection • uncertain compliance.			

RECOMMENDED EMPIRIC THERAPY OF SELECTED INFECTIONS IN ADULT PATIENTS[A]

Infection	Usual Pathogens	Recommended Empiric Therapy	Recommended Dose[B]	Recommended Duration	Comments
Genital					
Urethritis (male) (cont'd)					
Gonococcal* (cont'd) http://www.phac-aspc.gc.ca/std-mts/sti-its/pdf/506gonococca l-eng.pdf and http://www.phac-aspc.gc.ca/std-mts/sti-its/alert/2011/alert-gono-eng.php	Neisseria gonorrhoeae	**Cefixime** or **Ceftriaxone**** _Alternative_ **Azithromycin**	800mg PO 250mg IM 2g PO	1 dose 1 dose 1 dose	* All patients should also be treated for chlamydial infection unless treated with azithromycin. **Ceftriaxone is the preferred treatment in men who have sex with men. - Quinolones no longer recommended due to significant resistance. Ciprofloxacin 500mg PO x 1 dose may be considered if: • penicillin anaphylaxis or cephalosporin allergy AND • contraindications/intolerance/ failure of azithromycin AND • known ciprofloxacin susceptibility. Test of cure recommended.
Nonchlamydial/ nongonococcal		**Azithromycin** or **Doxycycline** _Alternative_ **Erythromycin base**	1g PO 100mg PO bid 500mg PO qid	1 dose 7 days 7 days	

- 338 -

RECOMMENDED EMPIRIC THERAPY OF SELECTED INFECTIONS IN ADULT PATIENTS[A]

Infection	Usual Pathogens	Recommended Empiric Therapy	Recommended Dose[B]	Recommended Duration	Comments
Genital					
Epididymo-orchitis*	http://www.phac-aspc.gc.ca/std-mts/sti-its/pdf/402epididymiti-eng.pdf - Usual presentation of acute epididymitis is unilateral testicular pain and tenderness of gradual onset +/- symptoms of urethritis or urethral discharge. * Important to rule out torsion of testis (surgical emergency) or tumour.				
Sexually transmitted - usually age < 35 years	Chlamydia trachomatis Neisseria gonorrhoeae Rare: • Enterobacteria-ceae • P. aeruginosa • M. tuberculosis	**Ceftriaxone** + **Doxycycline** Alternative **Ciprofloxacin**** + **Doxycycline**	250mg IM 100mg PO bid 500mg PO 100mg PO bid	1 dose 10-14 days 1 dose 10-14 days	- For suspected sexually transmitted infection, combination therapy for both gonorrhea & chlamydia recommended. **Quinolones no longer recommended due to significant gonococcal resistance. Ciprofloxacin regimen may be considered if: • penicillin anaphylaxis or cephalosporin allergy AND • known ciprofloxacin susceptibility. Test of cure recommended.
Non-sexually transmitted - usually age > 35 years	Enterobacteriaceae P. aeruginosa Rare: • N. gonorrhoeae • C. trachomatis • M. tuberculosis	**Ciprofloxacin** or **Ofloxacin** Severe/hospitalized **Ciprofloxacin IV/PO**[D] or **Piperacillin-tazobactam*****	500mg PO bid 200mg PO bid 400mg IV q12h/ 500mg PO bid 3.375g IV q6h	14 days 14 days 14 days 14 days	- Risk factors for non-sexually transmitted infections: • chronic bacterial prostatitis • recent urinary tract instrumentation or surgery • anatomical abnormalities of urinary tract. ***Piperacillin-tazobactam preferred if received quinolones in previous 3 months.

RECOMMENDED EMPIRIC THERAPY OF SELECTED INFECTIONS IN ADULT PATIENTS[A]

Infection	Usual Pathogens	Recommended Empiric Therapy	Recommended Dose[B]	Recommended Duration	Comments
Genital					
Pelvic inflammatory disease (PID) http://www.phac-aspc.gc.ca/std-mts/sti-its/pdf/404pelviinfla-eng.pdf and http://www.cdc.gov/std/treatment/2010/pid.htm	- Differential diagnosis of lower abdominal pain: • gynecologic disease or dysfunction (complications of pregnancy, acute infections, endometriosis, adnexal disorders, menstrual disorders) • gastrointestinal (appendicitis, gastroenteritis, inflammatory bowel disease) • genitourinary (cystitis, pyelonephritis, nephrolithiasis) • musculoskeletal • neurologic causes. - The most common infectious cause of lower abdominal pain in women is PID. - Only one-third of women with PID have temperature > 38°C. - Recommend pregnancy test to rule out ectopic pregnancy. - Screen for HIV and syphilis. Immunize against hepatitis B if not already immune.				

RECOMMENDED EMPIRIC THERAPY OF SELECTED INFECTIONS IN ADULT PATIENTS[A]

Infection	Usual Pathogens	Recommended Empiric Therapy	Recommended Dose[B]	Recommended Duration	Comments
Genital					
Pelvic inflammatory disease (PID) (cont'd) **Mild-moderate, non-hospitalized**	N. gonorrhoeae C. trachomatis Polymicrobial: • Enterobacteriaceae • Anaerobes • Streptococcus spp • Haemophilus spp • Gardnerella vaginalis • Mycoplasma spp • Ureaplasma urealyticum Rare: • Herpes simplex virus • Trichomonas vaginalis	**Ceftriaxone + Doxycycline** +/- **Metronidazole*** Alternative [**Levofloxacin** or **Ofloxacin**]** +/- [**Metronidazole** or **Clindamycin**]*	250mg IM 100mg PO bid 500mg PO bid 500mg PO daily 400mg PO bid 500mg PO bid 300mg PO qid	1 dose 14 days 14 days 14 days 14 days 14 days 14 days	- Test and treat, regardless of clinical signs/symptoms, all recent (60 days) sexual contacts. - If patient has IUD, remove soon after therapy is initiated. * Add metronidazole (clindamycin is an alternative but significant anaerobic resistance) for women at higher risk of anaerobic infection if: • adnexal mass/tubo-ovarian abscess • peritonitis • presence of IUD • previous history of PID • presence of bacterial vaginosis • HIV co-infection. **Quinolones no longer recommended due to significant gonococcal resistance. Ciprofloxacin regimen may be considered if: • penicillin anaphylaxis or cephalosporin allergy AND • known quinolone susceptibility. Test of cure recommended.

RECOMMENDED EMPIRIC THERAPY OF SELECTED INFECTIONS IN ADULT PATIENTS[A]

Infection	Usual Pathogens	Recommended Empiric Therapy	Recommended Dose[B]	Recommended Duration	Comments
Genital					

Pelvic inflammatory disease (PID) (cont'd)
Moderate-severe
		- Hospitalization should be considered if:
		  • severe illness or high fever present
		  • not responding to therapy (72 hours)
		  • unable to tolerate oral medications or noncompliant
		  • pregnant
		  • advanced HIV (CD_4 < 200)
		  • adnexal mass/tubo-ovarian abscess
		  • need for laparoscopy to clarify diagnosis i.e. to rule out acute appendicitis.			

RECOMMENDED EMPIRIC THERAPY OF SELECTED INFECTIONS IN ADULT PATIENTS[A]

Infection	Usual Pathogens	Recommended Empiric Therapy	Recommended Dose[B]	Recommended Duration	Comments
Genital					
Pelvic inflammatory disease (cont'd) **Moderate-severe** (cont'd)	N. gonorrhoeae C. trachomatis Polymicrobial: • Enterobacteriaceae • Anaerobes • Streptococcus spp • Haemophilus vaginalis • Gardnerella vaginalis • Mycoplasma spp • Ureaplasma urealyticum Rare: • Herpes simplex virus • Trichomonas vaginalis	[Ceftriaxone + Doxycycline + Metronidazole] or [Cefoxitin + Doxycycline][†] β-lactam allergy Clindamycin + Gentamicin Severe Piperacillin-tazobactam + Doxycycline Oral stepdown Doxycycline +/- Metronidazole* Alternative [Levofloxacin or Ofloxacin] + Azithromycin + [Metronidazole or Clindamycin]*	1-2g IV daily 100mg IV/PO bid 500mg IV/PO bid 2g IV q6h 100mg IV/PO bid 600mg IV q8h 5-7mg/kg IV q24h 4.5g IV q8h or 3.375g IV q6h 100mg IV/PO bid 100mg PO bid 500mg PO bid 500-750mg PO daily 400mg PO bid 2g PO 500mg PO bid 300mg PO qid	Until 24 hours after clinical improvement then switch to oral Until 24 hours after clinical improvement then switch to oral Until 24 hours after clinical improvement then switch to oral Until 24 hours after clinical improvement then switch to oral To complete at least 14 days To complete at least 14 days To complete at least 14 days 1 dose To complete at least 14 days	- If patient has IUD, remove soon after therapy is initiated. † Listed as alternative as anaerobic coverage not optimal and does not treat bacterial vaginosis. * Add metronidazole (clindamycin is an alternative but significant anaerobic resistance) for women at higher risk of anaerobic infection if: • adnexal mass/tubo-ovarian abscess • peritonitis • presence of IUD • previous history of PID • presence of bacterial vaginosis • HIV co-infection.

- 343 -

RECOMMENDED EMPIRIC THERAPY OF SELECTED INFECTIONS IN ADULT PATIENTS[A]

Infection	Usual Pathogens	Recommended Empiric Therapy	Recommended Dose[B]	Recommended Duration	Comments
Genital					
Pelvic inflammatory disease/ chorioamnionitis Pregnancy • **1st trimester*** (see PID) • **2nd/3rd trimester**		* PID in 1st trimester is rare. See PID section for management. After 1st trimester, should be considered as chorioamnionitis. - Hospitalization should be considered for all pregnant patients with suspect PID/chorioamnionitis. - Evacuation of uterus may be required for cure. Refer patient to specialist obstetrician. - If chlamydia or gonorrhea suspected/documented, refer to these sections for management. - If preterm labour with intact membranes and delivery imminent, give Group B Streptococcus (GBS) prophylaxis (see Intrapartum Antimicrobial Prophylaxis of GBS). - If premature rupture of membranes (PROM) and < 37 weeks and pregnancy to continue, give prophylactic erythromycin and amoxicillin (see Antimicrobial Prophylaxis for PROM).			
	1st trimester: N. gonorrhoeae C. trachomatis Mycoplasma spp Polymicrobial	**Clindamycin + Gentamicin**	600mg IV q8h 5-7mg/kg IV q24h	Until afebrile for 48-72 hours after evacuation/delivery of fetus.	
	2nd/3rd trimester: S. agalactiae (Group B Streptococcus)	_Alternative_ [**Ceftriaxone + Metronidazole + Erythromycin base***]	1-2g IV daily 500mg IV/PO bid 250mg PO qid	Until afebrile for 48-72 hours after evacuation/delivery of fetus.	* Do not use the estolate formulation in pregnancy as it may cause intrahepatic cholestasis.
	Rare : • S. pyogenes (Group A Streptococcus) • S. pneumoniae • Haemophilus spp	or [**Cefoxitin + Erythromycin base***]	2g IV q6h 250mg PO qid	Until afebrile for 48-72 hours after evacuation/delivery of fetus.	

RECOMMENDED EMPIRIC THERAPY OF SELECTED INFECTIONS IN ADULT PATIENTS[A]

Infection	Usual Pathogens	Recommended Empiric Therapy	Recommended Dose[B]	Recommended Duration	Comments
Genital					
Endometritis Postpartum Early (< 2 days)	Anaerobes S. agalactiae (Group B Streptococcus) S. pyogenes (Group A Streptococcus) Viridans Group Streptococci Enterobacteriaceae Chlamydia trachomatis Mycoplasma spp	[Ceftriaxone + Doxycycline + Metronidazole] or [Cefoxitin + Doxycycline] <u>Alternative</u> Clindamycin + Gentamicin <u>Oral therapy</u> Doxycycline + Metronidazole or Clindamycin alone	1-2g IV daily 100mg IV/PO bid 500mg IV/PO bid 2g IV q6h 100mg IV/PO bid 600mg IV q8h 5-7mg/kg IV q24h 100mg PO bid 500mg PO bid 450mg PO qid	IV +/- PO - until 48 hours after afebrile and clinical improvement. IV +/- PO - until 48 hours after afebrile and clinical improvement. IV +/- PO - until 48 hours after afebrile and clinical improvement.	- Early postpartum endometritis usually occurs after caesarean section.
Late (2 days - 6 weeks)	Chlamydia trachomatis Mycoplasma spp	Doxycycline	100mg PO bid	14 days	- Late postpartum endometritis usually occurs after vaginal delivery.
Septic pelvic vein thrombophlebitis (postpartum, post pelvic surgery, post abortion)	Polymicrobial: • Anaerobes • Viridans Group Streptococci • β-haemolytic Streptococci • Enterobacteriaceae	Ceftriaxone + [Metronidazole IV/PO[C] or Clindamycin] <u>Alternative</u> Imipenem or Ertapenem	2g IV daily 500mg IV/PO q12h 600mg IV q8h/ 300mg PO qid 500mg IV q6h 1g IV daily	4-6 weeks 4-6 weeks 4-6 weeks	- Check for pulmonary emboli. - Heparin therapy recommended along with antibiotics. - Ertapenem has not been studied in this clinical setting but has appropriate coverage of organisms involved.

RECOMMENDED EMPIRIC THERAPY OF SELECTED INFECTIONS IN ADULT PATIENTS[A]

Infection	Usual Pathogens	Recommended Empiric Therapy	Recommended Dose[B]	Recommended Duration	Comments
Genital					
Labial abscess	S. aureus/MRSA* β-haemolytic Strep (group A,B,C,G) Enterobacteriaceae Anaerobes	**Amoxicillin-clavulanate*** or [**Cephalexin +** **Metronidazole**]* β-lactam allergy* **Clindamycin +** **Ciprofloxacin**	875mg PO bid 500mg PO qid 500mg PO bid 300mg PO qid 500mg PO bid	5-7 days 5-7 days 5-7 days	- Recommend drainage of abscess. * If MRSA colonization/infection (in prior 12 mos) or high endemic rate of MRSA, add TMP/SMX or doxycycline.
Prostatitis	http://www.phac-aspc.gc.ca/std-mts/sti-its/pdf/405prostati-eng.pdf Prostatitis syndromes: • Acute bacterial prostatitis - severe symptoms, systemic infection. acute bacterial urinary tract infection. • Chronic bacterial prostatitis - chronic bacterial infection of prostate +/- signs/symptoms of prostatitis. Usually in setting of recurrent urinary tract infection (same strain). • Chronic pelvic pain syndrome - chronic pelvic pain +/- dysuria in absence of urinary tract infection. May be categorized as inflammatory or noninflammatory. • Asymptomatic inflammatory prostatitis - incidental finding (evaluation for infertility, elevated PSA) of inflammation of prostate in absense of genitourinary tract symptoms. Atypical causes of prostatitis to consider: - Chlamydia trachomatis - Trichomonas vaginalis - Ureaplasma urealyticum - Mycoplasma genitalium - Neisseria gonorrhoeae - Brucella spp (rare) - Mycobacterium tuberculosis - Fungal pathogens: • Candida spp • Coccidioides immitis • Blastomyces dermatiditis • Histoplasma capsulatum - Viral pathogens				

RECOMMENDED EMPIRIC THERAPY OF SELECTED INFECTIONS IN ADULT PATIENTS[A]

Infection	Usual Pathogens	Recommended Empiric Therapy	Recommended Dose[B]	Recommended Duration	Comments
Genital					
Prostatitis (cont'd) **Acute bacterial**	Enterobacteriaceae Enterococcus spp P. aeruginosa* Rare: • Staphylococcus spp • Streptococcus spp	Mild-moderate **Ciprofloxacin** or **Ofloxacin** or **TMP/SMX** or [**Ampicillin + Gentamicin**] Severe **Piperacillin-tazobactam**	500-750mg PO bid 400mg PO bid 1 DS tab PO bid 2g IV q6h 5-7mg/kg IV q24h 4.5g IV q6h	2-4 weeks** 2-4 weeks** 2-4 weeks** Switch to oral agents when clinical improvement to complete 2-4 weeks** Switch to oral agents when clinical improvement to complete 4 weeks	- In men with recurrent UTI due to the same organism, the prostate may be the source. - Submit urine for C. trachomatis and N. gonorrhoeae NAAT. * Nosocomial acquisition more likely to be P. aeruginosa. **Treat for 4 weeks if patient remains symptomatic at 2 weeks.
Chronic bacterial (symptoms > 3 months)	Enterobacteriaceae Enterococcus spp Pseudomonas aeruginosa* Rare: • Staphylococcus spp • Streptococcus spp	**Ciprofloxacin** or **Ofloxacin** or **TMP/SMX** or **Doxycycline**	500-750mg PO bid 400mg PO bid 1 DS tab PO bid 100mg PO bid	4-6 weeks* 4-6 weeks* 4-6 weeks* 4-6 weeks*	* If no response in 4-6 weeks, consult urologist. Occasionally infected prostatic calculi. Longer therapy (up to 12 weeks) may be required if patient remains symptomatic or non-quinolone therapy is used.
Chronic prostatitis/Chronic pelvic pain syndrome	- Symptoms of discomfort/pain in pelvic region for at least 3 months in the absence of uropathogenic bacteria. - The use of antibiotics in this condition is controversial. Some experts recommend a single 4 week course of antibiotics. Repeat courses of antibiotics are not indicated.				

- 347 -

RECOMMENDED EMPIRIC THERAPY OF SELECTED INFECTIONS IN ADULT PATIENTS[A]

Infection	Usual Pathogens	Recommended Empiric Therapy	Recommended Dose[B]	Recommended Duration	Comments
Genital					
Proctitis	N. gonorrhoeae C. trachomatis	See Urethritis			
	Herpes simplex virus (HSV)	Primary episode Severe **Acyclovir**	5mg/kg IV q8h	Switch to oral therapy when clinical improvement to complete course of therapy:	- No role for topical acyclovir.
		Mild-moderate **Valacyclovir** or **Acyclovir** or **Famciclovir**	1g PO bid 400mg PO tid 250mg PO tid	7-10 days 7-10 days 5-7 days	
		Recurrent See Genital Herpes - recurrent			
	Lymphogranuloma venereum (LGV)	See LGV			- Increasing incidence of LGV proctitis in men who have sex with men.
Genital ulcers/lesions	http://www.phac-aspc.gc.ca/std-mts/sti-its/pdf/405prostati-eng.pdf - For all patients presenting with genital ulcers, recommend testing for HIV and other STIs as appropriate. - Genital ulcers/lesions increase acquisition of HIV twofold.				

RECOMMENDED EMPIRIC THERAPY OF SELECTED INFECTIONS IN ADULT PATIENTS[A]

Genital Ulcers

[http://www.phac-aspc.gc.ca/std-mts/sti-its/pdf/403gud-ug-eng.pdf]

	Clinical	Diagnosis
Herpes simplex virus (HSV)	- multiple vesicular lesions that rupture, become painful shallow ulcers - constitutional symptoms/lymphadenopathy - atypical presentation includes: fissures, furuncles, patchy erythema, linear ulcerations or excoriations. Also consider HSV if lesions on lower abdomen, buttocks or thighs. - Increased incidence of HSV-1 genital ulcers.	- Ulcer scraping/vesicular lesion for Herpes culture/PCR. Unroof vesicle, rotate sterile Dacron/rayon swab firmly in base of lesion. Sample more than 1 lesion. Insert swab in viral transport medium.
Syphilis	- typically single painless well demarcated ulcer (chancre) with clean base/ indurated border - may be multiple/painful (up to 30% co-infected with HSV)	- Darkfield microscopy/direct fluorescent antibody test or serology (nontreponemal and treponemal tests) ± syphilis PCR (where available).
Chancroid	- nonindurated, painful with serpiginous border, friable base covered with necrotic/purulent exudate - tender, suppurative unilateral inguinal lymphadenopathy.	- Gram stain of lesion - Gram negative slender rod/coccobacilli in "school of fish" pattern. - H. ducreyi culture or PCR- consult microbiologist.
Lymphogranuloma venereum	- small shallow painless genital/rectal papule or ulcer - no induration - unilateral tender inguinal/femoral lymphadenopathy - rectal bleeding/pain/discharge - ulcerative proctitis	- CT NAAT or culture for Chlamydia - Positive Chlamydia NAAT or culture can be sent for typing for LGV serovars L1, L2, L3 - consult microbiologist.
Granuloma inguinale (donovanosis)	- persistent painless beefy red (highly vascular) papules/ulcers; may be hypertrophic/necrotic/sclerotic +/- subcutaneous granulomas - no lymphadenopathy	- Intracytoplasmic Donovan bodies on Wright stain or positive Giemsa stain - Biopsy of lesion - Consult microbiologist
Behcet's syndrome	- recurrent aphthous ulcers (> 3 per year) in association with recurrent genital ulcers +/- eye lesions (uveitis)/cutaneous lesions (erythema nodosum)	- Rheumatoid factor/antinuclear antibody testing - Biopsy demonstrating diffuse arteritis/venulitis. - Consult rheumatologist
Drug eruptions	- Ulcers resolve with discontinuation of drug (NSAIDS, antimalarials, ACE inhibitors, B-blockers, lithium, salicylates, corticosteroids)	- Careful drug history - Symptoms resolve when offending agent discontinued.

RECOMMENDED EMPIRIC THERAPY OF SELECTED INFECTIONS IN ADULT PATIENTS[A]

Infection	Usual Pathogens	Recommended Empiric Therapy	Recommended Dose[B]	Recommended Duration	Comments
Genital					
Genital ulcers/lesions (cont'd)					
Herpes		http://www.phac-aspc.gc.ca/std-mts/sti-its/pdf/504genherp-vhs-eng.pdf			
Primary episode	Herpes simplex II Herpes simplex I	Severe*/hospitalized **Acyclovir**	5mg/kg IV q8h	Switch to oral therapy when clinical improvement to complete course of therapy:	* Severe herpes infection: • disseminated • pneumonitis • hepatitis • meningitis/encephalitis • sacral radiculitis. <u>NB</u>: Therapy ideally should be initiated within 72 hours of onset of symptoms. - **No role for topical acyclovir.**
		Mild-moderate **Valacyclovir** or **Acyclovir** or **Famciclovir**	1g PO bid 400mg PO tid 250mg PO tid	7-10 days 7-10 days 5-7 days	

RECOMMENDED EMPIRIC THERAPY OF SELECTED INFECTIONS IN ADULT PATIENTS[A]

Infection	Usual Pathogens	Recommended Empiric Therapy	Recommended Dose[B]	Recommended Duration	Comments
Genital					
Genital ulcers/lesions (cont'd) **Herpes** (cont'd) **Recurrent**	Herpes simplex II Herpes simplex I	<u>Mild/infrequent*</u> No therapy			* For patients who have occasional mild recurrences.
		<u>Episodic</u> **Famciclovir** or **Valacyclovir**	125mg PO bid or 1000mg PO bid 500mg PO bid or 1000mg PO daily	5 days 1 day 3 days 3 days	- For patients with infrequent (< 6 episodes/year) moderate to severe recurrences with prodrome. **Must have:** • drug on hand • compliant patient • initiation of therapy within hours of prodromal symptoms (maximum 24 hours). **No proven efficacy if started after 24 hours.**
		<u>Alternative</u> **Acyclovir**	400mg PO tid or 800mg PO tid	5 days 2 days	
		<u>Suppressive**</u> **Acyclovir** or **Famciclovir** or **Valacyclovir**	400mg PO bid 250mg PO bid 6-9 episodes/year 500mg PO daily ≥10 episodes/year 1g PO daily	6-12 months 6-12 months 6-12 months 6-12 months	**For patients who have frequent (≥ 6 episodes/year) moderate to severe recurrences. - If symptom free for 6-12 months, reassess rate of recurrences and need for continuing suppressive therapy.

RECOMMENDED EMPIRIC THERAPY OF SELECTED INFECTIONS IN ADULT PATIENTS[A]

Infection	Usual Pathogens	Recommended Empiric Therapy	Recommended Dose[B]	Recommended Duration	Comments
Genital					
Genital ulcers/lesions (cont'd)					
Herpes (cont'd)					
Recurrent (cont'd)	Herpes simplex II	Episodic			
Immuno-compromised	Herpes simplex I	**Famciclovir**	500mg PO bid	5-10 days	
		or			
		Valacyclovir	1000mg PO bid	5-10 days	
		or			
		Acyclovir	400mg PO tid	5-10 days	
		<u>Suppressive</u>			
		Acyclovir	400-800mg PO bid-tid	6-12 months	
		or			
		Famciclovir	500mg PO bid	6-12 months	
		or			
		Valacyclovir	500mg PO bid	6-12 months	

- 352 -

RECOMMENDED EMPIRIC THERAPY OF SELECTED INFECTIONS IN ADULT PATIENTS[A]

Infection	Usual Pathogens	Recommended Empiric Therapy	Recommended Dose[B]	Recommended Duration	Comments
Genital					

Genital ulcers/lesions (cont'd)
Herpes (cont'd)
Pregnancy
	- Early pregnancy:
	  • no data that acyclovir will prevent congenital herpes (rare event).
	  • Infectious Diseases consult recommended.
	- Late pregnancy:
	  • Primary episode → 50% risk of transmission to infant.
	  • Recurrent → maximum 4% risk to infant.
	  • HSV infection in infant has 50% mortality.
	- If active lesions at time of labour, caesarean section recommended.				

Primary episode	Herpes simplex II Herpes simplex I	**Acyclovir** or **Acyclovir** or **Valacyclovir**	5mg/kg IV q8h 400mg PO tid 1g PO bid	Switch to oral therapy when clinical improvement to complete course of therapy: 7-10 days 7-10 days	- Acyclovir and valacyclovir are safe in pregnancy.
Recurrent	Herpes simplex II Herpes simplex I	**Acyclovir** or **Valacyclovir**	400mg PO tid 500mg PO bid	Continue until delivery Continue until delivery	- If previous recurrent disease but no outbreaks during pregnancy, suppressive therapy with acyclovir beginning at 36 weeks gestation until delivery is recommended to prevent recurrence at time of delivery, decrease risk of viral shedding and need for caesarean due to HSV. - Acyclovir and valacyclovir are safe in pregnancy.

RECOMMENDED EMPIRIC THERAPY OF SELECTED INFECTIONS IN ADULT PATIENTS[A]

Infection	Usual Pathogens	Recommended Empiric Therapy	Recommended Dose[B]	Recommended Duration	Comments
Genital					
Genital ulcers/ lesions (cont'd) **Syphilis**	http://www.phac-aspc.gc.ca/std-mts/sti-its/pdf/510syphilis-eng.pdf **Diagnosis** 1. Dark field microscopy/direct fluorescent antibody test of lesion exudate, lymph node aspirate, or tissue biopsy is recommended. Test sensitivity is poor and test may not be readily available. Syphilis PCR (where available) – sensitivity better than darkfield/DFA. 2. RPR, VDRL - These nontreponemal screening tests (NTT) may remain negative 1-4 weeks after chancre has formed and up to 90 days after exposure. • If RPR/VDRL negative, recommend repeat serology in 2-4 weeks. • RPR/VDRL can be helpful in staging infection, monitoring treatment response, and assessing for re-infection. 3. T. pallidum IgM/syphilis EIA - becomes positive earlier but false positives may occur and test availability limited. Refer to local testing algorithm. 4. Treponemal tests detect T. pallidum - specific antibodies, and usually remain positive lifelong even after successful therapy. - Ulcers should also be tested for herpes simplex virus (HSV) +/-: • Chancroid +/- • Lymphogranuloma venereum. - All patients with a diagnosis of syphilis should be tested for HIV. **Primary Syphilis** - Chancre – single painless genital ulcer (occasionally extragenital indurated ulcer) within 3 weeks of infection; may be multiple/painful (up to 30% co-infected with HSV) - Regional lymphadenopathy 70-80% - May resolve without treatment. **Secondary syphilis** - Highly infectious stage - Multiple organ systems can be involved including generalized lymphadenopathy, hepatosplenomegaly, hepatitis, alopecia, oral lesions, pharyngitis, anterior uveitis, optic neuritis, meningitis, glomerulonephritis, periostitis - Cutaneous manifestations include macular/maculopapular/scaly lesions of face, torso and flexor aspects of extremities. - Symptoms resolve without treatment within 6 months after primary infection.			

RECOMMENDED EMPIRIC THERAPY OF SELECTED INFECTIONS IN ADULT PATIENTS[A]

Infection	Usual Pathogens	Recommended Empiric Therapy	Recommended Dose[B]	Recommended Duration	Comments
Genital					
Genital ulcers/lesions (cont'd)					

Syphilis (cont'd)	Latent syphilis
	- Seroreactivity without clinical evidence of disease:
	  Early < 1 year
	  Late > 1 year
	
	Tertiary syphilis
	- Cardiovascular disease, neurosyphilis, gumma
	- Occurs years to decades after primary infection
	
	Treatment failure
	- Clinical progression or relapse of clinical symptoms or inadequate decline in RPR/VDRL titres.
	- RPR/VDRL should be negative at 1 year. NB: Treponemal test usually remains positive lifelong even after successful therapy.				

• **Primary** • **Secondary** • **Latent < 1 year duration (early)**	Treponema pallidum	**Benzathine Pen G** β-lactam allergy* **Doxycycline** Alternative in β-lactam allergic pregnant patients** Desensitization*** then **Benzathine Pen G**	2.4MU IM 100mg PO bid 2.4MU IM	1 dose 2 doses if pregnant 14 days 2 doses	- All sexual contacts of early syphilis should be tested and treated. - All HIV patients with early syphilis should receive benzathine Pen G 2.4MU IM weekly x 3 weeks. * Ceftriaxone 1g IV/IM daily x 10 days may be used but limited efficacy data; ensure patient follow-up. **Insufficient data to recommend ceftriaxone in pregnancy. ***Contact pharmacy for desensitization protocol.

RECOMMENDED EMPIRIC THERAPY OF SELECTED INFECTIONS IN ADULT PATIENTS[A]

Infection	Usual Pathogens	Recommended Empiric Therapy	Recommended Dose[B]	Recommended Duration	Comments
Genital					
Genital ulcers/ lesions (cont'd) **Syphilis** (cont'd) • **Latent > 1 year duration (late) or unknown duration** • **Cardiovascular**	Treponema pallidum	**Benzathine Pen G**	2.4MU IM weekly	3 doses	- Evaluation (including lumbar puncture) to rule out tertiary syphilis should be done in consultation with an Infectious Diseases/STI specialist prior to treatment.
		β-lactam allergy* **Doxycycline**	100mg PO bid	28 days	* Ceftriaxone 1g IV/IM daily x 10 days may be used but limited efficacy data; ensure patient follow-up.
		Alternative in β-lactam allergic pregnant patients** Desensitization*** then **Benzathine Pen G**	2.4MU IM	3 doses	**Insufficient data to recommend ceftriaxone in pregnancy. ***Contact pharmacy for desensitization protocol.
• **Neurosyphilis, including ocular syphilis**	Treponema pallidum	- Recommend LP if: • presence of neurologic or ophthalmic symptoms or signs • previously treated patients without adequate serological treatment response • tertiary syphilis • HIV patients with CD_4<350 or treated syphilis with suboptimal decline in VDRL/RPR titre • RPR ≥ 1:32 dilutions. - Test CSF for: • cell count and differential, protein • VDRL and FTA-ABS.			
		Penicillin G	3-4 MU IV q4h	10-14 days	* If severe allergy/anaphylaxis to penicillin consider: • desensitization (contact pharmacy for protocol) • infectious Diseases consult.
		β-lactam allergy* **Ceftriaxone**	2g IV daily	10-14 days	

RECOMMENDED EMPIRIC THERAPY OF SELECTED INFECTIONS IN ADULT PATIENTS[A]

Infection	Usual Pathogens	Recommended Empiric Therapy	Recommended Dose[B]	Recommended Duration	Comments
Genital					
Genital ulcers/ lesions (cont'd) **Chancroid** http://www.phac-aspc.gc.ca/std-mts/sti-its/pdf/501chancr-eng.pdf	Haemophilus ducreyi	**Azithromycin** or **Ciprofloxacin** or **Ceftriaxone** or **Erythromycin base**	1g PO 500mg PO 250mg IM 500mg PO tid	1 dose 1 dose 1 dose 7 days	- Must rule out HSV and syphilis. Also consider LGV and donovanosis (granuloma inguinale). - Test for HIV.
Lymphogranuloma venereum (LGV) http://www.phac-aspc.gc.ca/std-mts/sti-its/pdf/509lgv-eng.pdf	Chlamydia trachomatis serovars L1, L2, and L3	**Doxycycline** _Alternative_ **Erythromycin base** or **Azithromycin**[*] _Pregnancy_ **Erythromycin base**[**]	100mg PO bid 500mg PO qid 1g PO once weekly 500mg PO qid	21 days 21 days 3 weeks 21 days	- In patients with LGV, test for other STIs including HIV, syphilis, HSV, gonorrhea, hepatitis B & C. - Treat regardless of clinical signs/symptoms all recent (60 days) sexual contacts with: - azithromycin 1g PO single dose **or** - doxycycline 100mg PO bid x 7 days. * Should be effective but clinical data are lacking. **Do not use the estolate formulation in pregnancy as it may cause intrahepatic cholestasis.

Infection	Usual Pathogens	Recommended Empiric Therapy	Recommended Dose[B]	Recommended Duration	Comments
Genital					
Genital ulcers/lesions (cont'd)					

Genital Warts	http://www.phac-aspc.gc.ca/std-mts/sti-its/pdf/505hpv-vph-eng.pdf
	- Differential diagnosis:
	  • condyloma acuminata (HPV)
	  • molluscum contagiosum
	  • epidermoid cysts
	  • pearly penile papules
	  • condylomata lata (secondary syphilis)
	  • tumours.
	- Refer to specialist if:
	  • large/extensive warts
	  • resistant lesions
	  • internal lesions: vaginal, cervical, anal, urethral, meatal warts
	  • neoplasia suspected:
	    ○ pigmented lesions
	    ○ bleeding
	    ○ persistent ulceration
	    ○ persistent pruritus
	    ○ recalcitrant lesions.
	- Recommend testing for chlamydia, gonorrhea, hepatitis B&C, syphilis and HIV.
	- No therapy guarantees eradication of HPV.
	- Discuss HPV vaccination with patient.
	- Therapy is primarily to reduce lesion size - may reduce risk of transmission.				

RECOMMENDED EMPIRIC THERAPY OF SELECTED INFECTIONS IN ADULT PATIENTS[A]

Infection	Usual Pathogens	Recommended Empiric Therapy	Recommended Dose[B]	Recommended Duration	Comments
Genital					
Genital ulcers/lesions (cont'd)					
Genital Warts (cont'd)					
Condyloma acuminata	Human Papilloma Virus (HPV)	<u>Patient-applied</u> **Imiquimod 3.75% cream***†	Apply to warts daily, wash off in morning or 6-8 hours later	Up to 8 weeks	† Contraindicated in pregnancy. ‡ Contraindicated in: • pregnancy • cervical, meatal, vaginal and anal warts. * Dermatitis is the most common adverse event.
		or **Podofilox 0.5% solution**‡	Apply to warts (not contiguous skin) bid	3 days (4 days off) May repeat 3 day cycle up to 6 times	
		<u>Provider-applied</u> **Bi or tri chloracetic acid 50-80%***	Apply to warts (not contiguous skin) weekly	Once per week until resolved (6-8 weeks)	* Safe for use in pregnancy.
		or **Podophyllin 10-25%**†	Apply to warts (not contiguous skin) 1-2 times per week, wash off 1-4 hours later	Until resolved	† Contraindicated in: • pregnancy • cervical, meatal, vaginal and anal warts.
		<u>Other options</u> • **Cryotherapy** • **Electrocautery** • **Laser therapy**			

RECOMMENDED EMPIRIC THERAPY OF SELECTED INFECTIONS IN ADULT PATIENTS[A]

Infection	Usual Pathogens	Recommended Empiric Therapy	Recommended Dose[B]	Recommended Duration	Comments
Genital					
Scabies http://www.phac-aspc.gc.ca/std-mts/sti-its/pdf/503ectopara-eng.pdf	Sarcoptes scabiei	**Permethrin 5% cream*** (Nix®)	Apply from neck down, wash off after 8-14 hours	May be repeated in 7 days	* Permethrin is the only agent that should be used in pregnancy. **These options are less effective than permethrin. - Lindane has been discontinued from the Canadian market (Feb 2012) as it is a persistent organic pollutant. - Wash clothes and bedding in hot water/hot dryer or place in plastic bags for 3-7 days. Vacuum mattresses. - Treat all household contacts and sexual partners within last month. - Pruritus may persist for several weeks. Retreat after 1 week if no clinical improvement.
		<u>Alternative</u>** **Crotamiton 10% cream[1]** or **Sulphur 5% in petroleum**	Apply hs for 2 nights, wash off after 24 hours after last application Apply hs for 3 nights, wash off after 24 hours after last application.	2 doses 3 doses	
		<u>Resistant/Failure of above</u> **Ivermectin[1]**	200-400mcg/kg PO	1 dose. May be repeated in 2 weeks.	

1. Must be obtained through the TPD Special Access Program (Emergency Release). Contact pharmacy for assistance in ordering.

RECOMMENDED EMPIRIC THERAPY OF SELECTED INFECTIONS IN ADULT PATIENTS[A]

Infection	Usual Pathogens	Recommended Empiric Therapy	Recommended Dose[B]	Recommended Duration	Comments
Genital					
Pubic Lice* http://www.phac-aspc.gc.ca/std-mts/sti-its/pdf/503ectopara-eng.pdf	Phthirus pubis	**Permethrin 1% creme rinse (Nix®)** or **Pyrethin 0.33%-piperonyl butoxide 3% shampoo (R&C®)**	Apply, wash off after 10 minutes Apply, wash off after 10 minutes	May be repeated in 3-7 days May be repeated in 7 days	* Lice may also be found in chest, armpits, eyelashes or facial hair. If in eyelashes, recommend occlusive ophthalmic ointment to eyelid margins bid x 10 days. - Wash clothes, bedding and fomites in hot water (>50°C) and dry on hot cycle. If item can not be washed, place in plastic bags for 7 days. Vacuum mattresses. - Treat sexual partners within last month. - Pruritus may persist for several days or weeks. - Lindane has been discontinued from the Canadian market (Feb 2012) as it is a persistent organic pollutant.
		Alternative **Ivermectin[1]**	200-400mcg/kg PO	1 dose	

1. Must be obtained through the TPD Special Access Program (Emergency Release). Contact pharmacy for assistance in ordering.

RECOMMENDED EMPIRIC THERAPY OF SELECTED INFECTIONS IN ADULT PATIENTS[A]

Infection	Usual Pathogens	Recommended Empiric Therapy	Recommended Dose[B]	Recommended Duration	Comments
Urinary Tract					
	- In symptomatic (dysuria, frequency, urgency) premenopausal women, screening for pyuria (dipstick or microscopy) is highly sensitive and the preferred diagnostic technique.				
	- Cloudy/foul-smelling urine is NOT an indication for urine culture.				
	- If urine cultures indicated, submit for urinalysis and urine culture. Ensure proper urine collection:				
	• midstream urine (MSU) sample should be collected no sooner than 2 hours after last voiding				
	• cleansing prior to collection of MSU.				
	- $\geq 10^8$ cfu/L - significant colony count indicative of urinary tract infection WITH signs & symptoms				
	- $\geq 10^6$ cfu/L - may be significant in females with pyuria/dysuria syndrome, males, in/out catheter specimens, or suprapubic aspirate.				
	- $\geq 10^5$ cfu/L - significant colony count for suprapubic aspirate or cystoscopy specimens in patients with signs and symptoms.				
	- ≥ 3 mixed organisms - probable contamination. May be significant in adults with complicated UTI.				
	- Blood culture recommended if:				
	• febrile				
	• signs & symptoms of pyelonephritis				
	• immunocompromised.				
	- Amoxicillin and cephalexin are NOT recommended empirically due to unacceptably high E. coli resistance.				
	- Cefazolin susceptibility does not predict cephalexin susceptibility of E. coli, Proteus mirabilis and Klebsiella spp.				
	- Significant E. coli resistance to TMP/SMX and fluoroquinolones, and depending on geographic location, amoxicillin-clavulanate; knowledge of local susceptibility patterns and confirmation of susceptibility by culture is recommended.				
	- Quinolones – do not use moxifloxacin as inadequate urinary concentrations.				
	- Nitrofurantoin and fosfomycin should not be used for pyelonephritis or urosepsis as poor renal tissue and serum concentrations.				
	- Antifungal prophylaxis in women receiving antibiotic therapy for UTI is NOT routinely recommended.				

RECOMMENDED EMPIRIC THERAPY OF SELECTED INFECTIONS IN ADULT PATIENTS[A]

Infection	Usual Pathogens	Recommended Empiric Therapy	Recommended Dose[B]	Recommended Duration	Comments
Urinary Tract					

Asymptomatic Bacteriuria
 	
Adult males/females<ul><li>**community**</li><li>**hospitalized**</li><li>**institutionalized**</li><li>**long term catheterization**</li></ul>
	- Asymptomatic bacteriuria:
	<u>Definitions:</u>
	• asymptomatic females - <u>two</u> consecutive voided urine cultures with ≥ 10⁸ cfu/L of same organism +/- pyuria.
	• asymptomatic males - <u>one</u> voided urine culture with ≥ 10⁸ cfu/L of ≥ 1 organism +/- pyuria.
	• catheterized patients - catheter urine culture with ≥10⁸cfu/L of ≥ 1 organism +/- pyuria and no symptoms of UTI.
	<u>Incidence of asymptomatic bacteriuria:</u>
	• young adults: 1-3%
	• >65 years old: 20% females, 10% males
	• >80 years old: 50% females, 30% males
	• catheterized: - intermittent: 38-58%
	             - short-term (< 30 days) indwelling: 9-23%
	             - long-term (≥ 30 days) indwelling: 100%
	
	<u>Prevalence:</u>
	• Hospital > nursing home > community
	• most asymptomatic bacteriuria is intermittent.
	<u>Associated laboratory findings:</u>
	•>90% of elderly patients with asymptomatic bacteriuria have pyuria, hence pyuria is not a valid diagnostic criterion for UTI in this patient population; clinical correlation required.
	<u>Antibiotic therapy:</u>
	• Asymptomatic bacteriuria is **NOT** associated with incontinence, hypertension, or decreased renal function in the elderly.
	• **NO** evidence that antibiotic therapy of asymptomatic bacteriuria decreases symptomatic UTI.
	• **NO** evidence that antibiotic therapy of asymptomatic bacteriuria is of any benefit except as noted below.
	
	Antibiotic therapy NOT recommended unless:
	  • prior to urologic/gynecologic instrumentation/surgery, or surgery involving prosthetic material, or
	  • prior to catheter removal in patients catheterized for > 48 hours post surgery involving prosthetic material, or
	  • pregnant.
				- Routine screening cultures not recommended, unless prior to surgery or pregnant.
				NB: cloudy/foul smelling urine alone is not an indication for urine culture.

RECOMMENDED EMPIRIC THERAPY OF SELECTED INFECTIONS IN ADULT PATIENTS[A]

Infection	Usual Pathogens	Recommended Empiric Therapy	Recommended Dose[B]	Recommended Duration	Comments
Urinary Tract					
Asymptomatic Bacteriuria (cont'd)					- Pre-procedure cultures should be taken.
Prior to:	E. coli	Prophylactic regimens* (base on C&S results)			* Prophylaxis of asymptomatic bacteriuria in these settings is to prevent sepsis post-procedure, not to treat asymptomatic bacteriuria.
• urologic/ gynecologic instrumentation/ surgery	Other Enterobacter-iaceae Enterococcus spp**	**Cefixime** or	400mg PO	single dose 1-2 hours pre-op	
• surgery involving prosthetic material		**Ciprofloxacin** or	500mg PO	single dose 1-2 hours pre-op	**If C&S results unavailable, enterococcal coverage with ampicillin (in addition to Gram negative coverage) is recommended for high-risk patients:
• catheter removal in patients catheterized for > 48 hours post surgery involving prosthetic material		**Norfloxacin** or **TMP/SMX** or [**Gentamicin** +/- **Ampicillin**]	400mg PO 1 DS tab PO 1.5mg/kg IV/IM 1g IV/IM	single dose 1-2 hours pre-op single dose 1-2 hours pre-op single dose single dose	• elderly/institutionalized • catheterized • obstruction and/or anatomical abnormality of GU tract • diabetes.

RECOMMENDED EMPIRIC THERAPY OF SELECTED INFECTIONS IN ADULT PATIENTS[A]

Infection	Usual Pathogens	Recommended Empiric Therapy	Recommended Dose[B]	Recommended Duration	Comments
Urinary Tract					
Asymptomatic Bacteriuria (cont'd) Pregnancy	- Asymptomatic bacteriuria in pregnant women should be treated as associated with increased incidence of pyelonephritis, preterm labour, and low birthweight infants. - Screening for bacteriuria recommended at 12-16 weeks gestation, or first prenatal visit if later than 12-16 weeks gestation. - Post treatment urine cultures recommended 1 week after completion of treatment, as well as monthly urine cultures for remainder of pregnancy.				
	E. coli S. agalactiae (Group B Strep) S. saprophyticus	Options in pregnancy based on C&S results **Amoxicillin-clavulanate** or **Cefixime** or **Fosfomycin** or **Nitrofurantoin*** or **TMP/SMX**** or **Trimethoprim****	 875mg PO bid 400mg PO daily 3g PO once 50-100mg PO qid 1DS tab PO bid 100mg PO bid	 5-7 days 5-7 days 1 dose 5 days 3 days 3 days	* Nitrofurantoin should be avoided near term (36-42 weeks) due to potential for hemolytic anemia in the newborn. **TMP/SMX, trimethoprim should not be used in first trimester (potential for neural tube and cardiovascular defects) or after 32 weeks gestation (potential for jaundice, hemolytic anemia and kernicterus in the newborn).
Diabetes		- Increased incidence of asymptomatic bacteriuria and symptomatic UTI in diabetic women. However treatment of asymptomatic bacteriuria not recommended as does not reduce symptomatic UTIs, pyelonephritis, or hospitalization for UTI. - Optimal control of diabetes is best prevention.			
Cirrhosis		- Treatment of asymptomatic bacteriuria is controversial - may decrease incidence of spontaneous bacterial peritonitis. - Avoid urinary catheterization if possible. If catheterization is necessary, use prophylactic antibiotics. See previous page.			
Renal transplant		- Although screening and treatment of asymptomatic bacteriuria in renal transplant patients in initial (1 year) post-transplant period is advocated by some, this is controversial as recent studies show no association between asymptomatic bacteriuria and renal graft loss.			

RECOMMENDED EMPIRIC THERAPY OF SELECTED INFECTIONS IN ADULT PATIENTS[A]

Infection	Usual Pathogens	Recommended Empiric Therapy	Recommended Dose[B]	Recommended Duration	Comments
Urinary Tract					
Cystitis	\multicolumn 6 col: - Cystitis not typically associated with fever. If febrile, recommend blood culture and empiric therapy for pyelonephritis. - New onset or recurrent UTI in postmenopausal women may warrant investigation for structural abnormalities such as bladder diverticula or cystoceles.				
Females Sexually active, first episode	E. coli S. saprophyticus Other Enterobacter-iaceae	**Nitrofurantoin*** or **Fosfomycin**** Alternative **Cefixime** or **TMP/SMX**** or **Trimethoprim**** or **Ciprofloxacin****	50-100mg PO qid 3g PO 400mg PO daily 1 DS tab PO bid 100mg PO bid 250mg PO bid **or** XL 500mg PO daily	5 days 1 dose 5-7 days 3 days 3 days 3 days 3 days	* Nitrofurantoin - excellent activity against E. coli and S. saprophyticus. **Fosfomycin: • excellent activity against E. coli including multi-resistant strains (ESBL, Amp C, carbapenemases) • variable activity against other Enterobacteriaceae • no activity against S. saprophyticus. - Nitrofurantoin and fosfomycin NOT recommended if pyelonephritis suspected. ***Significant E. coli resistance; pre-treatment urine culture recommended.

Cell spanning across Usual Pathogens / Recommended Empiric Therapy / Recommended Dose / Recommended Duration for the Females row (upper portion):

- Screen for pyuria. Routine pre/post treatment urine cultures are not recommended when presenting with pyuria and typical symptoms of cystitis and adequate response to therapy.
  Exception: pre-treatment culture recommended in the following patients at risk of resistant uropathogens (e.g. ESBL-producing E. coli):
  - quinolone or cephalosporin use within last 6 months
  - travel outside Canada/U.S. within last 6 months
  - recent hospitalization.
- Lack of response after 48h of appropriate antibiotic therapy warrants urine culture (if not taken pre-treatment), treatment for pyelonephritis tailored to C&S results if available, and clinical evaluation for other genitourinary infections, including sexually transmitted infections (STIs).

RECOMMENDED EMPIRIC THERAPY OF SELECTED INFECTIONS IN ADULT PATIENTS[A]

Infection	Usual Pathogens	Recommended Empiric Therapy	Recommended Dose[B]	Recommended Duration	Comments
Urinary Tract (cont'd)					
Cystitis **Pregnant**	E. coli Other Enterobacter-iaceae S. agalactiae (Group B Strep) S. saprophyticus	- Pre/post treatment urine cultures recommended followed by monthly follow-up cultures during remainder of pregnancy			
		Nitrofurantoin*	50-100mg PO qid	7 days	* Nitrofurantoin should be avoided near term (36-42 weeks) due to potential for hemolytic anemia in the newborn.
		or **Cefixime**	400mg PO daily	7 days	** TMP/SMX, trimethoprim should not be used in first trimester (potential for neural tube and cardiovascular defects) or after 32 weeks gestation (potential for jaundice, hemolytic anemia and kernicterus in the newborn).
		or **Fosfomycin**	3g PO once	1 dose	
		Alternative **TMP/SMX****	1 DS tab PO bid	7 days	
		or **Trimethoprim****	100mg PO bid	7 days	- Quinolones are not recommended in pregnancy.

Recurrent cystitis		- Failure of cystitis to respond after 48 hours of appropriate antibiotic therapy warrants urine culture (if not taken pre-treatment), treatment as for pyelonephritis tailored to C & S results if available, and clinical evaluation for other genitourinary infections.
		- Within 1st month, it is difficult to differentiate between relapse and reinfection. Safest to treat for longer duration as for pyelonephritis. If different organism on culture, treat as cystitis.
		  1. Relapse (same organism) - usually occurs within 2 weeks after completion of therapy. Urologic investigation may be indicated. Treat as for pyelonephritis.
		  2. Re-infection - > 90% of recurrences are due to reinfection (different strain or species) usually after 2-4 weeks. Treat as cystitis.
		
		- Pre treatment urine cultures recommended.
		  • Isolation of certain organisms such as Proteus, Morganella, Providencia, and Corynebacterium urealyticum in non-catheterized patients may indicate structural abnormality and warrant investigation, especially if repeat isolation.
		  • Consultation with microbiologist or Infectious Diseases physician recommended for all culture negative recurrent UTIs.
		- Post treatment cultures not recommended unless symptoms persist or recur.			

RECOMMENDED EMPIRIC THERAPY OF SELECTED INFECTIONS IN ADULT PATIENTS[A]

Infection	Usual Pathogens	Recommended Empiric Therapy	Recommended Dose[B]	Recommended Duration	Comments
Urinary Tract					
Cystitis (cont'd) **Recurrent cystitis** (cont'd)	Prevention - Conflicting evidence for efficacy of cranberry juice/products in preventing recurrent UTIs. - No rationale for specific instructions regarding urinary hygiene (wiping patterns, douching, postcoital voiding, hot tub use, wearing of pantyhose/tight clothing).				
Females, Sexually active Early - < 1 month following therapy for UTI	E. coli S. saprophyticus Other Enterobacter-iaceae	- If different organism, see Cystitis, first episode. - If same organism, see Pyelonephritis.			
Late - > 1 month following therapy for UTI	E. coli S. saprophyticus Other Enterobacter-iaceae	- See Cystitis, first episode.			

RECOMMENDED EMPIRIC THERAPY OF SELECTED INFECTIONS IN ADULT PATIENTS[A]

Infection	Usual Pathogens	Recommended Empiric Therapy	Recommended Dose[B]	Recommended Duration	Comments
Urinary Tract					
Cystitis (cont'd), **Recurrent cystitis** (cont'd), **Females** (cont'd) **Frequent - ≥ 3 episodes/year**	- Pre treatment urine cultures recommended. - Isolation of certain organisms such as Proteus, Morganella, Providencia, and Corynebacterium urealyticum in non-catheterized patients may indicate structural abnormality and warrant investigation, especially if repeat isolation. - Consultation with microbiologist or Infectious Diseases physician recommended for all culture negative recurrent UTIs. - Post treatment cultures not recommended unless symptoms persist or recur. Prevention: - Conflicting evidence for efficacy of cranberry juice/products in preventing recurrent UTIs. - No rationale for specific instructions regarding urinary hygiene (wiping patterns, douching, postcoital voiding, hot tub use, wearing of pantyhose/tight clothing).				
• **related to coitus**	E. coli S. saprophyticus Other Enterobacter-iaceae	Pericoital prophylaxis* **TMP/SMX** or **Nitrofurantoin** Pregnant **Nitrofurantoin**** Alternative **Cefixime**	1 SS tab PO pericoitus* 50-100mg PO pericoitus* 50-100mg PO pericoitus* 400mg PO pericoitus*		* Antibiotic may be taken just before or after coitus. **Nitrofurantoin should be discontinued near term (36 weeks) due to potential for hemolytic anemia in the newborn.
• **unrelated to coitus**	E. coli S. saprophyticus Other Enterobacter-iaceae	Patient initiated therapy* **Same regimens as for Cystitis, First episode** OR Continuous prophylaxis **TMP/SMX** or **Trimethoprim**	 3 days 1 SS tab PO qhs or 3x/week 100mg PO qhs	 6 months 6 months	* Patients should have drug on hand and initiate therapy based on symptoms. NB: Patient initiated therapy recommended in pregnant women, rather than continuous prophylaxis, in order to decrease antibiotic exposure to the fetus.

- 369 -

RECOMMENDED EMPIRIC THERAPY OF SELECTED INFECTIONS IN ADULT PATIENTS[A]

Infection	Usual Pathogens	Recommended Empiric Therapy	Recommended Dose[B]	Recommended Duration	Comments
Urinary Tract					
Pyelonephritis Uncomplicated	E. coli Enterobacteriaceae S. saprophyticus	Office visit **Cefixime** Alternative **Amoxicillin-clavulanate*** or **Ciprofloxacin*** or **TMP/SMX*** ER/Hospitalized/Septic **Gentamicin**** or **Ceftriaxone****	400mg PO daily 875mg PO bid 500mg PO bid **or** XL 1g PO daily 1DS tab PO bid 5-7mg/kg IV q24h 1-2g IV q24h	10-14 days 10-14 days 7 days 7 days 14 days 10-14 days 10-14 days	- Pretreatment urine cultures recommended. Tailor antibiotics to C&S results. * Significant E. coli resistance; confirm susceptibility. ** Based on clinical response, switch to oral agent(s) as listed and/or according to C&S results.
Functional/ structural urinary abnormalities/ catheterized	See Complicated UTIs				
Pregnant	E. coli Other Enterobacteriaceae S. agalactiae (Group B Strep)	**Ceftriaxone** Alternative **Gentamicin + Ampicillin**	1-2g IV q24h 7mg/kg IV q24h 1-2g IV q6h	14 days 14 days	- Pre/post treatment urine cultures recommended followed by monthly follow-up cultures during remainder of pregnancy. - Tailor antibiotics to C&S results. - Based on clinical response, switch to oral agent(s) as listed under Uncomplicated pyelonephritis and/or according to C&S results.

RECOMMENDED EMPIRIC THERAPY OF SELECTED INFECTIONS IN ADULT PATIENTS[A]

Infection	Usual Pathogens	Recommended Empiric Therapy	Recommended Dose[B]	Recommended Duration	Comments
Urinary Tract					
Complicated UTI	Complicated UTI associated with functional and anatomical abnormalities of the genitourinary (GU) tract including: - Obstructive uropathies - strictures, tumors/cysts, stones, prostatic hypertrophy, congenital abnormalities. - Recent GU instrumentaion - cystoscopy/urologic procedures, catheterization, ureteric stent, nephrostomy tubes. - Delayed/impaired voiding - neurogenic bladder, vesicoureteral reflux, ileal conduit, cystocele. - Metabolic abnormalities - renal failure/dysfunction, nephrocalcinosis, poorly controlled diabetes. - Immunocompromised states - renal transplant, neutropenia, HIV Special Considerations: - Males - UTIs are typically considered complicated as functional or anatomical abnormalities are often present. Exception: young adult males with first time UTI related to sexual activity. Urologic work-up recommended in males with recurrent cystitis, pyelonephritis, and all young boys. - Postmenopausal women with new onset recurrent UTI should be investigated for impaired voiding. Investigations: - If febrile, do blood culture. - Pre and post treatment urine cultures recommended. Consultation with microbiologist or Infectious Diseases physician recommended for all culture negative recurrent UTIs. - Given the wide variety of potential pathogens and increased incidence of resistant organisms, modify empiric therapy to most narrow spectrum option based on C&S results.			

RECOMMENDED EMPIRIC THERAPY OF SELECTED INFECTIONS IN ADULT PATIENTS[A]

Infection	Usual Pathogens	Recommended Empiric Therapy	Recommended Dose[B]	Recommended Duration	Comments
Urinary Tract					
Complicated UTI (cont'd)	E. coli Other Enterobacter-iaceae Enterococcus spp S. agalactiae (Group B Strep)† P. aeruginosa Corynebacterium urealyticum Aerococcus urinae	<u>Afebrile, systemically well</u> **Cefixime**	400mg PO daily	7-14 days*	† Diabetics are predisposed to UTI with S. agalactiae (Group B Strep). * Continue antibiotic therapy for 3-5 days after defervescence or elimination of obstruction/infected focus. NB: Prolonged fever, renal function deterioration or septic presentation requires further investigation for abscess/undrained urine collection. If lower tract infection and prompt response (within 48h), treat for 7 days. If delayed response or structural abnormality, treat for 14 days. ** Significant E. coli resistance; confirm susceptibility. ***Add gentamicin if: • septic shock • recent antibiotic use • suspected ESBL, Amp C, or carbapenemase producing organism.
		<u>Alternative</u> **Amoxicillin-clavulanate**** or **Ciprofloxacin**** or **TMP/SMX*****	875mg PO bid 500mg PO bid **or** XL 1g PO daily 1DS tab PO bid	7-14 days* 7-14 days* 7-14 days*	
		<u>Febrile, systemically unwell</u> **Ampicillin** + **[Gentamicin]** or **Ceftriaxone]**	1-2g IV q6h 5-7mg/kg IV q24h 1-2g IV daily	7-14 days*	
		<u>Septic/Hemodynamically unstable</u> **Piperacillin-tazobactam** +/- **Gentamicin*****	3.375g IV q6h 5-7mg/kg IV q24h	7-14 days*	

RECOMMENDED EMPIRIC THERAPY OF SELECTED INFECTIONS IN ADULT PATIENTS[A]

Infection	Usual Pathogens	Recommended Empiric Therapy	Recommended Dose[B]	Recommended Duration	Comments
Urinary Tract					
Complicated UTI (cont'd)					
Catheter-associated UTI (CA-UTI)					

Definition of CA-UTI - catheter urine culture with ≥ 10⁶cfu/L of ≥ 1 organism(s) (infections may be polymicrobial) in a patient with urinary symptoms and/or signs (costovertebral tenderness, rigors, new onset delirium) who is currently catheterized (short-term [< 30 days], long-term [≥ 30 days])‡, intermittent, condom catheters) or has been catheterized within previous 48 hours.

‡ When a long-term catheterized patient has a symptomatic UTI, the catheter should be changed, and a urine specimen should be obtained through the newly placed catheter before starting antibiotics. Replacement of the catheter results in improved therapeutic outcomes, including decreased duration of fever and decreased likelihood of relapse.

NB: Neither fever nor pyuria are diagnostic for CA-UTI. Do not treat unless evidence of urinary tract symptoms or systemic infection as:

- catheter often colonized with bacteria
- significant risk associated with inappropriate use of antibiotics including development of resistance and C. difficile infection.

In patients with spinal cord injury, increased spasticity, autonomic dysreflexia, or sense of unease may indicate CA-UTI.

Prevention:

- Optimal hydration essential.
- Hand hygiene before and after patient care.
- Remove catheter as soon as not needed.
- Screening of urine (urinalysis or culture) NOT recommended unless prior to GU surgery/instrumentation.
- NB: cloudy/foul smelling urine alone is not an indication for urine culture.
- In catheterized patients, antibiotic prophylaxis is NOT recommended to reduce bacteriuria or UTI.
- Prophylactic antibiotics NOT recommended at time of catheter placement, replacement or removal except prior to catheter removal in patients catheterized for > 48 hours post surgery involving prosthetic material.
- Data inconclusive as to whether routine catheter change is effective in reducing CA-UTI.
- NO convincing evidence for efficacy of antibiotic coated catheters.

RECOMMENDED EMPIRIC THERAPY OF SELECTED INFECTIONS IN ADULT PATIENTS[A]

Infection	Usual Pathogens	Recommended Empiric Therapy	Recommended Dose[B]	Recommended Duration	Comments
Urinary Tract					
Complicated UTI (cont'd) **Catheter-associated UTI (CA-UTI)** (cont'd)	Enterobacteriaceae Enterococcus spp P. aeruginosa Coagulase negative Staphylococci Aerococcus urinae Corynebacterium urealyticum Candida spp* *See Recommended Empiric Therapy of Fungal Infections.	<u>Asymptomatic</u> None <u>Symptomatic</u>[†] **Cefixime** <u>Alternative</u> **Amoxicillin-clavulanate**** **or** **Ciprofloxacin**** <u>Febrile, systemically unwell</u> **Ampicillin + [Gentamicin]** or **Ceftriaxone**] <u>Septic/Hemodynamically unstable</u> **Piperacillin-tazobactam** +/- **Gentamicin**[‡]	 400mg PO daily 875mg PO bid 500 mg PO bid **or** XL 1g PO daily 1-2g IV q6h 5-7mg/kg IV q24h 1-2g IV daily 3.375g IV q6h 5-7mg/kg IV q24h	 7-14 days*** 7-14 days*** 7-14 days*** 7-14 days*** 7-14 days***	[†] Tailor empiric therapy to most narrow spectrum option based on C&S results. **Significant E. coli/Proteus mirabilis resistance; confirm susceptibility. ***If prompt response (within 72 hours), treat for 7 days. If delayed response, treat for 10-14 days. NB: 3 days may be sufficient in women ≤ 65 years old if: • no fever or upper urinary tract symptoms, and • short-term catheterization, and • catheter has been removed (and not replaced). [‡] Add gentamicin if: • septic shock • recent antibiotic use • suspected ESBL, Amp C, or carbapenemase producing organism.

- 374 -

RECOMMENDED EMPIRIC THERAPY OF SELECTED INFECTIONS IN ADULT PATIENTS[A]

Infection	Usual Pathogens	Recommended Empiric Therapy	Recommended Dose[B]	Recommended Duration	Comments
Central Nervous System					

Meningitis	- 95% of patients with bacterial meningitis will have at least 2 of 4 of the following signs & symptoms (S&S):
	   • fever
	   • stiff neck
	   • altered mental status
	   • headache.
	 NB: Absence of stiff neck does not rule out meningitis.
	 - Blood culture recommended.
	 - Lumbar puncture (LP) for cell count, glucose, protein, Gram stain* and culture recommended without neuroimaging prior to antibiotic therapy **unless:**
	   • S&S of increased intracranial pressure ((ICP): NB: normal CT scan does NOT rule out raised ICP.
	     ○ focal neurological deficit
	     ○ papilledema
	     ○ GCS < 11 or decrease in score of 3 or more
	     ○ relative bradycardia or hypertension
	   • uncorrected coagulopathy
	   • hemodynamically unstable
	   • extensive or spreading purpura
	   • new onset seizures.
	 * Sensitivity of Gram stain is organism-specific but generally 50-90% therefore cannot be used to rule out bacterial meningitis.
	 NB: Do not delay antibiotics if neuroimaging (CT/MRI) and/or LP cannot be performed expediently.
	 Typical CSF findings
	
	 Parameter Bacterial Viral
	 WBC count >500 x 10^6/L* <300 x 10^6/L (predominantly lymphocytes,
	            (predominantly neutrophils) although neutrophils may be significant early in illness)
	 Protein Elevated Normal
	 Glucose Reduced Normal
	 CSF:serum glucose ratio <0.4 >0.6
	 *Lower CSF WBC count may be seen in severe illness, septic shock, or meningitis due to Listeria or syphilis.
	 - Bacterial antigen test (latex agglutination) of CSF not recommended.
	 - Repeat LP should be considered if:
	   • patient not responding clinically after 48h of appropriate antibiotic therapy
	   • penicillin and/or cephalosporin intermediate/resistant S. pneumoniae.				

RECOMMENDED EMPIRIC THERAPY OF SELECTED INFECTIONS IN ADULT PATIENTS[A]

Infection	Usual Pathogens	Recommended Empiric Therapy	Recommended Dose[B]	Recommended Duration	Comments
Central Nervous System					
Meningitis (cont'd)	— see below				

Central Nervous System

Meningitis (cont'd)

- For prophylaxis of H. influenzae and N. meningitidis in close contacts, see Prophylaxis for Contacts of Communicable Diseases.
- Recommend droplet/contact precautions for 24 hours or until N. meningitidis ruled out.
- For organism - specific recommendations, see Recommended Therapy of Culture-Directed Infections Table 3.

Corticosteroid Therapy in Meningitis
- Dexamethasone **prior to administration of antibiotics** is an option in bacterial meningitis but remains controversial. [Lancet Neurol 2010;9:254–63]. The benefit of corticosteroids may depend on age, severity of presentation and pathogen. Corticosteroids have been shown to decrease mortality and hearing loss in adult patients with S. pneumoniae meningitis [Neurol 2010;75:1533-9].
- **Corticosteroids are not recommended if antibiotics have already been administered.**
- Dexamethasone 0.15mg/kg (maximum 10 mg/dose) IV q6h x 2-4 days. Give 15-20 minutes before, or with, the first dose of antibiotics, NOT AFTER.

Vancomycin has slow distribution and poor CSF penetration. It should be given AFTER the first dose of ceftriaxone and continued only if C&S results indicate ceftriaxone-resistant S. pneumoniae. Maintain trough vancomycin serum concentrations of 15-20mg/L.

Infection	Usual Pathogens	Recommended Empiric Therapy	Recommended Dose[B]	Recommended Duration	Comments
< 18 years old	See Paediatric Guidelines				
18-50 years old and immuno-competent	S. pneumoniae N. meningitidis H. influenzae	**Ceftriaxone** + **Vancomycin**[E*]	2g IV q12h 15mg/kg IV q8-12h	10 days	* Can discontinue vancomycin if ceftriaxone susceptible organism confirmed. **Alternatives to chloramphenicol are: TMP/SMX IV or moxifloxacin IV.
		Alternative **Meropenem** + **Vancomycin**[E*]	2g IV q8h 15mg/kg IV q8-12h	10 days	
		Severe ß-lactam allergy **Chloramphenicol**[**] + **Vancomycin**[E*]	12.5mg/kg IV q6h (max 4g/day) 15mg/kg IV q8-12h	10 days	

E. Desired vancomycin trough is 15-20 mg/L. Monitor renal function closely. See Vancomycin Dosing & Monitoring Guidelines.

RECOMMENDED EMPIRIC THERAPY OF SELECTED INFECTIONS IN ADULT PATIENTS[A]

Central Nervous System

Meningitis (cont'd)

Infection	Usual Pathogens	Recommended Empiric Therapy	Recommended Dose[B]	Recommended Duration	Comments

Adult > 50 years or **Immuno-compromised (including AIDS), Alcoholism, Debilitating illness, Pregnancy**	S. pneumoniae
	Listeria monocytogenes
	N. meningitidis
	Enterobacteriaceae
		Ceftriaxone + **Ampicillin** + **Vancomycin**[E]*	2g IV q12h
			
			2g IV q4h
			
			15mg/kg IV q8-12h
				S. pneumoniae - 10-14 days
				
				N. meningitidis - 5-7 days
				
				L. monocytogenes, Enterobacteriaceae - 21 days
					- Cephalosporins have no activity against Listeria
					- HIV individuals - need to rule out:
					  • Cryptococcosis
					  • M. tuberculosis
					  • Syphilis
					  • Toxoplasmosis.
					* Can discontinue vancomycin if ceftriaxone susceptible organism confirmed.
					**TMP/SMX should not be used in first trimester or after 32 weeks gestation.

		Alternative **Meropenem** + **Vancomycin**[E]*	2g IV q8h 15mg/kg IV q8-12h		
		<u>Severe ß-lactam allergy</u> **Vancomycin**[E] + **TMP/SMX****	15mg/kg IV q8-12h 15-20mg TMP/kg/day div q6-8h		
Post trauma or post operative	S. pneumoniae* S. aureus/MRSA S. epidermidis Enterobacteriaceae P. aeruginosa Propionibacterium spp (if foreign material)	**Meropenem** + **Vancomycin**[E] or **Vancomycin**[E] + **Ciprofloxacin**	2g IV q8h 15mg/kg IV q8-12h 15mg/kg IV q8-12h 400mg IV q8-12h	10-14 days 10-14 days	* Especially if CSF leak. - Send CSF for aerobic and anaerobic culture. - If no previous antibiotic therapy, no foreign material, and negative CSF cultures, can discontinue antibiotic therapy at 72 hours.

E. Desired vancomycin trough is 15-20 mg/L. Monitor renal function closely. See Vancomycin Dosing & Monitoring Guidelines.

RECOMMENDED EMPIRIC THERAPY OF SELECTED INFECTIONS IN ADULT PATIENTS[A]

Central Nervous System

Meningitis (cont'd)

Infection	Usual Pathogens	Recommended Empiric Therapy	Recommended Dose[B]	Recommended Duration	Comments
Shunt/External ventricular drain (EVD) (meningitis/ ventriculitis)	S. epidermidis S. aureus/MRSA Enterobacteriaceae Propionibacterium spp Corynebacterium spp Enterococcus spp	**Ceftriaxone** + **Vancomycin**[E]	2g IV q12h 15mg/kg IV q8-12h	14 days after shunt removal ≥ 21 days if Enterobacter-iaceae	- Send CSF for aerobic and anaerobic culture. If EVD, collect CSF from tubing, not collection bag. Tailor antibiotics to C&S results. - Shunt removal should be done ASAP. Before reimplantation: • give antibiotics for at least 7 days • repeat cultures: • if positive, continue antibiotic therapy until CSF cultures negative for 10 consecutive days before reimplanting shunt.
Basilar skull fracture	S. pneumoniae H. influenzae Group A strep <u>If prolonged hospitalization:</u> S. aureus/MRSA Enterobacteriaceae	**Ceftriaxone** + **Vancomycin**[E] Severe β-Lactam allergy [**Chloramphenicol**] or **Ciprofloxacin**] + **Vancomycin**[E]	2g IV q12h 15mg/kg IV q8-12h 12.5mg/kg IV q6h (max 4g/day) 400mg IV q8-12h 15mg/kg IV q8-12h	≥ 10 days ≥ 10 days	

E. Desired vancomycin trough is 15-20 mg/L. Monitor renal function closely. See Vancomycin Dosing & Monitoring Guidelines.

RECOMMENDED EMPIRIC THERAPY OF SELECTED INFECTIONS IN ADULT PATIENTS[A]

Infection	Usual Pathogens	Recommended Empiric Therapy	Recommended Dose[B]	Recommended Duration	Comments
Central Nervous System					

Recurrent Meningitis	- Recurrent meningitis requires evaluation of underlying cause:
	  • congenital anatomical defect (epidermoid/dermoid cysts, neural tube defects, asplenia)
	  • acquired anatomical defect (head injuries, basal skull fracture, malignancy)
	  • congenital immunodeficiencies (complement deficiency, agammaglobulinemia, IgG subclass deficiency, IRAK 4 deficiency)
	  • acquired immunodeficiencies - HIV
	  • chronic parameningeal infections (sinusitis, otitis media, mastoiditis)
	NB: - Anatomical defects most commonly cause recurrent S. pneumoniae or H. influenzae meningitis.
	  - Complement deficiency is associated with recurrent N. meningitidis meningitis. Vaccination for S. pneumoniae, N. meningitidis, H. influenzae recommended for asplenia or complement deficiency.
	-For chronic meningitis, recommend syphilis and Lyme serology.
	
	Bacterial:
	S. pneumoniae
	N. meningitidis
	H. influenzae
	S. aureus
	Enterobacteriaceae
	Listeria monocytogenes*
	Treponema pallidum
	Borrelia spp
	
	Other:
	Herpes Simplex virus 2 (HSV2) (Mollaret's syndrome)**
	
	Cryptococcus spp
	M. tuberculosis
		Vancomycin[E]
		+
		Ceftriaxone
		+/-
		Ampicillin*
			15mg/kg IV q8-12h
			
			2g IV q12h
			
			2g IV q4h
				S. pneumoniae, N. meningitidis, H. influenzae - 10 days
				S. aureus -14 days after last positive blood culture
				Enterobacteriaceae - 21 days
					* Add ampicillin if at risk for Listeria.
					
					**Consider HSV2 if ≥ 2 episodes of culture negative meningitis with lymphocytic predominance of CSF - send CSF for Herpes Simplex PCR.
					- Treatment of acute episodes with acyclovir is controversial, unless significant neurologic symptoms (urologic retention, weakness).
					- Prophylaxis with antivirals may prevent recurrences.

E. Desired vancomycin trough is 15-20 mg/L. Monitor renal function closely. See Vancomycin Dosing & Monitoring Guidelines.

RECOMMENDED EMPIRIC THERAPY OF SELECTED INFECTIONS IN ADULT PATIENTS[A]

Infection	Usual Pathogens	Recommended Empiric Therapy	Recommended Dose[B]	Recommended Duration	Comments
Central Nervous System					
Brain Abscess					
Contiguous 2° to sinusitis/otitis (usually single abscess)	- Surgical drainage often necessary if: • lesions > 3cm • gas present in abscess • risk of herniation or rupture into ventricles • no improvement with medical therapy.				
	Polymicrobial: • Viridans Group Streptococci • Streptococcus anginosus group • Anaerobes: Peptostreptococcus spp Bacteroides spp Prevotella spp Porphyromonas spp Fusobacterium spp	**Ceftriaxone** + **Metronidazole IV/PO**[C]* _Alternative_ **Penicillin** + **Metronidazole IV/PO**[C] _Temporal lobe_** **Meropenem**	2g IV q12h 500mg IV/PO q8h 4MU IV q4h 500mg IV/PO q8h 2g IV q8h	6 weeks*** 6 weeks*** 6 weeks*** ***If surgically excised, 3 weeks	* This regimen recommended if: • S&S of meningitis • history of recurrent otitis/sinusitis • MIC of Viridans Group Streptococci ≥ 0.1µg/mL. **Pseudomonas aeruginosa and Enterobacteriaceae may be pathogens in temporal lobe abscess.
Hematogenous 2° to endocarditis (usually multiple abscesses)	Viridans Group Streptococci S. aureus/MRSA	**Cloxacillin** + **Ceftriaxone** _MRSA colonized/ suspected*_ **Vancomycin**[E] + **Ceftriaxone**	2g IV q4h 2g IV q12h 15mg/kg IV q8-12h 2g IV q12h	6 weeks 6 weeks	- Blood cultures must be taken. * Tailor antibiotics to C&S results. Cloxacillin superior to vancomycin so preferred if susceptible.

E. Desired vancomycin trough is 15-20 mg/L. Monitor renal function closely. See Vancomycin Dosing & Monitoring Guidelines.

RECOMMENDED EMPIRIC THERAPY OF SELECTED INFECTIONS IN ADULT PATIENTS[A]

Infection	Usual Pathogens	Recommended Empiric Therapy	Recommended Dose[B]	Recommended Duration	Comments
Central Nervous System					
Brain Abscess (cont'd) **Post trauma Post neuro-surgery**	S. aureus Enterobacteriaceae P. aeruginosa	**Cloxacillin** + **Ceftriaxone*** or **Meropenem*** or **Cloxacillin** + **Ceftazidime*** Alternative **Vancomycin**[E] + 3rd **generation cephalosporin***	2g IV q4h 2g IV q12h 2g IV q8h 2g IV q4h 2g IV q8h 15mg/kg IV q8-12h as above	6 weeks 6 weeks 6 weeks 6 weeks 6 weeks	* Use meropenem alone, or ceftazidime in place of ceftriaxone. If increased risk of Pseudomonas: • prolonged ventilatory support • prolonged hospitalization • previous broad spectrum antibiotics • burns. Meropenem preferred if previous 3rd generation cephalosporin therapy.
HIV	Toxoplasma gondii	[**Pyrimethamine** + **Folinic acid** + **Sulfadiazine[1]**]* or **TMP/SMX** alone then follow with suppressive therapy **Pyrimethamine*** + **Folinic acid** + [**Sulfadiazine[1]** or **Clindamycin**] or **Atovaquone** alone	200mg PO loading dose then 50-75mg PO daily 10-25mg PO daily 1-1.5g PO q6h 5mg TMP/kg PO/IV q12h 25-50mg PO daily 10-25mg PO daily 0.5-1g PO q6h 600mg PO q8h 750mg PO q6-12h	Minimum 6 weeks after signs/ symptoms resolved Minimum 6 weeks after signs/ symptoms resolved Discontinue if CD4 count > 200 x 3 months.	* In sulfa-allergic patients, use clindamycin 600mg IV/PO q6h, azithromycin 0.9-1.2g PO daily, or atovaquone 1500mg PO bid, instead of sulfadiazine component. **Pyrimethamine + sulfadiazine prevents PCP and toxoplasmosis. Pyrimethamine + clindamycin prevents toxoplasmosis only.

E. Desired vancomycin trough is 15-20 mg/L. Monitor renal function closely. See Vancomycin Dosing & Monitoring Guidelines.
1. Not commercially available in Canada. Contact pharmacy for assistance in ordering.

- 381 -

RECOMMENDED EMPIRIC THERAPY OF SELECTED INFECTIONS IN ADULT PATIENTS[A]

Infection	Usual Pathogens	Recommended Empiric Therapy	Recommended Dose[B]	Recommended Duration	Comments
Central Nervous System					
Epidural abscess	- Infectious complication of: • endocarditis • vertebral osteomyelitis • psoas muscle abscess. Diagnosis - Classic triad of symptoms: • back pain • fever • neurologic deficit. - MRI				
		- Very little data on epidural penetration of antibiotics. Several case reports of success with cefazolin +/- gentamicin (however CSF penetration of antibiotic may be important especially in first few days due to risk of infection extending into dural sac).			
	S. aureus/MRSA Enterobacteriaceae Streptococci CoNS P. aeruginosa Anaerobes	**Cloxacillin** + **Ceftriaxone** + **Metronidazole IV/PO**[C]	2g IV q4h 2g IV q12h 500mg IV/PO q8h	6 weeks If osteomyelitis, 8 weeks	- Usually requires urgent surgical intervention. Medical therapy alone may be considered if the patient is not a surgical candidate AND has no neurologic deficit and/or shows improvement in symptoms.
		MRSA colonized/ suspected or implantable spinal or vascular devices **Vancomycin**[E] + **Ceftriaxone**[*] + **Metronidazole IV/PO**[C]	15mg/kg IV q8-12h 2g IV q12h 500mg IV/PO q8h	6 weeks If osteomyelitis, 8 weeks	- Treat according to C&S results of blood cultures or CT-guided aspirate of abscess. * IVDU - increased risk of P. aeruginosa; recommend using ceftazidime instead of ceftriaxone.

E. Desired vancomycin trough is 15-20 mg/L. Monitor renal function closely. See Vancomycin Dosing & Monitoring Guidelines.

RECOMMENDED EMPIRIC THERAPY OF SELECTED INFECTIONS IN ADULT PATIENTS[A]

Infection	Usual Pathogens	Recommended Empiric Therapy	Recommended Dose[B]	Recommended Duration	Comments
Central Nervous System					
Subdural empyema	Polymicrobial: • Viridans Group Streptococci • Streptococcus anginosus group • Anaerobes: Anaerobic Gram positive cocci Bacteroides fragilis Prevotella/ Porphyromonas spp Fusobacterium spp	**Cefriaxone + Metronidazole IV/PO**[C] or **Penicillin + Metronidazole IV/PO**[C]	2g IV q12h 500mg IV/PO q8h 4MU IV q4h 500mg IV/PO q8h	6 weeks 6 weeks	- Condition usually requires urgent surgical drainage. - If associated osteomyelitis, need to cover S. aureus (add cloxacillin or vancomycin).

Encephalitis	**Epidemiologic clues are important in directing investigation of meningoencephalitis and include:**
	• season of year • geographic locale
	• local prevalence of potential etiological agents • travel history
	• recreational activities • occupational exposure
	• insect contact • animal contact
	• vaccination history • immune status of patient
	• transfusion history.
	
	Initial Investigations
	CSF (NB: Collect at least 1mL of extra CSF for additional studies):
	- Gram stain and culture (Listeria monocytogenes, N. meningitidis)
	- Viral culture (Herpes/Enterovirus)
	- PCR:
	  • Herpes simplex virus (HSV) 1 and 2
	  • Enterovirus
	  • Meningococcus (if clinical suspicion)
	- VDRL				

RECOMMENDED EMPIRIC THERAPY OF SELECTED INFECTIONS IN ADULT PATIENTS[A]

Infection	Usual Pathogens	Recommended Empiric Therapy	Recommended Dose[B]	Recommended Duration	Comments
Central Nervous System					
Encephalitis (cont'd)	Blood: - Blood culture - HIV serology - Syphilis serology (Treponema pallidum) - Monospot - Blood smear (thick/thin) for malaria if travel history to endemic area Nasopharyngeal washing/swab: - Respiratory virus PCR (influenza, adenovirus, human metapneumovirus, enterovirus/rhinovirus) Stool: - Viral culture (Enterovirus) Chest X-ray EEG and MRI Tuberculin skin test: **Secondary Investigations** Blood: - Mycoplasma IgM (Mycoplasma spp) - Arbovirus serology (arthropod borne: Flaviviridae/Bunyaviridae/Togaviridae) - Lyme serology (Borrelia burgdorferi) - Epstein–Barr virus (EBV) VCA IgM - Cytomegalovirus (CMV) IgG/IgM - Herpes simplex (HSV) IgG/IgM - Human Herpes virus 6 (HHV6) IgM CSF/Blood: - Pan herpes PCR – HSV 1 & 2, HHV6, VZV, CMV, EBV - IgM for West Nile virus (depending on season/local prevalence) - Cryptococal antigen - Histoplasma antigen CSF: - Fungal cultures - Cryptococcus, Coccidioides spp, Histoplasma spp - Mycobacterial cultures/PCR (M. tuberculosis)				

- 384 -

RECOMMENDED EMPIRIC THERAPY OF SELECTED INFECTIONS IN ADULT PATIENTS[A]

Infection	Usual Pathogens	Recommended Empiric Therapy	Recommended DoseB	Recommended Duration	Comments
Central Nervous System					

Encephalitis (cont'd)	Respiratory sample:
	- Mycoplasma PCR
	Urine:
	- Coccidioides antigen
				Special considerations if initial/secondary investigations negative or deterioration on acyclovir
				NB: Initial Herpes PCR may be negative early in course of illness (1-3 days). **Repeat CSF for Herpes PCR at 3-7 days before discontinuing acyclovir.**
				
				Rare Etiologies:
				Viral
				- Arboviruses (arthropod-borne) - travel history, insect exposure
				  • Flaviviruses (St. Louis encephalitis, West Nile virus, Tick borne virus)
				  • Bunyaviruses (La Cross Virus, Toscana virus)
				  • Togaviruses (Eastern/Western/Venezuelan equine encephalitis virus, Chikungunya virus)
				- Rabies virus - animal/occupational exposure
				- Herpes B - monkey exposure
				- Parvovirus B19 - children/rash, anemia
				- JC viruses – immunocompromised
				- LCM virus - immunocompromised/ rodent exposure
				- Measles, mumps, rubella - post infectious/post vaccination (acute disseminated encephalomyelitis)
				Bacterial
				- Bartonella spp: B. henselae - cat exposure, B. bacilliformis - S. America travel
				- Tropheryma spp (Whipple's disease)
				Rickettsial
				- Coxiella burnetii (Q fever) - contact with sheep, goats, unpasteurized products
				- Rickettsia rickettsii (Rocky Mountain Spotted Fever) - travel to endemic areas of Americas
				- Ehrlichia chaffeensis - USA travel/coastal areas
				- Anaplasma phagocytophilum - travel to endemic area
				Protozoal:
				- Acanthamoeba spp – immunocompromised, chronic alcoholism
				- Naegleria fowleri - swimming in lakes/brackish waters
				- Toxoplasma gondii - reactivation in immunocompromised host/intrauterine infection
				- Trypanosoma spp - travel to endemic area

RECOMMENDED EMPIRIC THERAPY OF SELECTED INFECTIONS IN ADULT PATIENTS[A]

Infection	Usual Pathogens	Recommended Empiric Therapy	Recommended DoseB	Recommended Duration	Comments
Central Nervous System					
Encephalitis (cont'd)	**Helminths:** - Taenia solium - immigrants/travel to endemic areas (Mexico, Central/South America) - Gnathostoma spp - immigrants/travel to southeast Asia; eosinophilia (blood/CSF) - Baylisascaris procyonis - raccoon exposure (esp feces); eosinophilia (blood/CSF) - Strongyloides stercoralis - hyperinfection syndrome in immunocompromised host -Angiostrongyliasis cantonensis – exposure to/ingestion of snails, shrimp; eosinopilia (CSF) **Transmissible spongiform encephalopathy:** - sporadic/variant Creutzfeld-Jakob disease				
	Herpes simplex virus 1 * Enteroviruses Other causes – see Introduction above	**HSV** **Acyclovir** +/- Antibacterial: (if bacterial meningitis not ruled out) **Ceftriaxone** + **Vancomycin**E +/- **Ampicillin**** +/- **Doxycycline*****	10mg/kg (based on IBW or ABW, whichever is less) IV q8h 2g IV q12h 15mg/kg IV q8-12h 2g IV q4h 200mg IV†/PO once then 100mg IV†/PO bid	14-21 days for HSV 10-14 days for VZV	* Herpes simplex is most common cause of sporadic, fatal encephalitis and is one of the few treatable causes. - Infectious Diseases consult recommended. **If risk of Listeria and neutrophils/mononuclear cells and low glucose in CSF. NB: Also consider TB/fungal pathogens if low CSF glucose +/- increased CSF protein. ***If risk of Rickettsia/Borrelia infection, predominance of mononuclear cells, normal glucose +/- elevated protein in CSF.

E. Desired vancomycin trough is 15-20 mg/L. Monitor renal function closely. See Vancomycin Dosing & Monitoring Guidelines.
† Must be obtained through TPD Special Access Program (Emergency Release). Contact pharmacy for assistance in ordering.

RECOMMENDED EMPIRIC THERAPY OF SELECTED INFECTIONS IN ADULT PATIENTS[A]

Infection	Usual Pathogens	Recommended Empiric Therapy	Recommended Dose[B]	Recommended Duration	Comments
Cardiovascular					

Pericarditis	**Diagnostic criteria**
	• typical chest pain
	• pericardial friction rub
	• suggestive ECG charges (typically widespread ST-segment evaluation, PR depression)
	+/-
	• new or worsening pericardial effusion
	• increased CRP/ESR (supports diagnosis but neither sensitive nor specific for pericarditis)
	
	Investigations
	• cardiac auscultation
	• ECG
	• transthoracic echocardiogram (TTE)
	• ESR/CRP, CBC, creatinine, troponin, CK-MB
	• CXR
	• pericardial fluid for C&S and mycobacterial culture
	
	Differential diagnosis
	• infectious (viral, bacterial, mycobacterial, fungal, parasitic)
	• non-infectious:
	   o autoimmune
	   o neoplastic
	   o metabolic
	   o traumatic
	   o drug-related				

RECOMMENDED EMPIRIC THERAPY OF SELECTED INFECTIONS IN ADULT PATIENTS[A]

Infection	Usual Pathogens	Recommended Empiric Therapy	Recommended Dose[B]	Recommended Duration	Comments
Cardiovascular					
Pericarditis (cont'd)	Viral (~90%): • usually Enterovirus Rare: • M. tuberculosis • Ureaplasma spp • Mycoplasma spp • S. aureus/MRSA • β-haemolytic Streptococci • Enterobacteriaceae • S. pneumoniae	<u>Viral pericarditis</u> Self-limited. No antiviral therapy. <u>Purulent pericarditis</u>*† **Vancomycin**[E] + **Ceftriaxone**	15mg/kg IV q8-12h 2g IV daily	6 weeks	* Recommend urgent surgical drainage if purulent/bacterial etiology suspected. † Tailor antibiotics to C&S results. β-lactams superior to vancomycin so preferred if susceptible.

Endocarditis	- 10-20% of patients who develop endocarditis have no pre-existing heart disease.
	- Diagnosis includes: • multiple positive blood cultures
	  • new/worsening murmur
	  • definite emboli
	  • vegetations on echocardiogram.
	- For more specific diagnostic criteria, refer to Modified Duke Criteria www.circulationaha.org (Circulation 2005;111:e394-e433).
	- Blood cultures: • **NB:** in patients who are stable (no heart failure) with subacute presentation, wait for results of blood cultures before starting antibiotic therapy.
	  • draw maximum 2 sets/day
	  • adults – 8-10mL of blood/bottle
	  • consult microbiology laboratory if unusual/fastidious (Bartonella, Chlamydia/Chlamydophila, Coxiella, Brucella, Legionella, Tropheryma whippleii) organism suspected
	  • ensure clearance of bacteremia to guide duration of therapy.
	- For positive cultures or blood culture negative endocarditis, see Recommended Therapy of Culture-Directed Infections Tables 4 & 5, respectively.				

E. Desired vancomycin trough is 15-20 mg/L. Monitor renal function closely. See Vancomycin Dosing & Monitoring Guidelines.

RECOMMENDED EMPIRIC THERAPY OF SELECTED INFECTIONS IN ADULT PATIENTS[A]

Infection	Usual Pathogens	Recommended Empiric Therapy	Recommended Dose[B]	Recommended Duration	Comments
Cardiovascular					

Endocarditis (cont'd)		- Echocardiogram:
		• transthoracic echocardiogram (TTE) - 60-65% sensitivity
		transesophageal echocardiogram (TEE) - 85-95% sensitivity
		• TEE recommended if:
		  ○ prosthetic valves (TTE < 50% sensitivity)
		  ○ congenital heart disease
		  ○ previous endocarditis
		  ○ TTE negative AND:
		    ▪ new murmur
		    ▪ heart failure
		    ▪ stigmata of endocarditis
		• should be repeated following treatment for endocarditis to establish a new baseline.
		
		- For surgical indications and timing see Circulation 2010;121:1141-52.
		Duration of antibiotic therapy post-valve replacement:
		• negative valve cultures - 2 more weeks
		• positive valve cultures - full course of therapy starting from day of surgery.
		
		Vancomycin
		• Vancomycin is less rapidly bactericidal than ß-lactams so should only be used when β-lactams contraindicated (due to severe allergy, or resistance). Longer duration of therapy may be required.
		• Desired vancomycin trough is 15-20mg/L. Monitor renal function closely. See Vancomycin Dosing & Monitoring Guidelines.			

RECOMMENDED EMPIRIC THERAPY OF SELECTED INFECTIONS IN ADULT PATIENTS[A]

Infection	Usual Pathogens	Recommended Empiric Therapy	Recommended Dose[B]	Recommended Duration	Comments
Cardiovascular					
Endocarditis (cont'd)					
Native valve (non-IVDU)	Viridans Group Streptococci S. aureus/MRSA Enterococcus spp HACEK organisms Coagulase negative Staphylococci Streptococcus gallolyticus (S. bovis biotype I) Abiotrophia spp Granulicatella spp Gemella spp	**Vancomycin**[E] + **Ceftriaxone** _Severe penicillin/ cephalosporin allergy_ **Vancomycin**[E] + **Gentamicin***	15mg/kg IV q8-12h 2g IV daily 15mg/kg IV q8-12h 1mg/kg IV q8h	Culture negative - 6 weeks Culture positive - see Recommended Therapy of Culture-Directed Infections Table 4	- Tailor antibiotic therapy to C&S results. β-lactams superior to vancomycin so preferred if susceptible. * Desired gentamicin trough < 1mg/L. See Aminoglycoside Dosing & Monitoring Guidelines.
	Rare: • S. pneumoniae • S. pyogenes (Group A) • S. agalactiae (Group B) • β-haemolytic Streptococci group C&G • Enterobacteriaceae • Neisseria spp • Moraxella spp				

HACEK = Haemophilus parainfluenzae, Aggregatibacter actinomycetemcomitans/ aphrophilus, Cardiobacterium hominis, Eikenella corrodens, Kingella spp.
E. Desired vancomycin trough is 15-20 mg/L. Monitor renal function closely. See Vancomycin Dosing & Monitoring Guidelines.

RECOMMENDED EMPIRIC THERAPY OF SELECTED INFECTIONS IN ADULT PATIENTS[A]

Infection	Usual Pathogens	Recommended Empiric Therapy	Recommended Dose[B]	Recommended Duration	Comments
Cardiovascular					
Endocarditis (cont'd) **Intravenous Drug Users (right-sided)**	S. aureus/MRSA P. aeruginosa* Enterobacteriaceae, especially Serratia* Candida spp Enterococcus spp Viridans Group Streptococci Polymicrobial	**Vancomycin**[E] +/- **[Gentamicin*** or **Tobramycin*** or **Ciprofloxacin*]**	15mg/kg IV q8-12h 1.5-2mg/kg IV q8h 1.5-2mg/kg IV q8h 400mg IV q12h or 750mg PO bid	Culture negative - 6 weeks Culture positive - see Recommended Therapy of Culture-Directed Infections Table 4	* Include empiric therapy for P. aeruginosa/Enterobacteriaceae if: • left-side involved • multiple valves involved. - Tailor antibiotic therapy to C&S results. β-lactams superior to vancomycin so preferred if susceptible.

E. Desired vancomycin trough is 15-20 mg/L. Monitor renal function closely. See Vancomycin Dosing & Monitoring Guidelines.

RECOMMENDED EMPIRIC THERAPY OF SELECTED INFECTIONS IN ADULT PATIENTS[A]

Infection	Usual Pathogens	Recommended Empiric Therapy	Recommended Dose[B]	Recommended Duration	Comments
Cardiovascular					
Endocarditis (cont'd)					
Prosthetic valve					
• early (< 8 weeks)	S. aureus/MRSA Coagulase negative Staph Rare: Enterococcus spp Enterobacteriaceae S. gallolyticus (S. bovis biotype I) Fungi	**Vancomycin**[E] + **Gentamicin*** + **Rifampin**	15mg/kg IV q8-12h 1mg/kg IV q8h 300mg PO tid or 600mg PO bid	6 weeks 2 weeks 6 weeks	- Recommend urgent surgical consult if: • etiology is S. aureus, P. aeruginosa, fungi • heart failure • diabetes and/or renal failure • valve ring abscess • heart block. - Tailor antibiotic therapy to C&S results. β-lactams superior to vancomycin so preferred if susceptible. * Extended interval aminoglycoside dosing not recommended for synergy. Desired gentamicin trough < 1mg/L. See Aminoglycoside Dosing & Monitoring Guidelines.
• late (> 8 weeks)	S. aureus/MRSA Coagulase negative Staph Viridans Group Strep Enterococcus spp Rare: S. gallolyticus (S. bovis biotype I) Enterobacteriaceae Fungi				

E. Desired vancomycin trough is 15-20 mg/L. Monitor renal function closely. See Vancomycin Dosing & Monitoring Guidelines.

RECOMMENDED EMPIRIC THERAPY OF SELECTED INFECTIONS IN ADULT PATIENTS[A]

Infection	Usual Pathogens	Recommended Empiric Therapy	Recommended Dose[B]	Recommended Duration	Comments
Cardiovascular					
Cardiac device-related infections/endocarditis (CDRIE)	- CDRIE must be suspected if unexplained fever in a patient with a cardiac device.				
	Investigations • Cultures of blood, wound, drive line, device pocket, +/- pump • TTE/TEE - both may be falsely negative				
	- Complete device and lead removal is usually indicated, unless superficial infection. - When indicated, and where possible, device re-implantation should be postponed until 72 hours from first negative blood culture, or 14 days from device removal if valvular infection. - Long term suppressive therapy should be considered if complete device removal not possible.				
	Coagulase negative Staphylococcus S. aureus/MRSA Enterococcus spp Enterobacteriaceae P. aeruginosa Candida spp	**Vancomycin**[E] + **Ciprofloxacin IV/PO** +/- **Fluconazole IV/PO***	15mg/kg IV q8-12h 400mg IV q12h/ 750mg PO bid 800mg IV/PO daily	Until device removed, then: • additional 10-14 days for pocket-site infection • additional 14 days for bacteremia • 4-6 weeks for endocarditis, septic thrombophlebitis, osteomyelitis, or if bacteremia persists despite device removal	- Tailor antibiotic therapy to C&S results. β-lactams superior to vancomycin so preferred if susceptible. * Add fluconazole if: • recent positive fungal cultures. • recent broad-spectrum antibiotic use. • deterioration despite 24 hours of antibiotic therapy.

E. Desired vancomycin trough is 15-20 mg/L. Monitor renal function closely. See Vancomycin Dosing & Monitoring Guidelines.

RECOMMENDED EMPIRIC THERAPY OF SELECTED INFECTIONS IN ADULT PATIENTS[A]

Infection	Usual Pathogens	Recommended Empiric Therapy	Recommended Dose[B]	Recommended Duration	Comments
Sepsis	Typical findings of systemic inflammatory response syndrome (SIRS): • temperature >38.3°C or < 36°C • heart rate > 90 beats/min • respiratory rate > 20 breaths/min or $PaCO_2$ < 32mmHg • WBC > 12×10^9/L, < 4×10^9/L or > 10% immature forms Sepsis = SIRS + infection: • severe sepsis = sepsis + sepsis-induced organ dysfunction or hypoperfusion or hypotension • septic shock = sepsis-induced hypotension unresponsive to fluid resuscitation Investigations: • Blood cultures. For clinically significant Gram positive bacteremia or candidemia, repeat blood cultures 24-48 hours after starting antimicrobial therapy to ensure clearance. • Other cultures/investigations including imaging as appropriate according to presentation and suspected source of infection: • urine • wound • sputum for C&S and CXR if respiratory symptoms • CSF • thick/thin smear for malaria if relevent travel history. • Thorough physical examination to rule out septic emboli and other skin manifestations Antibiotic therapy: • Intravenous antibiotic therapy should be started within first hour of recognition of severe sepsis and septic shock. Other than for blood cultures, do NOT delay administration of antibiotics. • Avoid recently (≤ 3 months) used antibiotics. • Empiric Gram negative combination therapy recommended until C&S results available if: • septic shock • neutropenic patients with severe sepsis. See Febrile Neutropenia. • infections due to suspected multi-resistant organisms: ○ Pseudomonas aeruginosa ○ Acinetobacter ○ ESBL, Amp C, or carbapenemase producing Gram negative organisms.			

RECOMMENDED EMPIRIC THERAPY OF SELECTED INFECTIONS IN ADULT PATIENTS[A]

Infection	Usual Pathogens	Recommended Empiric Therapy	Recommended Dose[B]	Recommended Duration	Comments
Sepsis (cont'd)					

Antibiotic therapy (cont'd):
- Vancomycin recommended empirically if patient at risk of MRSA.
- Linezolid recommended empirically if patient immunocompromised and previous colonization/infection with VRE.
- Tailor/narrow antibiotic therapy according to C&S results. **NB:** maintain combination therapy for P. aeruginosa bacteremia as demonstrated mortality benefit over monotherapy.

- In general, recommended duration of therapy is 7-10 days; 14 days minimum for S. aureus pneumonia/bacteremia. Longer courses may be required in patients with persistent bacteremia (rule out endocarditis), slow clinical response, inadequate source control, or neutropenia.

- Source control critical in many causes of severe sepsis/septic shock including:
- toxic megacolon or C. difficile colitis with shock (discontinue inciting antibiotics)
- ischemic bowel
- perforated viscus
- any significant abscesses, e.g. intra-abdominal
- ascending cholangitis
- gangrenous cholecystitis
- necrotizing pancreatitis with infection
- bacterial empyema
- mediastinitis
- purulent tunnel or foreign body infections
- obstructive uropathy
- complicated pyelonephritis/perinephric abscess
- necrotizing soft tissue infections
- clostridial myonecrosis.
[Kumar Crit Care Clin 2009;25:745]

- Failure to clear blood cultures after 3 days of appropriate antimicrobial therapy indicative of:
- septic thrombophlebitis
- endocarditis or other endovascular source
- metastatic foci.

RECOMMENDED EMPIRIC THERAPY OF SELECTED INFECTIONS IN ADULT PATIENTS[A]

Infection	Recommended Empiric Therapy	Recommended Dose[B]	Recommended Duration	Comments
Sepsis				
Genitourinary/ Urosepsis	**Piperacillin-tazobactam** +/- **Gentamicin***	3.375g IV q6h 7mg/kg IV daily	7-10 days Assess need for continuation based on C&S results	* Add gentamicin if: • septic shock • recent antibiotic use • suspected ESBL, Amp C, carbapenemase producing organism.
	Severe penicillin allergy/ anaphylaxis **Ciprofloxacin** + **Gentamicin**	400mg IV q12h 7mg/kg IV daily	7-10 days Assess need for continuation based on C&S results	**Add vancomycin if: • recent antibiotic use • recent urinary tract instrumentation/stent. NB: If S. aureus isolated from the urine, rule out infection at a distal site; longer duration of therapy required.
	+/- **Vancomycin**[E]**	15mg/kg IV q8-12h	7-10 days	
Respiratory	**Ceftriaxone** + **Azithromycin** +/- **Vancomycin**[E]*	2g IV daily 500mg IV daily 25-30mg kg IV once then 15mg/kg IV q8-12h	7-10 days 3-5 days 7-10 days	* Add vancomycin if: • severe/necrotizing process on CXR • rapid deterioration • health-care associated • recent antibiotic use • previous (prior 12 months)/current MRSA colonization or infection - For organism - specific recommendations, see Recommended Therapy of Culture-Directed Infections Table 1.
	Severe penicillin/ cephalosporin allergy **Levofloxacin** +/- **Vancomycin**[E]*	750mg IV daily 25-30mg/kg IV once then 15mg/kg IV q8-12h	7-10 days 7-10 days	
Intra-abdominal	**Piperacillin-tazobactam** +/- **Gentamicin***	4.5g IV q8h or 3.375g IV q6h 7mg/kg IV daily**	Continue therapy until: • afebrile • normal WBC/ differential • no residual fluid collections • return of GI function.	* Add gentamicin if: • septic shock • recent antibiotic use • suspected ESBL, Amp C, carbapenemase producing organism. ** Assess need for continuation of gentamicin based on C&S results. ***Add vancomycin if: • ascending cholangitis • hemodynamically unstable/septic shock.
	Severe penicillin allergy/ anaphylaxis **Ciprofloxacin** + **Metronidazole** +/- **Vancomycin**[E]***	400mg IV q12h 500mg IV q12h 15mg/kg IV q8-12h		

E. Desired vancomycin trough is 15-20 mg/L. Monitor renal function closely. See Vancomycin Dosing & Monitoring Guidelines.

RECOMMENDED EMPIRIC THERAPY OF SELECTED INFECTIONS IN ADULT PATIENTS[A]

Infection	Recommended Empiric Therapy	Recommended Dose[B]	Recommended Duration	Comments
Sepsis				
Skin & Soft Tissue, Rapidly Progressive/ Necrotizing Fasciitis	**Ceftriaxone +** **Clindamycin***	2g IV daily 600-900mg IV q8h	10-14 days 10-14 days	* Inhibits toxin production of Streptococcal spp. Staphylococcal spp. and Clostridium spp. ** If S. aureus isolated, rule out infection at a distal site, e.g. osteomyelitis or endovascular infection; longer duration of therapy required.
	MRSA suspected** Add **Vancomycin**[E] to above or use **Ceftriaxone** **+** **Linezolid***	15mg/kg IV q8-12h 2g IV daily 600mg IV/PO q12h	10-14 days 10-14 days	
Polymicrobial skin & soft tissue • groin/peri-rectal • diabetic wound • severe bite/ traumatic wounds	[**Piperacillin-tazobactam** or **Imipenem**] **+/-** **Vancomycin**[E]*	3.375g-4.5g IV q6h 500mg-1g IV q6h 15mg/kg IV q8-12h	7-14 days 7-14 days MRSA: 14-21 days	* Add vancomycin to cover MRSA if: • previous (prior 12 months)/current MRSA colonization or infection • recent antibiotic use • recent hospitalization • intravenous drug use • health care worker. - If S. aureus isolated, rule out infection at a distal site, e.g. osteomyelitis or endovascular infection; longer duration of therapy required.
Severe immuno-suppression/ Neutropenia	Penicillin allergy/ anaphylaxis **Vancomycin**[E] **+** **Ciprofloxacin** **+** **Metronidazole**	15mg/kg IV q8-12h 400mg IV q12h 500mg IV q12h	7-14 days 7-14 days 7-14 days	

E. Desired vancomycin trough is 15-20 mg/L. Monitor renal function closely. See Vancomycin Dosing & Monitoring Guidelines.

RECOMMENDED EMPIRIC THERAPY OF SELECTED INFECTIONS IN ADULT PATIENTS[A]

Infection	Recommended Empiric Therapy	Recommended Dose[B]	Recommended Duration	Comments
Sepsis				
Central Nervous System* • **Adults 18- 50 years** • **Immuno-competent**	**Ceftriaxone** + **Vancomycin**[E**] _Alternative_ **Meropenem** + **Vancomycin**[E**] _Severe penicillin/ cephalosporin allergy_ **TMP/SMX** + **Vancomycin**[E**]	2g IV q12h 25-30mg/kg IV once then 15mg/kg IV q8-12h 2g IV q8h 25-30mg/kg IV once then 15mg/kg IV q8-12h 15-20mg TMP/kg/ day div q6-8h 25-30mg/kg IV once then 15mg/kg IV q8-12h	minimum 10 days Reassess based on C&S results** minimum 10 days Reassess based on C&S results** minimum 10 days Reassess based on C&S results**	* Dexamethasone (0.15mg/kg IV q6h x 2-4 days) **prior to administration of antibiotics** is an option in bacterial meningitis but remains controversial [Lancet Neurol 2010;9:254–63]. The benefit of corticosteroids may depend on age, severity of presentation and pathogen. Corticosteroids have been shown to decrease mortality and hearing loss in adult patients with S. pneumoniae meningitis [Neurol 2010:75:1533-9]. **Discontinue vancomycin if ceftriaxone or meropenem or TMP/SMX susceptible organism confirmed.
• **Adults > 50 years** • **Immunocompromised (including AIDS)** • **Alcoholism** • **Debilitating illness** • **Pregnancy**	**Ceftriaxone** + **Ampicillin** + **Vancomycin**[E*] _Severe penicillin/ cephalosporin allergy_ **TMP/SMX*** + **Vancomycin**[E*]	2g IV q12h 2g IV q4h 25-30mg/kg IV once then 15mg/kg IV q8-12h 15-20mg TMP/kg/ day div q6-8h 25-30mg/kg IV once then 15mg/kg IV q8-12h	minimum 10 days minimum 10 days Reassess based on C&S results* minimum 10 days Reassess based on C&S results*	*Discontinue vancomycin if ceftriaxone or ampicillin, or TMP/SMX susceptible organism confirmed. ** TMP/SMX should not be used in first trimester or after 32 weeks gestation.

E. Desired vancomycin trough is 15-20 mg/L.   Monitor renal function closely. See Vancomycin Dosing & Monitoring Guidelines.

RECOMMENDED EMPIRIC THERAPY OF SELECTED INFECTIONS IN ADULT PATIENTS[A]

Infection	Recommended Empiric Therapy	Recommended Dose[B]	Recommended Duration	Comments
Sepsis				
Central Nervous System (cont'd) **Post-trauma/neuro-surgery**	**Meropenem**[E] + **Vancomycin**[E]*	2g IV q8h 25-30mg/kg IV once then 15mg/kg IV q8-12h	10-14 days 10-14 days	- If no previous antibiotic therapy, no foreign material, and negative CSF cultures, can discontinue antibiotic therapy at 72 hours. * Discontinue vancomycin if meropenem susceptible organism confirmed.
	Severe penicillin allergy/ anaphylaxis **Ciprofloxacin** + **Vancomycin**[E]	400mg IV q8-12h 25-30mg/kg IV once then 15mg/kg IV q8-12h	10-14 days 10-14 days	
Suspected herpes encephalitis	Add: **Acyclovir** to above regimens	10mg/kg (based on IBW or ABW, whichever is less) IV q8h	Reassess/discontinue based on etiology.	
Sepsis Unknown Source	**Piperacillin-tazobactam** +/- **Gentamicin*** +/- **Vancomycin**[E]**	3.375-4.5g IV q6h 7mg/kg IV daily 15mg/kg IV q8-12h	7-10 days Reassess based on C&S results Reassess based on C&S results	* Add gentamicin if: • septic shock • recent antibiotic use • suspected ESBL, Amp C, carbapenemase-producing organism. **Add vancomycin if: • previous (prior 12 months/current MRSA colonization or infection • recent antibiotic use • recent hospitalization • medical device/vascular access-related infection. - If S. aureus isolated, rule out infection at a distal site, e.g. osteomyelitis or endovascular infection; longer duration of therapy required. ***Add metronidazole if elderly and vascular insufficiency, or anaerobic infection suspected.
	Severe penicillin allergy/ anaphylaxis **Ciprofloxacin**[E] + **Vancomycin**[E] +/- **Gentamicin*** +/- **Metronidazole*****	400mg IV q12h 15mg/kg IV q8-12h 7mg/kg IV daily 500mg IV q12h	7-10 days 7-10 days Reassess based on C&S results 7-10 days	
Splenectomized	**Ceftriaxone** + **Vancomycin**[E]	2g IV daily 15mg/kg IV q8-12h	7-10 days 7-10 days	

E. Desired vancomycin trough is 15-20 mg/L. Monitor renal function closely. See Vancomycin Dosing & Monitoring Guidelines.

RECOMMENDED EMPIRIC THERAPY OF SELECTED INFECTIONS IN ADULT PATIENTS[A]

Infection	Usual Pathogens	Recommended Empiric Therapy	Recommended Dose[B]	Recommended Duration	Comments
Sepsis					
Catheter-related bloodstream infection (CRBSI) [Clin Infect Dis 2009;49:1-45]	Prevention[Clin Infect Dis 2011;52:e1-32]: • Hand hygiene • Use maximal sterile barrier precautions (cap, mask, sterile gown and gloves, sterile full body drape) during catheter insertion. • Use skin antisepsis (chlorhexidine > 0.5% with alcohol for central venous catheters and arterial catheters). Peripheral venous catheters • If infection suspected, remove catheter. Send blood cultures (BCs) (2-4 bottles). • Start systemic antibiotic therapy. **NB**: For coagulase negative Staph (CoNS), catheter removal may be sufficient if patient not systemically ill. Short-term (<14 days) central venous catheters (CVC)/peripherally inserted central catheter (PICC)/arterial catheter (AC) Diagnosis: • Recommend two sets of BCs, one from the catheter* and one peripherally. • Differential time to positivity (DTP) > 2h between blood culture taken from CVC and peripherally suggests CRBSI. * Samples for BCs from all lumens may be required to establish the diagnosis of CRBSI. Management: • Remove CVC/PICC/AC if: - signs & symptoms of sepsis, septic thrombophlebitis, endocarditis, osteomyelitis - bacteremia that persists despite > 72h of appropriate antibiotic therapy - CRBSI due to Gram negative bacilli, S. aureus, enterococci, fungi, or mycobacteria - > 1 BC bottle positive for CoNS, Bacillus spp, Micrococcus spp. or Propionibacteria spp - erythema or purulence at CVC exit site - CVC tip (from line exchanged over a guidewire) has colony count ≥15 CFU. • If coagulase negative Staph (CoNS) – remove CVC and give systemic antibiotic therapy x 5-7 days, or retain CVC and give systemic antibiotic therapy + antibiotic lock therapy (see below) x 10-14 days. • If S. aureus, rule out endocarditis. Remove catheter and treat with systemic antibiotic therapy for ≥ 14 days. If persistent bacteremia or lack of clinical improvement > 3 days after catheter removal and appropriate antibiotic therapy, investigate for septic thrombophlebitis, endocarditis, or metastatic infection. • If Enterococcus spp or Gram negative bacilli, remove catheter and treat with systemic antibiotic therapy for 7-14 days. • If Candida spp. remove catheter and treat with systemic antifungal therapy for 14 days after first negative BC. Rule out endocarditis and/or endophthalmitis.			

RECOMMENDED EMPIRIC THERAPY OF SELECTED INFECTIONS IN ADULT PATIENTS[A]

Infection	Usual Pathogens	Recommended Empiric Therapy	Recommended Dose[B]	Recommended Duration	Comments
Sepsis					
Catheter-related bloodstream infection (CRBSI) (cont'd) [Clin Infect Dis 2009;49:1-45]	**Long-term/tunneled CVCs (e.g. Hickman, Broviac) & implantable vascular access devices (IVAD) (e.g. Port-a-cath)** • Complicated: tunnel infection, port abscess - Remove CVC/IVAD and treat with antibiotics x 7-10 days. • Uncomplicated: - CoNS - Retain CVC/IVAD: treat with systemic antibiotic therapy + antibiotic lock therapy* x 10-14 days. Remove CVC if clinical deterioration or persistent (> 72h) or relapsing bacteremia and work-up for complicated infection and treat accordingly. - S. aureus/MRSA/S. lugdunensis - Remove CVC/IVAD: treat with systemic antibiotic therapy x 14 days after first negative BC if TEE negative. If salvage of CVC/IVAD essential, give systemic + antibiotic lock therapy* x 4 weeks. Remove CVC if clinical deterioration or persistent (> 72h) or relapsing bacteremia and work-up for complicated infection and treat accordingly. If complicated infection not present, treat with systemic antibiotic therapy x 14 days. - Enterococcus spp - Retain CVC/IVAD: treat with systemic antibiotic therapy + antibiotic lock therapy* x 7-14 days. Remove CVC/IVAD if clinical deterioration or persistent (> 72h) or relapsing bacteremia and work-up for complicated infection and treat accordingly. - Gram negative organisms - Remove CVC/IVAD: treat with systemic antibiotic therapy x 7-14 days. If salvage of CVC/IVAD essential, give systemic + antibiotic lock therapy* x 10-14 days. Remove CVC if clinical deterioration or persistent (> 72h) or relapsing bacteremia and work-up for complicated infection and treat accordingly. If complicated infection not present, treat with systemic antibiotic therapy x 10-14 days. - Candida spp - Rule out endocarditis and/or endophthalmitis. Remove CVC/IVAD: treat with systemic antifungal therapy x 14 days after first negative BC. **Hemodialysis catheters** – increased risk of S. aureus/MRSA infection. *Antibiotic Lock Therapy NB: Always use in combination with systemic antibiotics. NB: Various concentrations have been studied. Further study is required to establish standard effective concentrations. Recommended concentrations based on available literature: • Gram positive - cefazolin: 10mg/mL, vancomycin: 5-10mg/mL • Gram negative - gentamicin: 5-10mg/mL, amikacin: 10mg/mL, ciprofloxacin: 5-10mg/mL Mix antibiotic with normal saline or 50-100 units of heparin (if compatible) to 2-5mL luminal volume (volume should be printed on outside of line; if not, contact manufacturer). Fill catheter lumen when not in use (e.g. 12h period overnight). Remove solution before infusion of next IV medication or solution. NB: Antibiotic lock therapy to prevent CRBSI is not generally recommended unless multiple episodes of CRBSI despite optimal adherence to aseptic technique [Clin Infect Dis 2011;52:e1-32].			

RECOMMENDED EMPIRIC THERAPY OF SELECTED INFECTIONS IN ADULT PATIENTS[A]

Infection	Usual Pathogens	Recommended Empiric Therapy	Recommended Dose[B]	Recommended Duration
Sepsis				
Catheter-related bloodstream infections (CRBSI) (cont'd) [Clin Infect Dis 2009;49:1-45]	Coagulase negative Staph (CoNS) S. aureus S. lugdunensis Enterococcus spp Corynebacterium spp Leuconostoc spp* Enterobacteriaceae Pseudomonas spp Yeast** * Leuconostoc spp are resistant to vancomycin and 3rd generation cephalosporins.	**Vancomycin**[E] +/- **Gentamicin**[†] +/- Antifungal therapy** **Anidulafungin** or **Caspofungin** or **Micafungin** or **Fluconazole*****	15mg/kg IV q8-12h 7mg/kg IV q24h 200mg IV once then 100mg IV daily 70mg IV once then 50mg IV daily 100mg IV daily 800mg IV loading dose then 400-800mg IV/PO daily	Duration dependent on: • ability to remove line • organism involved • uncomplicated/complicated (see below). Uncomplicated BC positive with: - CoNS - 5-7 days **Avoid treatment in response to single positive blood culture for CoNS. Repeat culture recommended.** - S. aureus & TEE negative - 14 days after first negative BC - Gram negative organisms - 7-14 days - Candida spp - 14 days after first negative BC. - If BC negative but catheter tip ≥15 CFU of S. aureus or Candida spp, consider 5-7 day course of therapy after line removal. Complicated - Septic thrombophlebitis - 4-6 weeks - Endocarditis - 4-6 weeks - Osteomyelitis - 6-8 weeks - Persistent bacteremia > 72h after catheter removal despite appropriate antimicrobial therapy - 4-6 weeks. † Add gentamicin if: • septic • neutropenic • femoral catheter • suspected infection/colonization with Gram negative organisms.

E. Desired vancomycin trough is 15-20 mg/L. Monitor renal function closely. See Vancomycin Dosing & Monitoring Guidelines.

RECOMMENDED EMPIRIC THERAPY OF SELECTED INFECTIONS IN ADULT PATIENTS[A]

Infection	Usual Pathogens	Recommended Empiric Therapy	Recommended Dose[B]	Recommended Duration
Sepsis				
Catheter-related bloodstream infections (CRBSI) (cont'd)				**Add antifungal therapy if: • patient receiving TPN • prolonged use of broad spectrum antibiotics • hematologic malignancy • stem cell or solid organ transplant • femoral catheter • Candida colonization at multiple sites. ***Use fluconazole if no azole exposure in past 3 months and risk of C. krusei or C. glabrata low.

RECOMMENDED EMPIRIC THERAPY OF SELECTED INFECTIONS IN ADULT PATIENTS[A]

Infection	Usual Pathogens	Recommended Empiric Therapy	Recommended Dose[B]	Recommended Duration	Comments
Febrile Neutropenia [Clin Infect Dis 2011;52:e56-93]	**Definitions** Febrile = oral temperature ≥ 38.3°C once or ≥ 38°C for ≥ 1 hour Neutropenia = absolute neutrophil count [ANC] < 0.5 x 10⁹/L **Investigations:** • Blood and urine cultures • CBC with differential, electrolytes, creatinine, AST, bilirubin • If respiratory symptoms: ○ CXR ○ Nasopharyngeal swab for viral respiratory panel PCR ○ Sputum for C&S and Mycoplasma/Chlamydophila/Legionella PCR Careful physical examination required including skin, oral mucosa, perianal area, respiratory system and abdomen. **Monotherapy** - Piperacillin-tazobactam monotherapy is recommended first-line in patients who are hemodynamically stable, and no evidence of catheter-related infection, skin & soft tissue infection (SSTI), or pneumonia. Ceftazidime monotherapy is not recommended as it: • has no reliable Gram positive (Enterococci, Streptococci, Staphylococci) activity compared to piperacillin-tazobactam • may promote antimicrobial resistance (extended-spectrum ß-lactamases (ESBL) and AmpC cephalosporinases) • **is not optimal in patients with profound (< 0.1 x 10⁹/L)/prolonged neutropenia.** - Cefepime monotherapy is an alternative to piperacillin-tazobactam: • good streptococcal activity • activity against methicillin-susceptible S. aureus • activity against Amp C cephalosporinase-producing Gram negative organisms (but not against ESBL) • lacks enterococcal coverage. - Carbapenem monotherapy is an alternative to piperacillin-tazobactam. In order to prevent the selection of carbapenem resistance, carbapenems should not be used first-line unless: • known/suspected infection with ESBL/Amp C cephalosporinase-producing organisms • penicillin allergy.			

RECOMMENDED EMPIRIC THERAPY OF SELECTED INFECTIONS IN ADULT PATIENTS[A]

Infection	Usual Pathogens	Recommended Empiric Therapy	Recommended Dose[B]	Recommended Duration	Comments
Febrile Neutropenia (cont'd)	**Combination therapy (β-lactam plus an aminoglycoside and vancomycin)** • provides increased coverage of potential pathogens, including resistant strains. • is recommended until C&S results available in patients who are hemodynamically unstable or with septic shock. **Recommendations for the Use of Vancomycin in Febrile Neutropenia** - Empiric vancomycin should not be used routinely in febrile neutropenic patients. - Empiric vancomycin therapy should be considered in: • clinically obvious central venous catheter-related infections (tunnel infection) • skin or soft tissue infection • pneumonia • hemodynamic instability • patients with positive blood culture for Gram positive organisms not yet identified (NB: Leuconostoc spp. Pediococcus spp are resistant to vancomycin) • known colonization with MRSA. - Vancomycin therapy should be discontinued on day 2-3 if cultures negative for β-lactam resistant Gram positive organisms. **Prophylaxis** - Quinolone prophylaxis may increase likelihood of Gram positive infections and Gram negative resistance.			

RECOMMENDED EMPIRIC THERAPY OF SELECTED INFECTIONS IN ADULT PATIENTS[A]

Infection	Usual Pathogens	Recommended Empiric Therapy	Recommended Dose[B]	Recommended Duration	Comments
Febrile Neutropenia **Low risk**	**Low risk:** • Adults < 60 years of age • No focal findings of infection • Cancer in partial or complete remission • Increasing ANC/anticipated neutropenia ≤ 7 days • Temperature <39°C • Normal chest x-ray • Absence of hypotension • Respiratory rate ≤24 • No chronic lung disease or diabetes • Absence of dehydration and confusion • No history of fungal infection or antifungal therapy in previous 6 months - Median time to defervescence for low risk patients treated with appropriate empiric antibiotic therapy is 2-3 days.				
	See Febrile Neutropenia, High Risk	Low risk (see above) **Amoxicillin-clavulanate** +/- **Ciprofloxacin***	875mg PO bid 500-750mg PO bid	• Afebrile and ANC ≥ 0.5 x 10⁹/L x ≥2 days: discontinue therapy after 3 days. • Afebrile but ANC < 0.5 x 10⁹/L: discontinue antibiotic therapy after 5-10 days if low risk.	* Ciprofloxacin NOT recommended in patients who have received quinolone prophylaxis or recent (within 3 months) quinolone therapy.

RECOMMENDED EMPIRIC THERAPY OF SELECTED INFECTIONS IN ADULT PATIENTS[A]

Infection	Usual Pathogens	Recommended Empiric Therapy	Recommended Dose[B]	Recommended Duration	Comments
Febrile Neutropenia **High risk**	**High risk:** • Profound neutropenia (ANC < 0.1 x 10^9/L) anticipated to be > 7 days • Significant comorbid conditions, including: ○ hemodynamic instability ○ oral or GI mucositis that impairs swallowing or causes severe diarrhea ○ new onset abdominal pain, nausea or vomiting, or diarrhea ○ neurologic changes/confusion ○ intravascular catheter infection ○ pneumonia/hypoxemia/chronic lung disease ○ hepatic insufficiency (AST > 5x normal value) ○ renal insufficiency (Clcr < 30mL/min). - Median time to defervescence for high risk patients treated with appropriate empiric antibiotic therapy is 5 days. - Antifungal therapy: using agent from a different class from that used for prophylaxis should be considered in patients who remain febrile and neutropenic at day 4-7 despite adequate antibiotic coverage. • Infectious Diseases consult recommended. • Repeat blood cultures plus ultrasound of abdomen recommended. or • If high risk for mould infections (hematologic malignancy, especially AML), repeat blood cultures including fungal blood cultures and CT chest/abdomen/sinuses. - Consider switch to oral therapy if: • non-septic presentation (no chills, hypotension or fluid resuscitation) • patient stable • mucositis resolving • neutrophils > 0.1x10^9/L. • adequate GI absorption.			

RECOMMENDED EMPIRIC THERAPY OF SELECTED INFECTIONS IN ADULT PATIENTS[A]

Infection	Usual Pathogens	Recommended Empiric Therapy	Recommended Dose[B]	Recommended Duration	Comments
Febrile Neutropenia High risk (cont'd)	<u>Gram positive</u> Coag neg Staph Enterococcus spp Viridans Grp Strep S. aureus/MRSA S. lugdunensis Corynebacterium spp Bacillus cereus Rothia spp β-haemolytic Strep S. pneumoniae Rhodococcus spp Abiotrophia spp Granulicatella spp Leuconostoc spp Pediococcus spp <u>Gram negative</u> Enterobacteriaceae Pseudomonas spp Stenotrophomonas maltophilia Achromobacter spp Acinetobacter spp Burkholderia spp Capnocytophaga spp Eikenella spp Anaerobes Polymicrobial (20-30%) Fungi (< 5%) Viruses	<u>Hemodynamically Stable#</u> **Piperacillin-tazobactam** Alternative **Cefepime** or **Imipenem*** or **Meropenem*** Severe β-lactam allergy/ anaphylaxis **Vancomycin**[E§] + **Ciprofloxacin** +/- **Metronidazole*** +/- [**Gentamicin**† or **Tobramycin**†] <u>Hemodynamically unstable</u> **Piperacillin-tazobactam*** + **Vancomycin**[E§] + [**Gentamicin** or **Tobramycin**] Severe β-lactam allergy/ anaphylaxis **Vancomycin**[E§] + **Ciprofloxacin** + **Metronidazole** + [**Gentamicin** or **Tobramycin**]	4.5g IV q6-8h** 2g IV q8h 500mg IV q6h 500mg IV q6h or 1g IV q8h 15mg/kg IV q12h 400mg IV q8-12h†] 750mg PO bid 500mg IV/PO q12h 7mg/kg IV daily 7mg/kg IV daily 4.5g IV q6-8h 15mg/kg IV q12h 7mg/kg IV daily 7mg/kg IV daily 15mg/kg IV q12h 400mg IV q8-12h†] 750mg PO q12h 500mg IV q12h 7mg/kg IV daily 7mg/kg IV daily	Tailor duration of therapy to identified organism and infection. Must be afebrile for at least 48hrs and neutrophil count > 0.5 x 10⁹/L before discontinuing antibiotic therapy. •Bacteremia, SSTI, pneumonia - 10-14 days. No focus: •If neutrophil count ≥ 0.5x10⁹/L – 7 days minimum. •If neutrophil count < 0.5x10⁹/L - 2 weeks minimum. Longer therapy may be required if: • neutrophil count < 0.1 x 10⁹/L • severe mucositis • unstable vital signs.	* Use imipenem or meropenem if: • known/suspected infection with ESBL or Amp C producing organism • nonsevere penicillin allergy. # Add vancomycin (alternative linezolid[†]) if: • suspected catheter-related infection, SSTI, pneumonia • previous/current colonization or infection with MRSA. Add linezolid instead of vancomycin if: • previous/current colonization or infection with VRE. **If P. aeruginosa documented, use 4.5g IV q6h and consider adding tobramycin. † Consider giving 7mg/kg gentamicin or tobramycin while awaiting culture results if: • previous quinolone therapy/ prophylaxis. • antibiotics in last 3 months • suspected infection with ESBL, Amp C, carbapenemase-producing organism. ‡ Use q8h if P. aeruginosa documented.

E. Desired vancomycin trough is 10-20 mg/L. Monitor renal function closely. See Vancomycin Dosing & Monitoring Guidelines.

RECOMMENDED EMPIRIC THERAPY OF SELECTED INFECTIONS IN ADULT PATIENTS[A]

Infection	Usual Pathogens	Recommended Empiric Therapy	Recommended Dose[B]	Recommended Duration	Comments
Febrile Neutropenia High risk (cont'd)					***Add metronidazole if: • abdominal symptoms • suspected anaerobic infection • severe mucositis/ neutropenic enterocolitis. [§]Use linezolid instead of vancomycin if previous/current colonization or infection with VRE.

RECOMMENDED EMPIRIC THERAPY OF SELECTED INFECTIONS IN ADULT PATIENTS[A]

FOOTNOTES:

A. These are empiric antibiotic recommendations based on current literature, national susceptibility patterns, and antimicrobials currently available on the Canadian market. Readers are encouraged to make antibiotic therapy choices based on usual pathogens and susceptibility patterns locally. Antibiotics listed for each condition are not all inclusive, nor are they all approved by Health Canada TPD for the listed indication. Choice of empiric antibiotic therapy should be based on the patient's age, allergies, co-morbidities, and clinical condition, as well as cost and convenience of the dosage regimen. Empiric antibiotic therapy should be modified to narrower spectrum antibiotic(s) according to culture and susceptibility (C&S) results.

B. Usual adult dose in patients with normal renal and hepatic function.

C. Oral clindamycin/metronidazole have excellent absorption. If intravenous therapy is deemed necessary, prompt switch to the oral formulation is recommended. (See IV to PO Switch Recommendations)

D. Linezolid and oral quinolones have excellent absorption and bioavailability. With equal/equivalent doses, the serum concentration attained with oral quinolones is comparable to that of the IV formulation. Therefore, unless the patient is strictly NPO, use oral formulation. (See IV to PO Switch Recommendations)

E. See Vancomycin Dosing & Monitoring Guidelines.

RECOMMENDED THERAPY OF CULTURE-DIRECTED INFECTIONS IN ADULT PATIENTS[A]

Table 1 - Treatment of Culture - proven Pneumonia

Pathogen	Recommended Therapy	Recommended Dose[B]	Recommended Duration
S. pneumoniae			
Penicillin Susceptible	**Penicillin G**	2MU IV q4h	5-7 days; 10-14 days if bacteremic
	or		
	Amoxicillin	1g PO tid	
Penicillin Intermediate/ Resistant	**Ceftriaxone**	1-2g IV q24h	
	or		
	Levofloxacin	750mg IV/PO daily	
S. aureus			
MSSA	**Cloxacillin**	2g IV q6h	14 days from first negative blood culture if bacteremic
	or		
	Cefazolin	2g IV q8h	
MRSA	**Vancomycin**[E]	25-30mg/kg IV once then 15mg/kg IV q8-12h	
	or		
	Linezolid[D]	600mg IV/PO q12h	
E. coli			
not ESBL or Amp C	**Ceftriaxone**	1-2g IV daily	7 days
	or		
	Ciprofloxacin (if susceptible)	400mg IV/PO q12h/ 500mg PO bid	7 days
ESBL or Amp C	**Ertapenem**	1g IV daily	7-10 days
	or		
	Ciprofloxacin (if susceptible)	400mg IV/PO q12h/ 500mg PO bid	7-10 days
Klebsiella pneumoniae	**Ceftriaxone**	2g IV q24h	≥ 14 days
	or		
	Ciprofloxacin	400mg IV/PO q12h/ 500mg PO bid	≥ 14 days

E. Desired vancomycin trough is 15-20 mg/L. Monitor renal function closely.
See Vancomycin Dosing & Monitoring Guidelines.

RECOMMENDED THERAPY OF CULTURE-DIRECTED INFECTIONS IN ADULT PATIENTS[A]

Table 1 - Treatment of Culture - proven Pneumonia (cont'd)

Pathogen	Recommended Therapy	Recommended Dose[B]	Recommended Duration
Enterobacter spp Serratia spp Citrobacter spp	**Meropenem**	500mg IV q6h or 1g IV q8h	7-10 days
Pseudomonas aeruginosa	**Ceftazidime** +/- **Tobramycin**	2g IV q8h 7mg/kg IV daily	14 days 5-7 days
Stenotrophomonas maltophilia	**TMP/SMX** +/- **Doxycycline**	15mg/kg/d IV/PO div q6h or 8h 200mg PO once then 100mg PO bid	14 days 14 days
Acinetobacter spp	**Meropenem** +/- **Rifampin**	500mg IV q6h or 1g IV q8h 300mg PO tid	14 days 14 days
Haemophilus influenzae Amoxicillin-susceptible	**Amoxicillin**	500mg PO tid	7 days
Amoxicillin-resistant, β- lactamase positive	**Amoxicillin-clavulanate**	875mg PO bid	7 days
Amoxicillin-resistant, β- lactamase negative	**Levofloxacin** or **Ceftriaxone**	750mg IV/PO daily 1-2g IV daily	7 days 7 days
Moraxella catarrhalis	**Ceftriaxone** or **Amoxicillin-clavulanate**	1-2g IV daily 875mg PO bid	7 days 7 days
Legionella spp	**Levofloxacin** or **Azithromycin**	750mg IV/PO daily 500mg IV/PO daily	7-14 days/if immuno- compromised 21 days 7-10 days/i if immuno- compromised 21 days

RECOMMENDED THERAPY OF CULTURE-DIRECTED INFECTIONS IN ADULT PATIENTS[A]

Table 1 - Treatment of Culture - proven Pneumonia (cont'd)

Pathogen	Recommended Therapy	Recommended Dose[B]	Recommended Duration
Mycoplasma pneumoniae	**Doxycycline** or	200mg PO once then 100mg PO bid	7-10 days
	Azithromycin or	500mg IV/PO daily	3 days
	Levofloxacin	750mg IV/PO daily	5 days
Chlamydophila pneumoniae	**Doxycycline** or	200mg PO once then 100mg PO bid	5-7 days
	Azithromycin or	500mg IV/PO daily	3 days
	Clarithromycin or	500mg PO bid	7 days
	Levofloxacin	750mg IV/PO daily	5-7 days
Nocardia spp	**TMP-SMX** +	15mg/kg/d IV/PO div q6h, 8h, or q12h	3 months/ if immuno-compromised 6 months
	Imipenem	500mg IV q6h	

RECOMMENDED THERAPY OF CULTURE-DIRECTED INFECTIONS IN ADULT PATIENTS[A]

Table 2 - Treatment of Culture - proven Peritoneal Dialysis (PD) Peritonitis

Pathogen	Recommended Empiric Therapy	Intermittent Dosing* Dwell time at least 6h	Continuous dosing* (per L bag)*	Recommended Duration
Coagulase negative Staph, methicillin-susceptible	Cefazolin IP	15mg/kg once per day**	500mg/L LD then 125mg/L MD***	14 days
Coagulase negative Staph, methicillin-resistant	Vancomycin IP	30mg/kg q 7 days‡ (max 2g/dose)	1000mg/L LD then 25mg/L MD***	At least 21 days
S. aureus, methicillin susceptible (MSSA)	Cefazolin IP +/- Rifampin PO[†]	15mg/kg once per day** 600mg PO daily Paediatric: 10-20mg/kg/d PO div bid	500mg/L LD then 125mg/L MD*** 600mg PO daily	21 days - Strongly recommend catheter removal for refractory infections. † Recommended x 1 week for tunnel or recurrent infection.
S. aureus, methicillin resistant (MRSA)	Vancomycin IP +/- Rifampin PO[†]	30mg/kg q 7 days‡ (max 2g/dose) 600mg PO daily Paediatric: 10-20mg/kg/d PO div bid	1000mg/L LD then 25mg/L MD*** 600mg PO daily	At least 21 days - Strongly recommend catheter removal for refractory infections. † Recommended x 1 week for tunnel or recurrent infection.
Consult Infectious Diseases				
Streptococcus spp. penicillin susceptible	Ampicillin IP or Cefazolin IP	500mg/L once per day 15mg/kg once per day**	125mg/L MD 500mg/L LD then 125mg/L MD***	14 days 14 days

IP=intraperitoneally; LD=loading dose; MD=maintenance dose
Refractory = cloudy effluent after 5 days of appropriate antibiotic therapy.

* Dosing recommendations for anuric (<100 mL urine/24 hours) patients. PD patients with residual renal function may require increased doses or more frequent dosing, especially when using intermittent regimens. See below and adult & paediatric treatment guidelines at www.ispd.org/

For nonanuric patients:
    ** > 100 mL urine/24 hours - use 20mg/kg cefazolin
    *** > 100 mL urine/24 hours - increase (maintenance) dose by 25%
    ‡ > 500 mL urine/24 hours - give every 5 days, or when serum level <15mg/L.

RECOMMENDED THERAPY OF CULTURE-DIRECTED INFECTIONS IN ADULT PATIENTS[A]
Table 2 - Treatment of Culture - proven PD Peritonitis (cont'd)

Pathogen	Recommended Empiric Therapy	Intermittent Dosing* Dwell time at least 6h	Continuous dosing (per L bag)*	Recommended Duration
Enterococcus spp, ampicillin-susceptible	Ampicillin IP[Φ] + Gentamicin IP[†] (if gent synergy susceptible)	500mg/L once per day 0.6mg/kg once per day***	125mg/L MD[Φ] 20mg/L once daily	21 days Φ Ampicillin incompatible with aminoglycosides in dialysis solution; do not add ampicillin to the bag containing the gentamicin given once daily, i.e. give ampicillin in 3 of 4 bags/day and gentamicin in 1 of 4 bags/day.
Enterococcus spp, ampicillin-resistant	Vancomycin IP +/- Gentamicin IP (if gent synergy susceptible)	15-30mg/kg q 7 days‡ (max 2g/dose) 0.6mg/kg once per day	1000mg/L LD then 25mg/L MD*** 20mg/L once daily	21 days
Enterococcus spp, vancomycin-resistant	Linezolid	600mg PO bid		21 days
Coryneform spp	Vancomycin IP	15-30mg/kg q 7 days‡ (max 2g/dose)	1000mg/L LD then 25mg/L MD***	21 days
Gram negative organisms (excluding Pseudomonas)	Based on C&S results: Gentamicin IP[†] or Ciprofloxacin or Cefazolin IP	0.6mg/kg once per day*** 500mg PO bid 15mg/kg once per day**	8mg/L LD then 4mg/L MD*** 50mg/L LD then 25mg/L MD 500mg/L LD then 125mg/L MD***	14-21 days

IP=intraperitoneally; LD=loadingdose; MD=maintenance dose
* Dosing recommendations for anuric (<100 mL urine/24 hours) patients. PD patients with residual renal function may require increased doses or more frequent dosing, especially when using intermittent regimens. See below and adult & paediatric treatment guidelines at www.ispd.org/
For nonanuric patients: ** > 100 mL urine/24 hours - use 20mg/kg cefazolin
   *** >100 mL urine/24 hours - increase (maintenance) dose by 25%
‡ > 500 mL urine/24 hours - give every 5 days, or when serum level <15mg/L.
† To optimize concentration-dependent activity of aminoglycosides and lessen potential for toxicity, intermittent dosing is recommended over continuous dosing.

Table 2 - Treatment of Culture - proven PD Peritonitis (cont'd)

Pathogen	Recommended Empiric Therapy	Intermittent Dosing* Dwell time at least 6h	Continuous dosing (per L bag)*	Recommended Duration
Pseudomonas spp	**Ceftazidime IP[†]** +	1-1.5g once per day Paediatric: 20mg/kg once per day	500mg/L LD then 125mg/L MD***	21-28 days If no response or associated with catheter infection, remove catheter.
	[Tobramycin IP[†] or **Ciprofloxacin]**	0.6mg/kg once per day*** 500mg PO bid	8mg/L LD then 4mg/L MD*** 50mg/L LD then 25mg/L MD	
Stenotrophomonas maltophilia	**TMP/SMX PO** +/- **Doxycycline**	1DS tab PO bid 100mg PO bid		21-28 days
Polymicrobial - suspect bowel perforation ⇒ consider surgical intervention	**Vancomycin IP** + **[Gentamicin IP[†]** or **Ciprofloxacin]** + **Metronidazole IV/PO[C]** or **Imipenem** monotherapy	15-30mg/kg q 7[‡] days 0.6mg/kg once per day*** 500mg PO bid 500mg IV/PO q12h 250mg IV q12h	1000mg/L LD then 25mg/L MD*** 8mg/L LD then 4mg/L MD*** 50mg/L LD then 25mg/L MD 500mg IV/PO q12h 250mg/L LD then 50mg/L MD	14- 21 days Consider catheter removal

IP=intraperitoneally; LD=loading dose; MD=maintenance dose

* Dosing recommendations for anuric (<100 mL urine/24 hours) patients. PD patients with residual renal function may require increased doses or more frequent dosing, especially when using intermittent regimens. See below and adult & paediatric treatment guidelines at www.ispd.org/

For nonanuric patients: ***> 100 mL urine/24 hours - increase (maintenance) dose by 25%

‡ > 500mL urine/24 hours - give every 5 days, or when serum level < 15mg/L

† To optimize concentration-dependent activity of aminoglycosides and lessen potential for toxicity, intermittent dosing is recommended over continuous dosing.

RECOMMENDED THERAPY OF CULTURE-DIRECTED INFECTIONS IN ADULT PATIENTS[A]

Table 2 - Treatment of Culture - proven PD Peritonitis (cont'd)

Pathogen	Recommended Empiric Therapy	Intermittent Dosing* Dwell time at least 6h	Continuous dosing* (per L bag)*	Recommended Duration
Candida spp	~25% mortality. Consult Infectious Diseases and/or pharmacist.			Catheter removal strongly recommended. Treat for 10-14 days after catheter removal. If immediate removal of catheter not possible, must be removed by 72 hours if patient not clinically improving.
	Anidulafungin or	200mg IV once then 100mg IV daily		‡ Some non-albicans Candida may be resistant to fluconazole. Intraperitoneal amphotericin B causes chemical peritonitis and pain.
	Caspofungin or	70mg IV once then 50mg IV daily		
	Micafungin	100mg IV daily		If clinically improving with catheter in place, treat for 4-6 weeks.
	Alternative[‡] **Fluconazole PO** or **IP** +	200mg PO or IP daily		
	Flucytosine PO[∞]	2g PO LD then 1g PO daily		
Mycobacteria spp	Consult Infectious Diseases and/or pharmacist			
Culture negative (see Diagnosis)	**Cefazolin IP** +	15mg/kg once per day**	500mg/L LD then 125mg/L MD***	- Continue empiric antibiotic therapy for 14 days if responding; repeat culture. - Refractory infections - recommend catheter removal and continue antibiotics for at least 14 days after catheter removal.
	Gentamicin IP[†]	0.6mg/kg once per day***	8mg/L LD then 4mg/L MD***	

IP=intraperitoneally; LD=loading dose; MD=maintenance dose

* Dosing recommendations for anuric (<100 mL urine/24 hours) patients. PD patients with residual renal function may require increased doses or more frequent dosing, especially when using intermittent regimens. See below and adult & paediatric treatment guidelines at www.ispd.org/

For nonanuric patients: ** > 100 mL urine/24 hours - use 20mg/kg cefazolin

                       *** > 100 mL urine/24 hours - increase (maintenance) dose by 25%

† To optimize concentration-dependent activity of AGs and lessen potential for toxicity, intermittent dosing is recommended over continuous dosing.

∞ Must be obtained through TPD Special Access Program (Emergency Release). Contact pharmacy for assistance in ordering.

RECOMMENDED THERAPY OF CULTURE-DIRECTED INFECTIONS IN ADULT PATIENTS[A]

Table 3 - Treatment of Culture - proven Meningitis

Pathogen	Recommended Therapy	Recommended Dose[B]	Recommended Duration	Comments
N. meningitidis Pen MIC ≤ 0.1 µg/mL	**Penicillin G**	4MU IV q4h	5 days	
	Alternative			
	Ceftriaxone	2g IV q12h	5 days	
Pen MIC > 0.1 µg/mL	**Ceftriaxone**	2g IV q12h	7 days	
	Alternative			
	Meropenem or	2g IV q8h	7 days	
	Chloramphenicol	12.5mg/kg IV q6h (max 4g/day)	7 days	
H. influenzae Amp MIC ≤ 1.0 µg/mL	**Ampicillin**	2g IV q4h	10 days	
Amp MIC > 1.0 µg/mL	**Ceftriaxone**	2g IV q12h	10 days	
	Alternative			
	Meropenem or	2g IV q8h	10 days	
	Chloramphenicol	12.5mg/kg IV q6h (max 4g/day)	10 days	
S. pneumoniae Pen MIC ≤ 0.1µg/mL	**Penicillin G**	4MU IV q4h	10-14 days	
	Alternative			
	Ceftriaxone	2g IV q12h	10-14 days	
Pen MIC > 0.1 - 1.0 µg/mL or	**Ceftriaxone**	2g IV q12h	10-14 days	
Ceftriaxone MIC < 0.5µg/mL	**Meropenem**	2g IV q8h	10-14 days	
Ceftriaxone MIC > 0.5µg/mL or Pen MIC ≥ 2.0 µg/mL	**Ceftriaxone** + **Vancomycin**[E] +/- **Rifampin***	2g IV q12h 15mg/kg IV q8-12h 600mg IV/PO daily	10-14 days	* If ceftriaxone MIC ≥ 2.0 µg/mL, recommend addition of rifampin. Consult Infectious Diseases.
	Alternative			
	Meropenem + **Vancomycin**[E] +/- **Rifampin**	2g IV q8h 15mg/kg IV q8-12h 600 mg IV/PO daily	10-14 days	

E. Desired vancomycin trough is 15-20 mg/L. Monitor renal function closely. See Vancomycin Dosing & Monitoring Guidelines.

RECOMMENDED THERAPY OF CULTURE-DIRECTED INFECTIONS IN ADULT PATIENTS[A]

Table 3 - Treatment of Culture - proven Meningitis (cont'd)

Pathogen	Recommended Therapy	Recommended Dose[B]	Recommended Duration	Comments
Group A Streptococci	**Penicillin G**	4MU IV q4h	14-21 days	- Often associated with otitis media or sinusitis.
	Alternative			
	Ceftriaxone	2g IV q12h	14-21 days	
Group B Streptococci	**Penicillin G +**	4MU IV q4h	14-21 days	
	Gentamicin	1mg/kg IV q8h		
	Alternative			
	Ceftriaxone	2g IV q12h	14-21 days	
S. aureus				
Cloxacillin sensitive (MSSA)	**Cloxacillin**	2g IV q4h	14 days*	- Rule out endocarditis, unless related to recent neurosurgical procedure.
	B-lactam allergy			* If S. aureus bacteremia, treat for 14 days after first negative blood culture.
	Vancomycin[E]	15mg/kg IV q8-12h	14 days*	
Cloxacillin resistant (MRSA)	**Vancomycin**[E] +/-	15mg/kg IV q8-12h	14 days*	
	Rifampin	600mg IV/PO daily		
	Alternative			
	TMP/SMX	15-20mg TMP/kg/day IV div q6-8h	14 days*	
	or			
	Linezolid	600mg IV q12h	14 days*	
S. epidermidis	**Vancomycin**[E] +/-	15mg/kg IV q8-12h	14 days	
	Rifampin	600mg IV/PO daily		
	Alternative			
	Linezolid	600mg IV q12h	14 days	

E. Desired vancomycin trough is 15-20 mg/L. Monitor renal function closely. See Vancomycin Dosing & Monitoring Guidelines.

RECOMMENDED THERAPY OF CULTURE-DIRECTED INFECTIONS IN ADULT PATIENTS[A]

Table 3 - Treatment of Culture - proven Meningitis (cont'd)

Pathogen	Recommended Therapy	Recommended Dose[B]	Recommended Duration	Comments
Enterococcus spp Amp S, Gent synergy S	**Ampicillin** + **Gentamicin***	2g IV q4h 1mg/kg IV q8h	14 days 14 days	* Do not use extended interval aminoglycoside dosing. Desired gentamicin trough < 1mg/L.
Amp R, Gent synergy S**	**Vancomycin**[E] + **Gentamicin***	15mg/kg IV q8-12h 1mg/kg IV q8h	14 days 14 days	**Consider ampicillin 3g IV q4h if MIC16-64 μg/mL, but not if >128 μg/mL.
Amp R, Vancomycin resistant	**Linezolid** or **Chloramphenicol*****	600mg IV/PO q12h 12.5mg/kg IV q6h (max 4g/day)	14 days 14 days	***Use only if susceptibility has been confirmed. - Daptomycin is an alternative if other options are not appropriate but CSF penetration is poor and only a few case reports of success with daptomycin (6-12mg/kg IV daily) in combination with linezolid or gentamicin.
Listeria monocytogenes	**Ampicillin** β-lactam allergy **TMP/SMX** Alternative **Meropenem***	2g IV q4h 15-20mg TMP/kg/day IV div q6-8h 2g IV q8h	≥ 21 days ≥ 21 days ≥ 21 days	* Some clinical failures noted with meropenem.
E. coli Klebsiella spp Salmonella spp	**Ceftriaxone** Alternative **Meropenem** Severe penicillin allergy/anaphylaxis **Ciprofloxacin*** or **Moxifloxacin*** or **TMP/SMX**	2g IV q12h 2g IV q8h 400mg IV q8-12h 400mg IV daily 15-20mg TMP/kg/day IV div q6-8h	21 days 21 days 21 days 21 days 21 days	* Consult microbiology for MIC testing: Ciprofloxacin has better Gram negative activity than moxifloxacin but moxifloxacin has better CSF penetration than ciprofloxacin. Clinical data for quinolones in meningitis is limited.

E. Desired vancomycin trough is 15-20 mg/L. Monitor renal function closely. See Vancomycin Dosing & Monitoring Guidelines.

RECOMMENDED THERAPY OF CULTURE-DIRECTED INFECTIONS IN ADULT PATIENTS[A]

Table 3 - Treatment of Culture - proven Meningitis (cont'd)

Pathogen	Recommended Therapy	Recommended Dose[B]	Recommended Duration	Comments
Enterobacter spp Citrobacter spp Serratia spp	**Meropenem** Alternative TMP/SMX or **Ciprofloxacin**	2g IV q8h 15-20mg TMP/kg/day IV div q6-8h 400mg IV q8-12h	21 days 21 days 21 days	
Pseudomonas aeruginosa	**Ceftazidime** + **Tobramycin** Alternative **Meropenem** + **Tobramycin** Severe β-lactam allergy **Ciprofloxacin** + **Tobramycin**	2g IV q8h 2mg/kg IV q8h 2g IV q8h 2mg/kg IV q8h 400mg IV q8h 2mg/kg IV q8h	≥ 21 days ≥ 21 days ≥ 21 days	
Acinetobacter baumannii	**Meropenem** +/- [**Amikacin** or **Gentamicin**] Alternative **Colistin IV*** + **Colistin Intraventricular**	2g IV q8h 30mg intraventricular daily 5mg intraventricular daily 5mg/kg/day IV div q8h 10mg intraventricular daily	≥ 21 days ≥ 21 days	- Due to multiple mechanisms of resistance, ensure susceptibility of antibiotics chosen and do not extrapolate/assume susceptibility between antibiotics in the same class. * 5mg colistin base/kg/day = 13.3mg colistimethate sodium (CMS)/Kg/day. Each vial contains 150mg colistin base or 400mg CMS.

RECOMMENDED THERAPY OF CULTURE-DIRECTED INFECTIONS IN ADULT PATIENTS[A]

Table 4 - Treatment of Culture - proven Endocarditis

Pathogen	Recommended Therapy	Recommended Dose[B]	Recommended Duration Native*	Recommended Duration Prosthetic	Comments
Viridans Group Streptococci[†] Streptococcus gallolyticus (S. bovis biotype I)[†] Penicillin MIC ≤ 0.12 µg/mL	**Penicillin** or	3MU IV q4h	4 weeks	NA	[†] All isolates of viridans group/nonhaemolytic streptococci should be identified to species level.
	Ceftriaxone or	2g IV daily	4 weeks	NA	• S. gallolyticus - strong association with colorectal cancer. Recommend colonoscopy.
	[**Penicillin** + **Gentamicin**] or	3MU IV q4h 3mg/kg IV q24h** or 1mg/kg IV q8h**	2 weeks 2 weeks	6 weeks 2 weeks	• S. anginosus group (S. anginosus, S. constellatus S. intermedius) - increased tendency to form abscesses and disseminated infections. Longer therapy may be required.
	[**Ceftriaxone** + **Gentamicin**]	2g IV daily 3mg/kg IV q24h** or 1mg/kg IV q8h**	2 weeks 2 weeks	6 weeks 2 weeks	
	Severe penicillin/ cephalosporin allergy **Vancomycin**[E]	15mg/kg IV q8-12h	4 weeks	6 weeks	* 4 week regimens recommended in patients with pre-existing renal dysfunction, or with cardiac or extra cardiac abscesses.
Penicillin MIC > 0.12 - < 0.5 µg/mL	[**Penicillin** + **Gentamicin**] or	4MU IV q4h 3mg/kg IV q24h** or 1mg/kg IV q8h**	4 weeks 2 weeks	6 weeks 6 weeks	**Synergy aminoglycoside dosing. Monitor trough only to rule out toxicity; desired gentamicin trough < 1mg/L.
	[**Ceftriaxone** + **Gentamicin**]	2g IV daily 3mg/kg IV q24h** or 1mg/kg IV q8h**	4 weeks 2 weeks	6 weeks 6 weeks	- For penicillin MIC > 0.1 µg/mL, ensure MIC to ceftriaxone ≤ 1µg/mL.
	Severe penicillin/ cephalosporin allergy **Vancomycin**[E]	15mg/kg IV q8-12h	4 weeks	6 weeks	
Penicillin MIC ≥ 0.5 µg/mL	[**Ceftriaxone** + **Gentamicin**]	2g IV daily 3mg/kg IV q24h** or 1mg/kg IV q8h**	4 weeks[‡] 4 weeks[‡]	6 weeks 6 weeks	- If ceftriaxone MIC ≥ 2µg/mL, use vancomycin. Consult Infectious Diseases. [‡] If symptoms > 3 months, recommend 6 weeks of therapy.
	Severe penicillin/ cephalosporin allergy **Vancomycin**[E]	15mg/kg IV q8-12h	4 weeks[‡]	6 weeks	

E. Desired vancomycin trough is 15-20 mg/L. Monitor renal function closely. See Vancomycin Dosing & Monitoring Guidelines.

RECOMMENDED THERAPY OF CULTURE-DIRECTED INFECTIONS IN ADULT PATIENTS[A]

Table 4 - Treatment of Culture - proven Endocarditis (cont'd)

Pathogen	Recommended Therapy	Recommended Dose[B]	Recommended Duration Native	Recommended Duration Prosthetic	Comments
S. pneumoniae Penicillin MIC ≤ 0.12 µg/mL	**Ceftriaxone*** or Penicillin	3MU IV q4h 2g IV daily**	4 weeks 4 weeks	6 weeks 6 weeks	- Early surgical intervention often required. * Ensure ceftriaxone MIC ≤ 1µg/mL (≤ 0.5 µg/mL if concomitant meningitis). **If concomitant meningitis; use ceftriaxone 2g IV q12h.
Penicillin MIC >0.12 - 2.0 µg/mL	**Ceftriaxone***	2g IV daily**	4 weeks	6 weeks	
Ceftriaxone MIC ≥ 2.0 µg/mL	**Ceftriaxone +** **Vancomycin[E] +** **Rifampin**	2g IV daily 15mg/kg IV q8-12h 300mg PO bid	4 weeks 4 weeks 4 weeks	6 weeks 6 weeks 6 weeks	
β-haemolytic Streptococci S. pyogenes	**Penicillin** or **Ceftriaxone**	3MU IV q4h 2g IV daily	4 weeks 4 weeks	6 weeks 6 weeks	- Early surgical intervention improves survival.
S. agalactiae Group C, G	**Penicillin +** **Gentamicin** or **Ceftriaxone +** **Gentamicin**	4MU IV q4h 3mg/kg IV daily* or 1mg/kg IV q8h* 2g IV daily 3mg/kg IV daily* or 1mg/kg IV q8h*	4-6 weeks 2 weeks 4-6 weeks 2 weeks	6 weeks 2 weeks 6 weeks 2 weeks	* Synergy aminoglycoside dosing. Monitor trough only to rule out toxicity; desired gentamicin trough < 1mg/L.
Abiotrophia spp, Gemella spp **Granulicatella spp** Penicillin MIC ≤ 0.5 µg/mL	**Penicillin +** **Gentamicin**	4MU IV q4h 3mg/kg IV daily* or 1mg/kg IV q8h*	4 weeks** 4 weeks**	6 weeks 6 weeks	* Synergy aminoglycoside dosing. Monitor trough only to rule out toxicity; desired gentamicin trough < 1mg/L. ** If symptoms > 3 months, recommend 6 weeks of therapy.
Penicillin MIC > 0.5 µg/mL	**Ceftriaxone +** **Gentamicin**	2g IV daily 3mg/kg IV daily* or 1mg/kg IV q8h*	4 weeks** 4 weeks**	6 weeks 6 weeks	
Severe penicillin/ cephalosporin allergy	**Vancomycin[E]**	15mg/kg IV q8-12h	4 weeks**	6 weeks	

E. Desired vancomycin trough is 15-20 mg/L. Monitor renal function closely. See Vancomycin Dosing & Monitoring Guidelines.

RECOMMENDED THERAPY OF CULTURE-DIRECTED INFECTIONS IN ADULT PATIENTS[A]

Table 4 - Treatment of Culture - proven Endocarditis (cont'd)

Pathogen	Recommended Therapy	Recommended Dose[B]	Recommended Duration	Comments
Enterococcus spp				
Amp S, Gent synergy S	[Ampicillin + Gentamicin**]	2g IV q4h 1mg/kg IV q8h	4 weeks‡ 4 weeks‡	* If gent synergy R, check streptomycin synergy susceptibility.
Amp S, Gent synergy R*, Strep synergy S	[Ampicillin + Streptomycin**]	2g IV q4h 7.5mg/kg IV/IM q12h	4 weeks‡ 4 weeks‡	**Synergy aminoglycoside dosing. Monitor trough only to rule out toxicity; desired gentamicin trough < 1mg/L, streptomycin trough < 10 mg/L.
Amp S, Gent/Strep synergy R	Ampicillin or [Ampicillin + Ceftriaxone]	3g IV q4h 2g IV q4h 2g IV q12h	8-12 weeks 6 weeks 6 weeks	‡ If symptoms > 3 months or prosthetic valve endocarditis, recommend 6 weeks of therapy.
Amp R, Gent synergy S - high level resistance > 128 µg/mL	[Vancomycin[E] + Gentamicin**]	15mg/kg IV q8-12h 1mg/kg IV q8h	6 weeks 6 weeks	†High dose ampicillin (3g IV q4h) + gentamicin or streptomycin may achieve therapeutic levels if gent synergy S or strep synergy S.
- low level resistance 16-64 µg/mL†	[Vancomycin[E] + Gentamicin**] or [Ampicillin† + Gentamicin]	15mg/kg IV q8-12h 1mg/kg IV q8h 3g IV q4h 1mg/kg IV q8h	6 weeks 6 weeks ≥ 6 weeks 4-6 weeks	
Amp R, Vanco R, Gent/Strep synergy R E. faecium	Linezolid* or Daptomycin**	600mg IV/PO q12h 6mg/kg IV daily***	≥ 8 weeks ≥ 8 weeks	Consult Infectious Diseases. * NB: bacteriostatic agent; 40% relapse rate **Rifampin may have synergistic activity but clinical data lacking. ***Dosages of 8-12mg/kg daily can be considered.

E. Desired vancomycin trough is 15-20 mg/L. Monitor renal function closely. See Vancomycin Dosing & Monitoring Guidelines.

RECOMMENDED THERAPY OF CULTURE-DIRECTED INFECTIONS IN ADULT PATIENTS[A]

Table 4 - Treatment of Culture - proven Endocarditis (cont'd)

Pathogen	Recommended Therapy	Recommended Dose[B]	Recommended Duration	Comments
Enterococcus spp (cont'd) Amp R, Vanco R, Gent/ Strep synergy R (cont'd) E. faecalis - Amp MIC 16-64 µg/mL	**Ampicillin*** + [**Ceftriaxone** or **Imipenem*+**]	2g IV q4h 2g IV q12h 500mg IV q6h	≥ 8 weeks ≥ 8 weeks	Consult Infectious Diseases. * Combination of two β-lactam agents has been successful in a small number of patients.
	Severe penicillin/ cephalosporin allergy **Linezolid**	600mg IV/PO q12h	≥ 8 weeks	* NB: bacteriostatic agent; 40% relapse rate.
- Amp MIC > 128 µg/mL	**Linezolid*** or **Daptomycin****	600mg IV/PO q12h 6mg/kg IV daily***	≥ 8 weeks ≥ 8 weeks	**Rifampin may have synergistic activity but clinical data lacking. ***Dosages of 8-12mg/kg daily can be considered.
S. aureus (right-sided/ tricuspid valve) Cloxacillin sensitive	**Cloxacillin**	2g IV q4h	2 weeks*	- Tricuspid valve involvement - rule out septic pulmonary emboli. - Surgical consult if persistent (≥ 3 weeks) fever and no pulmonary emboli. - No longer recommend addition of gentamicin for native valve S. aureus endocarditis as: • no difference in clinical cure, mortality, or relapse • increased risk of nephrotoxicity. - Oral regimen can be considered if patient unwilling to complete IV course of antibiotics; must confirm susceptibility of MSSA. Two randomized controlled trials of quinolone (e.g. ciprofloxacin 750mg PO bid) + rifampin 300mg PO tid or 600mg PO bid × 4 weeks. Levofloxacin and moxifloxacin have better in vitro S. aureus activity.
	Severe penicillin allergy/ anaphylaxis **Vancomycin**[E]	15mg/kg IV q8-12h	4-6 weeks*	

E. Desired vancomycin trough is 15-20 mg/L. Monitor renal function closely. See Vancomycin Dosing & Monitoring Guidelines.

RECOMMENDED THERAPY OF CULTURE-DIRECTED INFECTIONS IN ADULT PATIENTS[A]

Table 4 - Treatment of Culture - proven Endocarditis (cont'd)

Pathogen	Recommended Therapy	Recommended Dose[B]	Recommended Duration	Comments

S. aureus (right-sided/ tricuspid valve)				- Tricuspid valve involvement - rule out septic pulmonary emboli.
				 - Surgical consult if persistent (≥ 3 weeks) fever and no pulmonary emboli.
				 - No longer recommend addition of gentamicin for native valve S. aureus endocarditis as:
				   • no difference in clinical cure, mortality, or relapse
				   • increased risk of nephrotoxicity.

Cloxacillin sensitive (MSSA)	**Cloxacillin**	2g IV q4h	2 weeks*	- Oral regimen can be considered if patient unwilling to complete IV course of antibiotics: must confirm susceptibility of MSSA. Two randomized controlled trials of quinolone (e.g. ciprofloxacin 750mg PO bid) + rifampin 300mg PO tid or 600mg PO bid x 4 weeks. Levofloxacin and moxifloxacin have better in vitro S. aureus activity.
				 * Treat for 4-6 weeks if:
				   • agents other than cloxacillin used
				   • metastatic infection or empyema
				   • left side involved
				   • prosthetic valve (urgent surgical consult required)
				   • vegetations >2cm
				   • lack of clinical or bacteriologic response at 96h.
				   • cardiac or extracardiac complications (e.g. ARF)
				   • severe immunosuppression/CD4 < 200.

	Severe penicillin allergy/ anaphylaxis **Vancomycin**[E]	15mg/kg IV q8-12h	4-6 weeks*	
Cloxacillin resistant (MRSA)	**Vancomycin**[E]	15mg/kg IV q8-12h	6 weeks	*Dosages of 8-12mg/kg daily can be considered. Rule out pulmonary site of infection (emboli or empyema) as daptomycin not effective in pulmonary infections.
	Alternative **Daptomycin**	6mg/kg IV daily*	6 weeks	

E. Desired vancomycin trough is 15-20 mg/L. Monitor renal function closely. See Vancomycin Dosing & Monitoring Guidelines.

RECOMMENDED THERAPY OF CULTURE-DIRECTED INFECTIONS IN ADULT PATIENTS[A]

Table 4 - Treatment of Culture - proven Endocarditis (cont'd)

Pathogen	Recommended Therapy	Recommended Dose[B]	Recommended Duration	Comments

S. aureus (left-sided/mitral and/or aortic valve)	- Urgent surgical consult required if:
	  • evidence of abscess on echocardiogram
	  • prosthetic valve
	  • lack of defervescence within 72 hours of appropriate antibiotic therapy
	  • persistent (≥ 7 days) bacteremia on appropriate antibiotic therapy.			

Cloxacillin sensitive (MSSA) Native Valve[*]	**Cloxacillin** or **Cefazolin** Severe penicillin/ cephalosporin allergy **Vancomycin**[E]	2g IV q4h 2g IV q8h 15mg/kg IV q8-12h	4-6 weeks[†] 4-6 weeks[†] 6 weeks	* NB: Rifampin is not routinely recommended in native valve endocarditis but may be considered in patients who do not respond to therapy. † 6 weeks recommended for perivalvular or septic emboli.
Prosthetic Valve	**Cloxacillin** + **Gentamicin*** + **Rifampin** Severe penicillin/ cephalosporin allergy **Vancomycin**[E] + **Gentamicin*** + **Rifampin**	2g IV q4h 1mg/kg IV q8h 300mg PO tid or 600mg PO bid 15mg/kg IV q8-12h 1mg/kg IV q8h 300mg PO tid or 600mg PO bid	≥ 6 weeks 2 weeks ≥ 6 weeks ≥ 6 weeks 2 weeks ≥ 6 weeks	* Synergy aminoglycoside dosing. Monitor trough only to rule out toxicity; desired gentamicin trough < 1mg/L.
Cloxacillin resistant (MRSA) Native Valve	- Consult Infectious Diseases. - Increased incidence of recurrence. **Vancomycin**[E]	15mg/kg IV q8-12h	6 weeks	
Prosthetic Valve	**Vancomycin**[E] + **Gentamicin*** + **Rifampin**	15mg/kg IV q8-12h 1mg/kg IV q8h 300mg PO tid or 600mg PO bid	≥ 6 weeks 2 weeks ≥ 6 weeks	* Synergy aminoglycoside dosing. Monitor trough only to rule out toxicity; desired gentamicin trough <1mg/L. Use only if organism susceptible in vitro to gentamicin. Call Microbiology.

E. Desired vancomycin trough is 15-20 mg/L. Monitor renal function closely. See Vancomycin Dosing & Monitoring Guidelines.

RECOMMENDED THERAPY OF CULTURE-DIRECTED INFECTIONS IN ADULT PATIENTS[A]

Table 4 - Treatment of Culture - proven Endocarditis (cont'd)

Pathogen	Recommended Therapy	Recommended Dose[B]	Recommended Duration	Comments
S. lugdunensis	**Cloxacillin** _Severe penicillin allergy/ anaphylaxis_ **Vancomycin**[E]	2g IV q4h 15mg/kg IV q8-12h	6 weeks 6 weeks	- Increased risk of perivalvular extension and metastatic infection. Early surgical intervention required.
Coagulase negative Staph S. epidermidis Native Valve[*]	**Vancomycin**[E,***] +/- **Gentamicin****	15mg/kg IV q8-12h 1mg/kg IV q8h	6 weeks 3-5 days	* Usually have underlying valvular abnormality. Rule out S. lugdunensis. **Synergy aminoglycoside dosing. Monitor trough only to rule out toxicity; desired gentamicin trough < 1mg/L. Use only if organism susceptible in vitro to gentamicin. Call Microbiology. ***If organism susceptible, switch to/use cloxacillin 2g IV q4h as superior to vancomycin.
Prosthetic Valve	**Vancomycin**[E,***] + **Gentamicin**** + **Rifampin**	15mg/kg IV q8-12h 1mg/kg IV q8h 300mg PO q8h	6 weeks 2 weeks 6 weeks	
HACEK organisms	**Ceftriaxone** _Alternative_ **Ciprofloxacin**	2g IV daily 750mg PO bid or 400mg IV q12h	4 weeks[*] 4 weeks[*]	- Tailor antibiotics to C&S results. * 6 weeks if prosthetic valve.
Enterobacteriaceae	[**Ceftriaxone** + **Gentamicin**] _ESBL/AmpC producing organism_ **Imipenem** or **Meropenem**	2g IV daily 1.5-2mg/kg IV q8h 500mg IV q6h 500mg IV q6h or 1g IV q8h	≥ 6 weeks ≥ 6 weeks ≥ 6 weeks ≥ 6 weeks	- Consult Infectious Diseases. - Valve replacement often necessary depending on organism.
Pseudomonas aeruginosa	[**Ceftazidime** or **Piperacillin**] + **Tobramycin**	2g IV q8h 3g IV q4h 7mg/kg IV q24h	≥ 6 weeks ≥ 6 weeks	- Consult Infectious Diseases. - Increased risk of perivalvular extension and metastatic infection. Early surgical intervention required. Valve replacement recommended if left sided involvement.

E. Desired vancomycin trough is 15-20 mg/L. Monitor renal function closely. See Vancomycin Dosing & Monitoring Guidelines.
HACEK = Haemophilus parainfluenzae, Aggregatibacter actinomycetemcomitans/aphrophilus, Cardiobacterium hominis, Eikenella corrodens, Kingella spp

RECOMMENDED THERAPY OF CULTURE-DIRECTED INFECTIONS IN ADULT PATIENTS[A]

Table 4 - Treatment of Culture - proven Endocarditis (cont'd)

Pathogen	Recommended Therapy	Recommended Dose[B]	Recommended Duration	Comments
Candida spp	**Anidulafungin**	200mg IV once then 100mg IV daily	Minimum 6 weeks after valve replacement	- Consult Infectious Diseases. - Valve replacement almost always necessary. If valve cannot be replaced, consider long term suppressive antifungal therapy.
	or			
	Caspofungin	70mg IV once then 50mg IV daily	Minimum 6 weeks after valve replacement	
	or			
	Micafungin	100-150mg IV daily	Minimum 6 weeks after valve replacement	
	or			
	[Amphotericin B + Flucytosine]	0.6-1mg/kg IV daily 25-37.5mg/kg PO qid	Minimum 6 weeks after valve replacement	

RECOMMENDED THERAPY OF CULTURE-DIRECTED INFECTIONS IN ADULT PATIENTS[A]

Table 5 - Blood Culture Negative Endocarditis (BCNE)

Definition: endocarditis without etiology following 3 sets of blood cultures with negative results after 5 days of incubation. Consult microbiologist and Infectious Diseases physician in all cases of BCNE.
- Cultures are negative for 2 major reasons:
  - previous administration of antibiotics - in these cases, viridans group streptococci most likely pathogen and should be treated empirically - see relevant Empiric Therapy recommendations (native valve, IVDU, prosthetic valve)
  - infection with highly fastidious bacteria (see below) or nonbacterial pathogens.

Pathogen	Clinical	Diagnosis	Recommended Empiric Therapy	Recommended Dose[B]	Recommended Duration
Bartonella spp [European Heart J 2009;30:2369-2413.]	**B. quintana** - associated with alcoholism, homelessness, body lice. **B. henselae** -contact with cats, previous valvular disease - valve surgery required in > 50% of patients	• Blood cultures - only occasionally positive • Serology - antibody titre ≥ 1:800 • Culture, immuno-histology and PCR of surgical material	**Ceftriaxone** + **Doxycycline*** + **Gentamicin**** *Alternative for doxycycline: **Azithromycin** **Gentamicin synergy dosing. Monitor trough only to rule out toxicity; desired gentamicin trough < 1mg/L. Alternative for gentamicin: **Rifampin**	2g IV daily 100mg PO bid 3mg/kg IV daily or 1mg/kg IV q8h 500mg PO daily 300mg PO bid	6 weeks 6 weeks 2 weeks 6 weeks Optimal duration of therapy unknown. Some recommend continuing doxycycline (or azithromycin) for 3-6 months, especially if all affected cardiac tissue not removed. 2 weeks

RECOMMENDED THERAPY OF CULTURE-DIRECTED INFECTIONS IN ADULT PATIENTS[A]
Table 5 - Blood Culture Negative Endocarditis (BCNE) (cont'd)

Pathogen	Clinical	Diagnosis	Recommended Therapy	Recommended Dose[B]	Duration
Brucella spp [Lancet Infect Dis 2007;7:775, MMWR 2008:57 :603, European Heart J 2009;30:2369-2413.]	**B. melitensis** and **B. abortus** most common. - associated with exposure to cattle, sheep, pigs, goats, dogs & unpasteur-ized dairy products. Notify microbiology if suspect (Level 3 pathogen). - Almost always require valve surgery. - Treatment success: antibody titre < 1:60.	• Blood cultures • Serology • Culture, immuno-histology and PCR of surgical material	**Doxycycline** + **TMP/SMX** + **Rifampin** +/- **Gentamicin**	100mg PO bid 1DS tab PO bid 300mg PO bid 7mg/kg IV daily	≥ 3 months ≥ 3 months ≥ 3 months 2 weeks
Coxiella burnetii (Q fever) [Clin Infect Dis 2011;52:1431, Lancet Infect Dis 2010:10:527, European Heart J 2009;30:2369-2413, J Antimicrob Chemother 2012;67:269-89.]	- Associated with previous valve disease, prosthetic valve, or immunosuppres-sion and contact with cattle, sheep, goats, cats, & dogs. - Endocarditis most common manifestation of chronic (> 6 months) infection. - Peripheral manifestations common: splenomegaly, digital clubbing, purpuric rash, hepatomegaly, immune complex glomerulonephritis, pulmonary/pleural emboli. - Treatment success predicted if: IgG titre < 1:800, IgA and IgM titres < 1:50.	• Serology - phase 1 IgG titre > 1:800 • Culture, immuno-histology and PCR of surgical material.	**Doxycycline** + **Hydroxychloroquine** Alternative **Doxycycline** + [**Ciprofloxacin** or **Levofloxacin**]	100mg PO bid 200mg PO tid 100mg PO bid 750mg PO bid 750mg PO daily	≥ 18 months* ≥ 18 months* *24 months if prosthetic valve endocarditis 36 months 36 months 36 months If possible, at least 3 weeks of therapy should be given prior to valve surgery.

Table 5 - Blood Culture Negative Endocarditis (BCNE) (cont'd)

Pathogen	Clinical	Diagnosis	Recommended Therapy	Recommended Dose[B]	Duration
Legionella spp	- Almost always requires valve surgery.	• Blood cultures • Urine for Legionella antigen • Serology • Culture, immuno-histology and PCR of surgical material	**[Erythromycin + Rifampin]** or **Levofloxacin** Alternative **Doxycycline**	500mg PO/IV q6h 300mg PO bid 750mg IV/PO daily 200mg PO bid	≥ 6 weeks ≥ 6 weeks ≥ 6 weeks ≥ 6 weeks Optimal duration of therapy unknown; may be at least 5 months.
Tropheryma whipplei (Whipple's disease) [European Heart J 2009;30:2369-2413.]	- Peripheral manifestations common: polyarthralgias, chronic diarrhea, weight loss, abdominal pain, neurologic symptoms. - Almost always requires valve surgery.	• Culture, immuno-histology and PCR of surgical material	**Ceftriaxone** or **Penicillin** then **TMP/SMX** Alternative in sulfa-allergy **Doxycycline + Hydroxychloroquine**	2g IV daily 2MU IV q4h 1DS tab PO bid 100mg PO bid 200mg PO tid	2-4 weeks 2-4 weeks 1-2 years ≥ 18 months ≥ 18 months Optimal duration of therapy unknown.

FOOTNOTES:

A. These antibiotic recommendations are based on current literature, national susceptibility patterns, and antimicrobials currently available on the Canadian market. Antibiotics listed for each condition are not all inclusive, nor are they all approved by Health Canada TPD for the listed indication. Choice of antibiotic therapy should be based on the patient's age, allergies, co-morbidities, and clinical condition, as well as cost and convenience of the dosage regimen.

B. Usual adult dose in patients with normal renal and hepatic function.

RECOMMENDED EMPIRIC THERAPY OF SELECTED OPHTHALMIC INFECTIONS

Infection	Usual Pathogens	Recommended Empiric Therapy	Recommended Dose[A]	Recommended Duration	Comments
Blepharitis	- Bilateral inflammation of eyelid margin with irritation, burning, and itching. - Dry scales can be seen on the lashes of the upper and lower lids. Lids may become thick and irregular.				
	S. aureus S. epidermidis Moraxella lacunata P. acnes Corynebacterium spp	Warm compresses + Wash off debris, then apply **Bacitracin-Polymyxin B** or **Erythromycin 0.5%**	qhs qhs	6-8 weeks 6-8 weeks	- Infectious etiology suspected but not proven. - Often associated with seborrhea. - Difficult to eradicate. - Eyelid hygiene is key to therapy. - Patients with associated rosacea may benefit from doxycycline 100mg PO bid x 3-4 weeks.
Hordeolum (sty)	- Pain, redness, and tenderness of the eyelid margin followed by an area of induration.				
External (adjacent to eyelash follicles)	S. aureus	Hot compresses	10-15 min tid or qid	Until a yellowish point is formed that ruptures and drains	- Self-limiting condition; antibiotics not necessary. - Often associated with blepharitis.
Internal (on conjunctival side of lid)	S. aureus	Hot compresses If cellulitis is present: **Cloxacillin** or **Cephalexin**	10-15 min tid or qid 500mg PO qid 500mg PO qid	 7 days 7 days	- Rarely drains spontaneously. - Recurrence is common. - Often associated with blepharitis.
Chalazion	- Sterile, nontender, chronic granulomatous inflammation of the meibomian gland. - At onset may be indistinguishable from a sty. Resolves after a few days, leaving a painless, slowly growing round mass in the lid. - Most chalazia disappear after a few months; incision and curettage may be indicated if there is no resolution after 6-8 weeks.				
		Hot compresses	10-15 min tid or qid	6-8 weeks or until resolved	

RECOMMENDED EMPIRIC THERAPY OF SELECTED OPHTHALMIC INFECTIONS

Infection	Usual Pathogens	Recommended Empiric Therapy	Recommended Dose[A]	Recommended Duration	Comments
Canaliculitis	- Nasal conjunctival redness, swollen and pouting punctum, and a mucopurulent discharge with itching, tearing, and irritation. - Digital pressure over the punctum results in a greenish-yellow exudate often followed by yellowish concretions.				
	A. israelii	Remove granules + **Penicillin G 100,000U/mL**[B] **ophthalmic solution** + **Erythromycin**	qid 500mg PO qid	1 week 10 days	- Gram stain of the exudate confirms diagnosis. - Surgical drainage may be necessary if curettage fails. - Definitive treatment is surgical; antibiotics may play a 2° role.
Dacryocystitis	- Unilateral inflammation of lacrimal sac due to obstruction of the flow of tears from the sac. - May progress to periorbital/orbital cellulitis.				

Acute	S. aureus
	S. pneumoniae
	H. influenzae
	S. pyogenes
	P. aeruginosa
		Infants
		Massage lacrimal sac
		
		Adults
		Warm compresses +
		Cloxacillin or
		Cephalexin
			
			500mg PO qid
			500mg PO qid
				
				7 days
				7 days
					- Collect exudate from lacrimal punctum for C&S.
					- Infants:
					  • 50% resolve spontaneously by 12-18 months.
					  • If chronic consider probing (after 1 year of age).
					- Adults (usually > 40 years):
					  • Usually requires systemic therapy.
					  • Chronic or recurrent cases usually require dacryocystorhinostomy.

RECOMMENDED EMPIRIC THERAPY OF SELECTED OPHTHALMIC INFECTIONS

Infection	Usual Pathogens	Recommended Empiric Therapy	Recommended Dose[A]	Recommended Duration	Comments
Conjunctivitis **Viral** (pink eye)	- Unilateral with 30-50% of cases spreading to the other eye. - Clear watery discharge, mild foreign-body sensation, burning, red eyelid, preauricular lymphadenopathy and follicular reaction. - Onset of photophobia and ocular pain after 10-14 days in adults suggests corneal involvement (rare). Visual loss should **not** be present in conjunctivitis. Slit lamp examination recommended if photophobia or decreased visual activity present. - Prevent transmission by counseling on handwashing and avoiding personal contact. Virus viable on dry surfaces for ≥ 2 weeks.				
	Adenovirus Enterovirus Coxsackie virus	Cold compresses ± Decongestants ± Lubricants			- Typically lasts 2 to 4 weeks; highly contagious for the first 2 weeks. - Topical corticosteroids are not recommended.
Bacterial **Hyperacute**	- Usually unilateral with a fulminant onset (< 24 hours) - Copious purulent discharge, conjunctival hyperemia, redness, and irritation. Preauricular lymphadenopathy commonly seen. - Corneal perforation can occur in up to 10% of cases. **Refer to an ophthalmologist promptly.**				
	N. gonorrhoeae N. meningitidis	**Ceftriaxone** or **Ciprofloxacin*** + **Doxycycline** or **Azithromycin**	1g IM 500mg PO 100mg PO bid 1g PO	1 dose 1 dose 7 days 1 dose	- Obtain Gram stain and culture of conjunctival scrapings. - Frequent association with chlamydial disease (up to 33%). - Consider adjunctive topical antibiotic therapy (bacitracin-polymyxin or erythromycin). * Significant quinolone resistance in N. gonorrhoeae; only use ciprofloxacin in severe penicillin allergy.

RECOMMENDED EMPIRIC THERAPY OF SELECTED OPHTHALMIC INFECTIONS

Infection	Usual Pathogens	Recommended Empiric Therapy	Recommended Dose[A]	Recommended Duration	Comments
Conjunctivitis (cont'd) **Bacterial** (cont'd) **Acute**	- Usually begins unilaterally with involvement of the second eye within 24 to 48 hours. - Moderate purulent discharge, conjunctival hyperemia, and eyelid swelling/redness. Preauricular lymphadenopathy usually absent. - Cultures are not recommended unless infection is not resolving with standard therapy.				
	S. pneumoniae H. influenzae S. aureus Group A Strepto- cocci Moraxella spp Proteus spp	Warm compresses + Ophthalmic Solution (adults)* **Gramicidin-Polymyxin B** or **Gentamicin 0.3%**[C] **Tobramycin 0.3%** Ophthalmic Ointment (infants/ children) **Bacitracin-Polymyxin B** or **Erythromycin 0.5%** or **Gentamicin 0.3%**[C]	qid qid qid qid qid qid	7-10 days 7-10 days 7-10 days 7-10 days 7-10 days 7-10 days	- Often self-limiting. - Oral antibiotics not indicated. - Topical corticosteroids not recommended. - Avoid eye patching. * If contact lens wearer, Pseudomonas coverage is essential; use ciprofloxacin 0.3% or gentamicin 0.3% or tobramycin 0.3% ophthalmic solutions.
Chronic	- Redness, irritation, lid excoriation, scant mucopurulent discharge, or morning crusting for > 4 weeks.				
	Staphylococcus spp Moraxella spp Enterobacteriaceae	Ophthalmic Solution **Gramicidin-Polymyxin B** or Ophthalmic Ointment **Bacitracin-Polymyxin B** or **Erythromycin 0.5%**	qid qid qid	7-10 days 7-10 days 7-10 days	- Eyelid hygiene is important. - If persists for > 10 days, do not repeat treatment. Look for 2° causes such as chronic nasolacrimal obstruction or chronic blepharitis.

RECOMMENDED EMPIRIC THERAPY OF SELECTED OPHTHALMIC INFECTIONS

Infection	Usual Pathogens	Recommended Empiric Therapy	Recommended Dose[A]	Recommended Duration	Comments
Conjunctivitis (cont'd) **Newborn**	- In 1st 36 hours, conjunctivitis often clinically induced by silver nitrate; self-resolving in 1-2 days.				
	N. gonorrhoeae	Prophylaxis **Erythromycin 0.5% ophthalmic ointment**	both eyes	once only	- Hyperpurulent conjunctivitis that appears 2 to 4 days after birth. - If severe, irrigate eye hourly with normal saline until discharge eliminated. - The mother and her sexual partner(s) should also be treated.
		Treatment **Ceftriaxone**	25-50mg/kg IV/IM once (max 125mg)	single dose	
	C. trachomatis	Prophylaxis **Erythromycin 0.5% ophthalmic ointment**	both eyes	once only	- Hyperpurulent conjunctivitis that appears 3 to 10 days after birth. - The mother and her sexual partner(s) should also be treated.
		Treatment **Erythromycin**	40mg/kg/d PO/IV div q6h	14 days	
Adult Inclusion	- Onset usually 1-2 weeks after inoculation. - Usually unilateral with mild discomfort, minimal conjunctival injection and no exudate.				
	C. trachomatis	**Doxycycline**	100mg PO bid	2-3 weeks	- Can remain undetected for a long time. - Sexual partner(s) should also be treated.
		Alternative **Erythromycin** or **Azithromycin**	250mg PO qid 1g PO	2-3 weeks 1 dose	

RECOMMENDED EMPIRIC THERAPY OF SELECTED OPHTHALMIC INFECTIONS

Infection	Usual Pathogens	Recommended Empiric Therapy	Recommended Dose[A]	Recommended Duration	Comments
Keratitis	- A serious and potentially sight-threatening infection of the cornea (ocular pain, photophobia, conjunctival injection, tearing, decreased vision, foreign body sensation, corneal infiltrate or opacity and purulent discharge). - **Refer to an ophthalmologist promptly.** - Contact lens wearers have 10 fold risk of developing infectious keratitis.				
Viral	Herpes simplex	Ophthalmic Solution **Trifluridine 1%** or Ophthalmic Ointment **Acyclovir 3%** (SAP)	q1h, 9x/day 5x/day	10-14 days (up to 21 days) 7-10 days	- Debridement recommended. - Addition of oral acyclovir is controversial. - Topical corticosteroids are restricted to specific clinical presentations. Consult an ophthalmologist. - 30-50% rate of recurrence within 2 years.
	Varicella zoster	**Acyclovir** or **Famciclovir** or **Valacyclovir**	800mg PO 5x/day 500mg PO tid 1g PO tid	10 days 10 days 10 days	- Therapy ideally should be initiated within 72 hours of onset of skin lesions. - Skin lesions on tip of nose generally result in corneal involvement.

RECOMMENDED EMPIRIC THERAPY OF SELECTED OPHTHALMIC INFECTIONS

Infection	Usual Pathogens	Recommended Empiric Therapy	Recommended Dose[A]	Recommended Duration	Comments
Keratitis (cont'd)					
Bacterial					
• Contact Lens Wearer	P. aeruginosa Staphylococcus spp Streptococcus spp B. cereus Enterobacteriaceae Moraxella spp H. influenzae P. acnes	Ophthalmic Solutions **Tobramycin 15mg/mL**[B] + [**Piperacillin 6mg/mL**[B] or **Ceftazidime 50mg/mL**[B]] or **Ciprofloxacin 0.3%** (alone)	q5min for first hour, then q15-60min around the clock for 24-72 hours, then slowly reduce frequency.	3-4 weeks (dependent on clinical picture)	- Rapid onset of symptoms. - Ciprofloxacin 0.3% solution may form a white precipitate on the cornea.
• Non-Contact Lens Wearer	Staphylococcus spp Streptococcus spp B. cereus Enterobacteriaceae Moraxella spp H. influenzae P. acnes	Ophthalmic Solutions[B] **Cefazolin 50mg/mL** + [**Gentamicin 15mg/mL** or **Tobramycin 15mg/mL**] Alternative[B] **Vancomycin 50mg/mL + Ceftazidime 50mg/mL**	q5min for first hour, then q15-60min around the clock for 24-72 hours, then slowly reduce frequency.	3-4 weeks (dependent on clinical picture)	- Risk factors: • diabetes • immunosuppression • dry cornea. - Quinolones may not provide optimal Staph and Strep coverage.

RECOMMENDED EMPIRIC THERAPY OF SELECTED OPHTHALMIC INFECTIONS

Infection	Usual Pathogens	Recommended Empiric Therapy	Recommended Dose[A]	Recommended Duration	Comments
Keratitis (cont'd) **Fungal**	Aspergillus spp Fusarium spp Candida spp	<u>Ophthalmic Solutions</u> **Voriconazole 1%**[B] or **Amphotericin B 0.15%**[B] or **Natamycin 5%** *(SAP)*	q1h, then slowly reduce frequency q2-3h, then slowly reduce frequency q2-3h, then slowly reduce frequency	Up to 6 weeks	- Risk factors: • trauma due to vegetation • chronic topical steroid use. - Very resistant to topical therapy; debridement usually required. May need corneal transplant. - **Topical/oral corticosteroids are contraindicated.** - Consider adjunctive systemic antifungal therapy.
Protozoan	Acanthamoeba spp	<u>Ophthalmic Solutions</u> **Propamidine 0.1%** *(SAP)* + **[Polyhexamethylene biguanide 0.02%** and/or **Chlorhexidine 0.02%**[B]] +/- **Neomycin-gramicidin-polymyxin B**	q1h while awake, then slowly reduce frequency	Dependent on clinical picture	- Risk factors: • trauma • soft contact lens use (overnight use increases risk). - Severe pain is a predominant symptom. - Consult ophthalmology and microbiology for diagnosis.
Nontuber-culous mycobac-teria*	M. chelonae M. fortuitum	**Moxifloxacin 0.5%** ophthalmic solution + **Systemic antimycobacterial agent(s)** according to susceptibility results	qid	Dependent on clinical picture	* Most commonly cultured organisms post-LASIK.

RECOMMENDED EMPIRIC THERAPY OF SELECTED OPHTHALMIC INFECTIONS

Infection	Usual Pathogens	Recommended Empiric Therapy	Recommended Dose[A]	Recommended Duration	Comments
Endophthalmitis	- Inflammation of the vitreous is an urgent and severe ocular infection (ocular pain, decreased vision, headache, photophobia, hazy cornea, eyelid swelling, conjunctival injection, decreased red reflex and hypopyon). - **Refer to an ophthalmologist immediately.** - Anterior chamber tap and vitreous biopsy for culture should be performed prior to initiating therapy. - Intravitreal administration of antimicrobials is essential (intravitreal ophthalmic preparations are not commercially available; manufactured by pharmacy).				
Post-Surgical Acute	S. epidermidis S. aureus Streptococcus spp Pseudomonas spp	Ophthalmic Preparations[B] **Vancomycin 1mg/0.1mL + Ceftazidime 2.25mg/0.1mL** β-lactam Allergy[B] **Vancomycin 1mg/0.1mL + [Gentamicin 0.2mg/0.1mL[D] or Amikacin 0.4 mg/0.1mL[D]]**	0.1mL intravitreally 0.1mL intravitreally 0.1mL intravitreally 0.1mL intravitreally 0.1mL intravitreally	Dependent on clinical picture Dependent on clinical picture	- Fulminant onset 2-7 days postoperatively. - Vitrectomy may be required. - IV antibiotics usually not needed unless infection is outside globe. - Intravitreal dexamethasone 0.4mg/0.1mL may be beneficial.
Chronic	P. acnes S. epidermidis Fungi (see next page)	Ophthalmic Preparation[B] **Vancomycin 1mg/0.1mL**	0.1mL intravitreally	Dependent on clinical picture	- Low grade infection occurring 1 month to 1 year post-op.
Post-Trauma	B. cereus S. epidermidis Enterobacteriaceae Pseudomonas spp Anaerobes Fungi (see next page)	Ophthalmic Preparations[B] **Vancomycin 1mg/0.1mL + Ceftazidime 2.25mg/0.1mL** β-lactam Allergy[B] **Vancomycin 1mg/0.1mL + [Gentamicin 0.2mg/0.1mL[D] or Amikacin 0.4 mg/0.1mL[D]]**	0.1mL intravitreally 0.1mL intravitreally 0.1mL intravitreally 0.1mL intravitreally 0.1mL intravitreally	Dependent on clinical picture Dependent on clinical picture	- Fulminant onset 2-7 days following penetrating trauma. - Vitrectomy may be required. - Consider adjunctive systemic antibiotics. - Intravitreal dexamethasone 0.4mg/0.1mL may be beneficial.

RECOMMENDED EMPIRIC THERAPY OF SELECTED OPHTHALMIC INFECTIONS

Infection	Usual Pathogens	Recommended Empiric Therapy	Recommended Dose[A]	Recommended Duration	Comments
Endophthalmitis (cont'd) **Hematogenous**	Streptococcus spp N. meningitidis S. aureus B. cereus* Candida spp* *(see below)*	Ophthalmic Preparations[B] **Vancomycin 1mg/0.1mL + Ceftazidime 2.25mg/0.1mL**	0.1mL intravitreally 0.1mL intravitreally	Dependent on clinical picture	- Insidious onset. - Risk factors: • endocarditis • immunosuppression • *chronic IV drug abuser • *TPN. - Blood cultures should be taken. - Vitrectomy may be required. - IV antibiotics required for systemic infection (tailor antibiotics according to C&S results).
		β-lactam Allergy[B] **Vancomycin 1mg/0.1mL + [Gentamicin 0.2mg/0.1mL[D] or Amikacin 0.4 mg/0.1mL[D]]** plus Systemic Antibiotics **Ceftriaxone + Vancomycin[E]**	0.1mL intravitreally 0.1mL intravitreally 0.1mL intravitreally 2g IV q12h 15mg/kg IV q8-12h	Dependent on clinical picture 6 weeks, dependent on culture results	
Fungal	Candida spp Aspergillus spp Fusarium spp	Systemic therapy* **Fluconazole** or **Voriconazole** or **Amphotericin B** plus Ophthalmic Preparation[B] **Voriconazole 100mcg/0.1mL** or **Amphotericin B 5mcg/0.1mL**	6-12mg/kg IV/PO daily 200mg IV/PO q12h 0.7-1mg/kg IV daily 0.1mL intravitreally 0.1mL intravitreally	4-12 weeks dependent on clinical picture Single dose; repeat dosing highly controversial	- Etiologies include: • chronic post-surgical • penetrating ocular trauma due to vegetation • hematogenous. - Vitrectomy may be required. * Systemic antifungal therapy recommended if hematogenous source. - Neither posaconazole nor echinocandins achieve adequate therapeutic concentrations in the vitreous.

E. Desired vancomycin trough is 15-20 mg/L. Monitor renal function closely. See Vancomycin Dosing & Monitoring Guidelines.

RECOMMENDED EMPIRIC THERAPY OF SELECTED OPHTHALMIC INFECTIONS

Infection	Usual Pathogens	Recommended Empiric Therapy	Recommended Dose[A]	Recommended Duration	Comments
Periorbital/Pre-septal Cellulitis 2° to paranasal sinusitis	S. aureus/MRSA Group A Streptococci S. pneumoniae H. influenzae	- Marked hyperemia and edema of eyelids and facial subcutaneous tissues. - No impairment of eye movement, vision or pupillary response.			
		<u>Mild/Afebrile</u> **Amoxicillin-clavulanate**	<u>Paediatric</u> 40 mg/kg/d PO div tid <u>Adult</u> 875 mg PO bid	7-10 days 7-10 days	- Consider otolaryngology consult.
		If MRSA suspected Add **TMP/SMX**	<u>Paediatric</u> 8-12mg TMP/kg/d PO div bid <u>Adult</u> 1-2 DS tabs PO bid	7-10 days 7-10 days	
		<u>Moderate-Severe</u> **Cefuroxime**	<u>Paediatric</u> 100-150 mg/kg/d IV div q8h <u>Adult</u> 750mg IV q8h	7-10 days 7-10 days	- Stepdown to oral agents when clinically improved.
		or **Ceftriaxone**	<u>Paediatric</u> 50-75mg/kg IV q24h <u>Adult</u> 1-2g IV daily	7-10 days 7-10 days	
		If MRSA suspected Add **Vancomycin**[E]	<u>Paediatric</u> 60mg/kg/d IV div q6h <u>Adult</u> 15mg/kg IV q8-12h	7-10 days 7-10 days	

E. Desired vancomycin trough is 15-20 mg/L. Monitor renal function closely. See Vancomycin Dosing & Monitoring Guidelines.

RECOMMENDED EMPIRIC THERAPY OF SELECTED OPHTHALMIC INFECTIONS

Infection	Usual Pathogens	Recommended Empiric Therapy	Recommended Dose[A]	Recommended Duration	Comments
Periorbital/Pre-septal Cellulitis (cont'd) **2° to skin trauma**	S. aureus/MRSA Group A Streptococci Anaerobes	<u>Mild-moderate</u> **Amoxicillin-clavulanate** +	<u>Paediatric</u> 40mg/kg/d PO div tid <u>Adult</u> 875mg PO bid	7-10 days 7-10 days	- Types of trauma include: • puncture wounds • lacerations • insect bites • animal bites.
		TMP/SMX	<u>Paediatric</u> 8-12mg TMP/kg/d PO div bid <u>Adult</u> 1-2 DS tabs PO bid	7-10 days 7-10 days	
		<u>Severe</u> **Vancomycin**[E] +	<u>Paediatric</u> 60mg/kg/d IV div q6h <u>Adult</u> 15mg/kg IV q8-12h	7-10 days 7-10 days	
		Ceftriaxone +	<u>Paediatric</u> 50-75mg/kg IV q24h <u>Adult</u> 1-2g IV daily	7-10 days 7-10 days	
		Metronidazole	<u>Paediatric</u> 30mg/kg/d IV/PO div q12h <u>Adult</u> 500mg IV/PO q12h	7-10 days 7-10 days	

E. Desired vancomycin trough is 15-20 mg/L. Monitor renal function closely. See Vancomycin Dosing & Monitoring Guidelines.

RECOMMENDED EMPIRIC THERAPY OF SELECTED OPHTHALMIC INFECTIONS

Infection	Usual Pathogens	Recommended Empiric Therapy	Recommended Dose[A]	Recommended Duration	Comments
Orbital Cellulitis	- Initial soft tissue swelling, redness, and increased warmth of the eyelids. - Progresses to impairment of extraocular motility, globe proptosis, ocular pain, diplopia and/or decreased vision. - **Consult Ophthalmology, Otolaryngology and Infectious Diseases.** - Obtain urgent CT scan of orbit and sinuses and blood cultures. - Surgical intervention recommended if: • ≥ 8 years of age • abscess > 1cm • marked fever on admission • lack of response to medical therapy • concern for optic nerve or retinal compromise. - Complications include visual loss from optic neuropathy, cavernous sinus thrombosis, meningitis, and intracranial infections.				
2° to paranasal sinusitis	S. pneumoniae M. catarrhalis H. influenzae S. aureus/MRSA Group A Strepto-cocci Anaerobes*	**Paediatric**** **Cloxacillin** + **Ceftriaxone** +/- **Metronidazole** **Adult**** **Cloxacillin***** + **Ceftriaxone** + **Metronidazole**	200mg/kg/d IV div q6h 100mg/kg/d IV div q12h 30mg/kg/d IV div q8h 2g IV q4h 2g IV q12h 500mg IV q8h	10-14 days 10-14 days	- Consider P. aeruginosa in recently hospitalized, instrumented, or immunocompromised patients. Use ceftazidime instead of ceftriaxone. * Anaerobes are more prominent pathogens in adults. **Stepdown to oral therapy when clinically appropriate. ***Use vancomycin instead of cloxacillin if abscess on CT or MRSA suspected.

RECOMMENDED EMPIRIC THERAPY OF SELECTED OPHTHALMIC INFECTIONS

Infection	Usual Pathogens	Recommended Empiric Therapy	Recommended Dose[A]	Recommended Duration	Comments
Orbital Cellulitis (cont'd) **2° to immuno-suppression**	Mucor spp Rhizopus spp P. aeruginosa* S. aureus/MRSA*	**Amphotericin B**	0.8mg/kg IV daily; if tolerated increase up to 1.5mg/kg/d	3g total dose	* For bacterial causes, see Orbital Cellulitis, 2° to paranasal sinusitis. - Risk factors: • diabetic ketoacidosis • neutropenia. - Surgical debridement necessary. - Treat underlying condition. - Consult ophthalmologist re: need for intravitreal antifungal.
2° to trauma	S. aureus Group A Streptococci Bacillus spp Anaerobes	<u>Paediatric</u> **Vancomycin**[E] + **Ceftriaxone** + **Metronidazole PO/IV** <u>Adult</u> **Vancomycin**[E] + **Ceftriaxone** + **Metronidazole PO/IV**	60mg/kg/d IV div q6h 100mg/kg/d IV div q12h 30mg/kg/d PO/IV div q8h 15mg/kg IV q8-12h 2g IV q12h 500mg PO/IV q8h	10-14 days 10-14 days	- Tailor antibiotic therapy to C&S results.

FOOTNOTES:
SAP = TPD Special Access Program (formerly Emergency Release)
A. Usual **adult** dose in patients with normal renal and hepatic function, unless otherwise noted. Mg/kg/d = milligrams per kilogram per day.
B. Not commercially available, manufactured by Pharmacy.
C. Ocular toxicity may occur with prolonged use of aminoglycoside ophthalmic solutions (> 7-10 days).
D. Retinal toxicity related to intravitreal use of aminoglycosides (gentamicin > amikacin).
E. Desired vancomycin trough is 15-20 mg/L. Monitor renal function closely. See Vancomycin Dosing & Monitoring Guidelines.

RECOMMENDED EMPIRIC THERAPY OF FUNGAL INFECTIONS

Infection	Usual Pathogens	Recommended Empiric Therapy	Recommended Dose[1]	Recommended Duration	Comments
Non-hair bearing skin **Tinea pedis*** **(athlete's foot)** **Tinea corporis** **(ring worm)** **Tinea cruris** **(jock itch)** **Tinea manuum** **Tinea facei**	Trichophyton spp Epidermophyton spp Microsporum spp	Topical therapy with one of: **Ciclopirox 1%** **Clotrimazole 1%** **Ketoconazole 2%** **Miconazole 2%** **Terbinafine 1%** **Tolnaftate 1%**	Apply bid Apply bid Apply daily Apply daily Apply daily - bid Apply bid	2-4 weeks 2-4 weeks 2-4 weeks 2-4 weeks 2-4 weeks** 2-4 weeks * 4-6 weeks for T. pedis	- Oral therapy is effective, but topical therapy is preferred. * Tinea pedis prone to recurrence; prolonged therapy (4-6 weeks) recommended. **Shorter course of therapy with terbinafine (1-2 wks) may be adequate for mild cases of Tinea pedis.
Hair bearing skin **Tinea capitis** (scalp, eyebrows, eyelashes) **Tinea barbae** (beard, mustache)	Trichophyton spp Microsporum spp	Adult **Terbinafine*** **Itraconazole** Alternative **Fluconazole** **Griseofulvin** Paediatrics **Terbinafine*** or **Itraconazole** or **Griseofulvin**	250mg PO daily 100mg PO bid 150mg PO weekly 250mg PO daily **<20kg** 62.5mg PO daily **20-40kg** 125mg PO daily **>40kg** 250mg PO daily 5mg/kg PO daily 15-20mg/kg/d PO in divided doses	2-4 weeks 4-8 weeks 4-8 weeks 6-12 weeks 4 weeks 4 weeks 4 weeks 4 weeks 8-10 weeks	- Topical therapy not recommended. - For severe inflammatory disease (kerion), adjunctive prednisone is sometimes used. * Poor response with M. canis. Continue therapy for 6-8 weeks.

RECOMMENDED EMPIRIC THERAPY OF FUNGAL INFECTIONS

Infection	Usual Pathogens	Recommended Empiric Therapy	Recommended Dose[1]	Recommended Duration	Comments
Tinea versicolor (**Pityriasis versicolor**)	Malassezia furfur (Pityrosporum orbiculare)	Topical **Clotrimazole 1%** **Ketoconazole 2%** **Miconazole 2%** **Selenium sulfide 2.5%**	Apply bid Apply daily Apply bid Apply daily (lather, then wash off after 10 minutes)	7 days 7 days 7 days 7 days	- Oral therapy recommended for: • extensive involvement • recurrent infections • failure of topical agents. - Oral terbinafine (Lamisil®) is not effective.
		Terbinafine 1%	Apply daily - bid	7 days	
		Oral **Itraconazole** or **Fluconazole** or **Ketoconazole**	400mg PO daily 400mg PO 400mg PO **or** 200mg PO daily	3-7 days 1 dose 1 dose 7 days	
Onychomycosis (**Tinea unguium**)	Trichophyton spp	**Terbinafine**	250mg PO daily	6 weeks (fingers) 12 weeks (toes)	- Terbinafine is more effective than fluconazole, itraconazole or oral griseofulvin. - Terbinafine cream is NOT effective. - 25-30% relapse rate.
		Alternative **Itraconazole**	200mg PO daily	8 weeks (fingers) 12 weeks (toes)	

RECOMMENDED EMPIRIC THERAPY OF FUNGAL INFECTIONS

Infection	Usual Pathogens	Recommended Empiric Therapy	Recommended Dose[1]	Recommended Duration	Comments
Sporotrichosis [Clin Infect Dis 2007;45:1255–65]					
• lympho-cutaneous	Sporothrix schenckii	**Itraconazole**	200mg PO daily	3-6 months*	* Give for 2-4 weeks after all lesions have resolved, usually for a total of 3-6 months.
		Unresponsive **Itraconazole**	200mg PO bid	Continue until 2-4 weeks after all lesions resolved.*	
		or **Terbinafine**	500mg PO bid	Continue until 2-4 weeks after all lesions resolved.*	
• extra-cutaneous	Sporothrix schenckii	Osteoarticular **Itraconazole**	200mg PO bid	12 months	
		Pulmonary Severe **Amphotericin B**	0.7- 1mg/kg IV daily	Until response then switch to itraconazole for total of 12 months	
		Less severe **Itraconazole**	200mg PO bid	12 months	* For HIV-positive or immuno-compromised patients, suppressive therapy with itraconazole 200mg PO daily is recommended, life-long if continuing immunosuppression. Consult Infectious Diseases.
		Meningeal* or Disseminated* **Amphotericin B**	0.7- 1mg/kg IV daily	Until response then switch to itraconazole for total of 12 months	

RECOMMENDED EMPIRIC THERAPY OF FUNGAL INFECTIONS

Infection	Usual Pathogens	Recommended Empiric Therapy	Recommended Dose[1]	Recommended Duration	Comments
Candida					
Vaginal candidiasis	See Recommended Empiric Therapy, Adult, Genital, Vulvovaginitis, Candidiasis.				
Oropharyngeal candidiasis [Clin Infect Dis 2009;48:503-35.]	Candida albicans Occasionally non-albicans spp	**Nystatin** susp or **Clotrimazole** vag insert used orally	500,000 U (5mL) qid 100mg PO daily	7-14 days 7-14 days	- Screen for HIV unless: • infant • known immunodeficiency/ immunosuppression • recent use of inhaled steroids. - For immunosuppressed patients, fluconazole 200mg/ day is recommended. Maintenance therapy may be necessary. * For fluconazole - refractory disease, see Esophageal Candidiasis.
		Alternative **Fluconazole*** Infants (Thrush) **Nystatin**	100-200mg (3mg/kg) PO daily 100,000 U (1mL) qid	7-14 days 7-10 days	
Esophageal candidiasis [Clin Infect Dis 2009;48:503-35.]	Candida albicans Occasionally non-albicans spp	**Fluconazole*** Refractory – based on susceptibility results **Itraconazole** or **Voriconazole** or **Posaconazole**	200-400mg (3-6mg/kg) PO daily 200mg PO daily** 200mg PO bid 400mg PO bid	14-21 days 14-21 days 14-21 days 14-21 days	- Always indicative of immuno-suppression. * Oral suspension available. **Oral solution given without food has better absorption than capsules. - For recurrent infections, suppressive therapy with fluconazole 100-200mg PO 3x/week recommended. ***Echinocandins have higher relapse rates than fluconazole.
		Alternative **Amphotericin B**[2] or **Anidulafungin*** or **Caspofungin*** or **Micafungin***	0.3-0.7mg/kg IV daily 200mg IV once then 100mg IV daily 70mg IV once then 50mg IV daily 150mg IV daily	14-21 days 14-21 days 14-21 days 14-21 days	

RECOMMENDED EMPIRIC THERAPY OF FUNGAL INFECTIONS

Infection	Usual Pathogens	Recommended Empiric Therapy	Recommended Dose[1]	Recommended Duration	Comments
Candida (cont'd) **Candiduria** [Clin Infect Dis 2009;48:503-35.]	- Usually associated with foreign body in urinary tract. Removal of urinary catheter or stent results in ~40% eradication of candiduria but only 20% eradication if catheter/stent subsequently reinserted. - Persistent candiduria in immunocompromised patients warrants ultrasound or CT of kidney. ***Bladder irrigation with amphotericin B has been used to treat candidal cystitis but does not treat infections beyond the bladder and has a high relapse rate. May be useful for fluconazole resistant Candida species, e.g. C. krusei or C. glabrata. - Use of echinocandins should be avoided for candiduria due to poor urinary concentrations and limited clinical data.				
	Candida spp*	**Asymptomatic** Treatment not recommended unless high risk[†] **Symptomatic/High risk[†]** Cystitis **Fluconazole** Alternative **Amphotericin B**[‡,***,‡] Pyelonephritis **Fluconazole** Alternative **Amphotericin B**[‡]	200mg (3mg/kg) PO daily 0.3-0.6mg/kg IV daily 200-400mg (3-6mg/kg) PO daily 0.5-0.7mg/kg IV daily	 14 days 1-7 days 14 days 14 days	* Fluconazole may not be effective against C. krusei and some strains of C. glabrata. C. lusitaniae may be resistant to amphotericin B. **Repeat urine culture to rule out contamination. If candiduria is confirmed, screen for diabetes, renal dysfunction, metabolic abnormalities, and genito-urinary structural abnormalities, including imaging of kidneys and collecting system to rule out abscess or fungal ball. [†] High risk: • neutropenia • low birth weight infants • renal transplant patients • patients undergoing urological procedures. [‡] Lipid formulations of amphotericin B should not be used due to low renal tissue concentrations.

RECOMMENDED EMPIRIC THERAPY OF FUNGAL INFECTIONS

Infection	Usual Pathogens	Recommended Empiric Therapy	Recommended Dose[1]	Recommended Duration	Comments
Candida (cont'd) **Invasive candidiasis/ Candidemia** [Clin Infect Dis 2009;48:503-35.] and [Can J Infect Dis Med Microbiol 2010;21:e122-50.]	General Management - Removal of central venous and/or peritoneal dialysis catheters generally recommended in non-neutropenic patients but controversial for neutropenic patients as source often from GI tract. - Discontinue broad spectrum antibiotics if possible. - Serial blood cultures (minimum daily x 3) to ensure sterilization. - Fundoscopic examination should be considered. - For positive Candida spp cultures: • C. glabrata – some resistance with low dose fluconazole; may be overcome with high dose therapy. • C. krusei - resistant to fluconazole • C. lusitaniae, C. guiliermondii - usually resistant to amphotericin B.				
	Candida albicans Candida tropicalis* Candida parapsilosis* Candida glabrata Candida krusei	<u>Hemodynamically stable, no azole exposure in past 3 months</u> **Fluconazole**	800mg (12mg/kg) IV loading dose then 400mg (6mg/kg) IV/PO daily		* Usually associated with prosthetic device, especially central venous catheters.
		<u>Hemodynamically unstable or azole exposure in past 3 months</u> **Anidulafungin** or **Caspofungin** or **Micafungin** or **Amphotericin B**[2]	200mg IV once then 100mg IV daily 70mg IV once then 50mg IV daily 100mg IV daily 0.5-1mg/kg IV daily	minimum 14 days after first negative blood culture and resolution of signs & symptoms minimum 14 days after first negative blood culture and resolution of signs & symptoms	

RECOMMENDED EMPIRIC THERAPY OF FUNGAL INFECTIONS

Infection	Usual Pathogens	Recommended Empiric Therapy	Recommended Dose[1]	Recommended Duration	Comments
Candida (cont'd) **Hepatosplenic candidiasis/ Chronic disseminated candidiasis** [Clin Infect Dis 2009;48:503-35.]	Candida spp	**Fluconazole** or **Amphotericin B*** _Alternative_ **Anidulafungin** or **Caspofungin** or **Micafungin**	400mg (6mg/kg) IV/PO daily 0.5-0.7mg/kg IV daily 200mg IV once then 100mg IV daily 70mg IV once then 50mg IV daily 100mg IV daily	3-6 months and resolution or calcification of radiologic lesions 3-6 months and resolution or calcification of radiologic lesions	* Fluconazole may be given after 1-2 weeks of amphotericin B if clinically stable and improved. - Patients receiving ongoing chemotherapy or stem cell transplantation should continue antifungal therapy throughout high risk period to prevent relapse.
Aspergillosis	[Clin Infect Dis 2008;46:327-60.]				
Aspergilloma	- Aspergilloma is a fungal mass that develops in a pre-existing lung cavity. - Embolization/surgical resection, if feasible, is recommended in cases of persistent hemoptysis. - The role of antifungal therapy is uncertain.				
Chronic cavitary pulmonary aspergillosis (CCPA)	- Typically occurs in patients with chronic underlying lung diseases +/- comorbidities (e.g. diabetes, malnutrition) and/or inhaled/systemic corticosteroids but without severe immunosuppression. - Surgical resection of CCPA not recommended as associated with high morbidity and mortality.				
	Aspergillus spp	**Itraconazole** or **Voriconazole**	200mg PO bid 200mg PO bid	4-12 months, possibly lifelong 4-12 months, possibly lifelong	
Allergic broncho-pulmonary aspergillosis (ABPA)	- Allergic response to fungal hyphae in bronchial tree, manifesting as sinusitis and asthma and characterized by wheezing and pulmonary infiltrates, leading to bronchiectasis and fibrosis. - Corticosteroids are primary therapy.				
	Aspergillus spp	**Itraconazole*** _Alternative_ **Voriconazole**	200mg PO bid 200mg PO bid	3-6 months 3-6 months	* Itraconazole has corticosteroid-sparing effect as it decreases number of exacerbations.

RECOMMENDED EMPIRIC THERAPY OF FUNGAL INFECTIONS

Infection	Usual Pathogens	Recommended Empiric Therapy	Recommended Dose[1]	Recommended Duration	Comments
Aspergillosis (cont'd)					
Invasive aspergillosis (IA)	- Typically occurs in patients with severe immunosuppression; e.g. neutropenic, post-transplantation, post chemotherapy, advanced AIDS, chronic granulomatous disease. - IA is classified as proven, probable, or possible based on host factors, clinical manifestations and mycological evidence [Clin Infect Dis 2008;46:1813-21.].				
	Aspergillus fumigatus Aspergillus flavus Other Aspergillus spp	<u>Histologically proven or probable IA</u> **Voriconazole**	6mg/kg IV q12h first day then 4mg/kg IV q12h or 200mg PO bid*	Until clinical/ radiographic resolution**	- Infectious Diseases consult recommended. * If <40kg, use oral dose of 10mg/kg/d PO bid (max 300mg/day). **Itraconazole (200mg PO bid) or voriconazole may be used as stepdown oral agents. - For central nervous system infection, voriconazole recommended and neuro-surgery often required. ***Combination antifungal therapy may have a role but clinical data lacking. Consult Infectious Diseases. - Anidulafungin not listed as limited clinical experience in IA.
		or **Amphotericin B**[2]	1-1.5mg/kg IV daily	Until clinical/ radiographic resolution**	
		<u>Refractory***</u> **Caspofungin**	70mg IV first day then 50mg IV daily	Until clinical/ radiographic resolution**	
		or **Micafungin**	100-150mg IV daily	Until clinical/ radiographic resolution**	

RECOMMENDED EMPIRIC THERAPY OF FUNGAL INFECTIONS

Infection	Usual Pathogens	Recommended Empiric Therapy	Recommended Dose[1]	Recommended Duration	Comments
Fungal sinusitis	Aspergillus spp Rhizopus spp** Mucor spp**	- In immunocompetent host, fungi in sinuses may be associated with nasal polyposis and do not routinely require antifungal therapy. - In immunocompromised patients/diabetic ketoacidosis, a fungal infection can present as a cellulitis that may rapidly progress and be fatal. Surgical debridement is necessary.			* Use the higher dose if neutropenic. **Echinocandins not active against Rhizopus/Mucor spp.**
		<u>Immunocompetent</u> Antifungal therapy not routinely recommended			
		<u>Immunocompromised/ diabetic ketoacidosis</u>			
		<u>Aspergillus</u> **Voriconazole**	6mg/kg IV q12h first day then 4mg/kg IV q12h or 200mg PO bid	Until clinical and radiographic resolution and reversal of immunosuppression, if possible.	
		or **Amphotericin B**[2]	1-1.25mg/kg IV daily*	Suppressive therapy then usually continued for at least 3-6 months, or life-long if continuing immunosuppression.	
		<u>Rhizopus/Mucor****</u> **Amphotericin B**[2]	1-1.5mg/kg IV daily		
		<u>Alternative</u> **Posaconazole**	400mg PO bid		

RECOMMENDED EMPIRIC THERAPY OF FUNGAL INFECTIONS

Infection	Usual Pathogens	Recommended Empiric Therapy	Recommended Dose[†]	Recommended Duration	Comments
Pneumocystis pneumonia (PCP) Treatment[†]	Pneumocystis jirovecii	**TMP/SMX**	2DS tab PO q8h **or** 15-20mg TMP/kg/day IV div q8h	21 days	- Always test for HIV if not known to be positive.
		or			[†]After 21 days therapy, PCP prophylaxis is indicated in HIV (+) patients (see below).
		[**Trimethoprim** +	15mg/kg/d PO div tid	21 days	* Check G6PD status in selected patients (individuals of African, Mediterranean, or southern Chinese descent).
		Dapsone[*]] Alternative	100mg PO daily	21 days	**Watch for dysglycemia and pancreatitis.
		Pentamidine[**] or	4mg/kg IV daily	21 days	
		[**Clindamycin IV/PO**[C] +	600mg IV q8h/ 300-450mg PO qid	21 days	
		Primaquine[*]] or	15mg PO daily	21 days	
		Atovaquone susp	750mg PO bid with food	21 days	
		PLUS if indicated[***] Adjunctive Corticosteroid			[***]For all listed regimens, indications for adjunctive corticosteroid therapy:
		Prednisone then	40mg PO bid	5 days	• PaO₂ < 70mmHg (on room air)
		Prednisone then	40mg PO daily	5 days	• D(A-a)O₂ > 35mmHg.
		Prednisone	20mg PO daily	11 days	NB: best evidence of benefit in AIDS patients.
		or Adjunctive *Parenteral* Corticosteroid			
		Methylprednisolone then	30mg IV bid	5 days	
		Methylprednisolone then	30mg IV daily	5 days	
		Methylprednisolone	15mg IV daily	11 days	

RECOMMENDED EMPIRIC THERAPY OF FUNGAL INFECTIONS

Infection	Usual Pathogens	Recommended Empiric Therapy	Recommended Dose[†]	Recommended Duration	Comments
Pneumocystis pneumonia (PCP) (cont'd)					

Prophylaxis and post-treatment suppression	- PCP prophylaxis recommended for:
	  • HIV patients with CD_4 < 200 cells/mm^3 (0.2 x 10^9/L) or <14% or history of oropharyngeal candidiasis or AIDS-defining illness
	  • solid organ or stem cell transplant in past 12 months.
	Consider for other patients with prolonged high dose corticosteroids (> 20mg/day prednisone or equivalent for > 4 weeks)/TNF inhibitors/immunosuppression.				

	Pneumocystis jirovecii	**TMP/SMX**	1 DS tab PO daily* **or** 1 SS tab PO daily**	chronic***	* TMP/SMX DS or dapsone combination regimen also provide prophylaxis of toxoplasmosis (prophylaxis recommended if CD_4 < 100 cells/mm^3 (0.1 x 10^9/L and toxoplasma antibody positive). - TMP/SMX also provides prophylaxis of some bacterial infections. **Can be used if toxoplasma antibody negative; may be better tolerated than 1 DS tab daily ***Discontinue when CD_4 > 200 cells/mm^3 or > 14% x 3 months. † Check G6PD status in selected patients (individuals of African, Mediterranean, or southern Chinese descent). ‡ Watch for dysglycemia and pancreatitis.
		Alternative **Dapsone**[†] or	100mg PO daily	chronic***	
		[Dapsone[†] + **Pyrimethamine** + **Leucovorin** (Folinic acid)]*	200mg PO once per week 75mg once per week 25mg once per week	chronic***	
		or **Atovaquone**	1500mg PO daily with food	chronic***	
		or **Pentamidine**[‡]	300mg in 6mL SWI by aerosol every 4 weeks	chronic***	

- 457 -

RECOMMENDED EMPIRIC THERAPY OF FUNGAL INFECTIONS

Infection	Usual Pathogens	Recommended Empiric Therapy	Recommended Dose[1]	Recommended Duration	Comments
Endemic mycoses	- Infectious Diseases consult strongly recommended.				
Blastomyces spp	- Clin Infect Dis 2008;46:1801-12.				
Coccidioides spp	- Clin Infect Dis 2005;41:1217-23.				
Cryptococcus spp	- Echinocandins not active against Cryptococcus spp. - Clin Infect Dis 2010;50:291-322.				
Histoplasma spp	- Fluconazole less effective than itraconazole against Histoplasma spp. - Clin Infect Dis 2007;45:807-25.				

Footnotes:
1. Unless otherwise indicated, usual **adult** dose in patients with normal renal and hepatic function. mg/kg = milligrams per kilogram
2. Amphotericin B IV (see algorithm following)
   Test doses and **incremental dosing** are no longer recommended for the following reasons:
   a. hypersensitivity reactions and anaphylaxis are rare
   b. fever and chills associated with amphotericin B administration are not dose- or time-dependent
   c. commercial formulation now in use is of high purity
   d. causes unnecessary delays in patient receiving therapeutic dose.

The routine use of **premedication** (e.g. acetaminophen + diphenhydramine +/- corticosteroid +/- meperidine) is also no longer recommended prior to the initial dose of amphotericin B IV but may be administered promptly if an adverse reaction does occur, and then as pretreatment with subsequent amphotericin B doses.

Management of Adult Patients on Amphotericin B

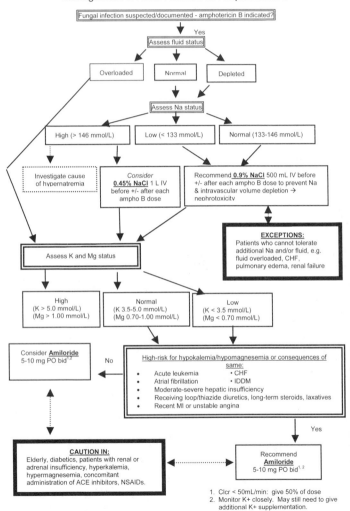

Fungal infection suspected/documented - amphotericin B indicated?

Yes

Assess fluid status

Overloaded | Normal | Depleted

Assess Na status

High (> 146 mmol/L) | Low (< 133 mmol/L) | Normal (133-146 mmol/L)

Investigate cause of hypernatremia

Consider **0.45% NaCl** 1 L IV before +/- after each ampho B dose

Recommend **0.9% NaCl** 500 mL IV before +/- after each ampho B dose to prevent Na & intravascular volume depletion → nephrotoxicity

EXCEPTIONS:
Patients who cannot tolerate additional Na and/or fluid, e.g. fluid overloaded, CHF, pulmonary edema, renal failure

Assess K and Mg status

High (K > 5.0 mmol/L) (Mg > 1.00 mmol/L) | Normal (K 3.5-5.0 mmol/L) (Mg 0.70-1.00 mmol/L) | Low (K < 3.5 mmol/L) (Mg < 0.70 mmol/L)

Consider **Amiloride** 5-10 mg PO bid[1,2]

No

High-risk for hypokalemia/hypomagnesemia or consequences of same:
- Acute leukemia
- Atrial fibrillation
- Moderate-severe hepatic insufficiency
- Receiving loop/thiazide diuretics, long-term steroids, laxatives
- Recent MI or unstable angina
- CHF
- IDDM

Yes

CAUTION IN:
Elderly, diabetics, patients with renal or adrenal insufficiency, hyperkalemia, hypermagnesemia, concomitant administration of ACE inhibitors, NSAIDs.

Recommend **Amiloride** 5-10 mg PO bid[1,2]

1. Clcr < 50mL/min: give 50% of dose
2. Monitor K+ closely. May still need to give additional K+ supplementation.

Management of Adult Patients on Amphotericin B

Administration of Amphotericin B	
Infusion	
Peripheral line	- infuse dose over 4-6 hours
	- max. concentration 0.1 mg/mL
Central line	- infuse dose over 2-4 hours
	- max. concentration 0.25 mg/mL*
	(*concentrations up to 1.4 mg/mL are soluble in D5W and may be considered in fluid-restricted pts)
Premedication	
Routine premedication NOT recommended.	
May be given if infusion-related reaction occurs & then as pretreatment with subsequent doses.	
Fever/chills/rigors	Meperidine 25-50 mg IV
Fever	Acetaminophen 650mg PO
	(max 4 g/day)
Nausea/Vomiting	Diphenhydramine 25-50 mg PO/IV
Give premedication 30 min. prior to ampho B	
AVOID OTHER NEPHROTOXINS (e.g. aminoglycosides, calcineurin inhibitors [cyclosporine, tacrolimus], cisplatin, foscarnet, pentamidine, tenofovir)	

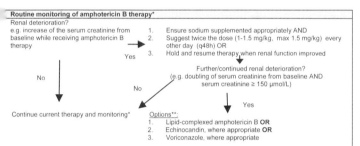

Routine monitoring of amphotericin B therapy*

Renal deterioration?
e.g. increase of the serum creatinine from baseline while receiving amphotericin B therapy

Yes →
1. Ensure sodium supplemented appropriately AND
2. Suggest twice the dose (1-1.5 mg/kg, max 1.5 mg/kg) every other day (q48h) OR
3. Hold and resume therapy when renal function improved

No ↓

Further/continued renal deterioration?
(e.g. doubling of serum creatinine from baseline AND serum creatinine ≥ 150 µmol/L)

No ← / Yes ↓

Continue current therapy and monitoring*

Options**:
1. Lipid-complexed amphotericin B OR
2. Echinocandin, where appropriate OR
3. Voriconazole, where appropriate

***Routine monitoring**	** **Continuous Infusion of amphotericin B - NOT ROUTINELY RECOMMENDED:**
<ul><li>Cardiovascular status (HR, BP)</li><li>Respiratory status (RR < 20/minute dependent upon baseline and underlying illness)</li><li>Body weight (assess fluid status)</li><li>Fluid intake and output (Ins/Outs)</li><li>CBC with differential</li><li>Serum K/Na/Ca/Mg</li><li>Renal function (i.e. Scr/BUN)</li><li>Liver function tests</li></ul>	<ul><li>A study [BMJ 2001;322:1-6] compared continuous infusion of amphotericin B with 4h infusion (n=80). ⇒ Continuous infusion had fewer side effects, significantly reduced nephrotoxicity, and decreased mortality (p<0.05). ⇒ However, the study was not powered to show equivalent efficacy and few (n=3/80) patients had documented fungal infections.</li><li>In addition, ampho B has concentration dependent antifungal activity; as concentrations increase, activity goes from fungistatic to fungicidal with maximal activity at peak serum concentration: MIC ratio of ≥ 10:1.</li><li>Therefore continuous infusion cannot be recommended routinely until more clinical evidence is available but perhaps as an alternative if patients experience nephrotoxicity.</li></ul>

TREATMENT OF ENTERIC PARASITIC INFECTIONS

This section includes the most common intestinal parasites (acquired locally or abroad) along with recommended therapy.

Parasite	Symptoms	Recommended Drug	Recommended Dose[A]	Recommended Duration	Comments
• Ova and parasite exam recommended if: ⟹ diarrhea > 14 days duration or ⟹ recent travel or immigration from endemic area. NB: If applicable, specify above on lab requisition. • **Collect one sample initially.** Use SAF fixative transport system. Multiple (3) stool samples on alternate days (collected within 10 days) indicated if any of: ⟹ chronic, persistent or relapsing diarrhea ⟹ illness in person with recent travel history or immigration from endemic areas ⟹ food handler ⟹ suspected helminthic infection. NB: If applicable, specify above on lab requisition. • Post treatment ova and parasite exam indicated for: ⟹ food handlers ⟹ institutionalized/long term care patients ⟹ post treatment amebiasis.					
HELMINTHS					
Nematodes **Ascaris lumbricoides (roundworm)**	• usually asymptomatic* • not usually a cause of diarrhea	**Mebendazole** **or** _Alternative_ **Albendazole**[1] or **Ivermectin**[2]	100mg PO bid **or** 500mg PO 400mg PO 150-200mcg/kg PO	3 days 1 dose 1 dose 1 dose	*A history of passing a large round worm is often the presenting complaint. Submit worm to lab if available. • May cause eosinophilia during acute infection. • Common in developing countries.

1. Available as 200mg tablet through Therapeutic Products Directorate (TPD) Special Access Program (Emergency Release). Contact pharmacy for assistance in ordering.

TREATMENT OF ENTERIC PARASITIC INFECTIONS

Parasite	Symptoms	Recommended Drug	Recommended Dose[A]	Recommended Duration	Comments
HELMINTHS					
Nematodes (cont'd) Enterobius vermicularis (pinworm)	• perianal pruritus	**Mebendazole**	100mg PO	Repeat in 2 weeks (2 doses total)	• Most common human helminth in Canada. • Common in children and household contacts. • Treatment of the entire household is recommended.
		Pyrantel pamoate	11mg/kg PO (max 1g)	Repeat in 2 weeks (2 doses total)	
		Alternative **Albendazole**[1]	400mg PO	Repeat in 2 weeks (2 doses total)	
	Pregnancy • Treatment of pinworms in the first trimester of pregnancy is NOT recommended due to the lack of safety experience with recommended antiparasitics in the first trimester. If possible, treatment should be delayed until after delivery. • Worm infestations do not require treatment during pregnancy unless they are considered a threat to the health of the mother or her fetus. • All antiparasitics discussed below are pregnancy risk category C (See Antimicrobials in Pregnancy/Lactation sections): ○ If treatment is required during pregnancy (2nd or 3rd trimester), use either: ▫ **Pyrantel pamoate** 11mg/kg PO once then repeat in 2 weeks (2 doses total) or ▫ **Pyrvinium pamoate** 5mg/kg PO (after a meal) once then repeat in 2 weeks (2 doses total) ○ Drug of choice FOLLOWING DELIVERY: ▫ **Mebendazole** 100mg PO once then repeat in 2 weeks (2 doses total). Can be given to breastfeeding women since only 2-10% of a dose is absorbed and levels in the breast milk are undetectable.				
Trichuris trichiura (whipworm)	• diarrhea may occur with heavy infections	**Mebendazole**	100mg PO bid	3 days	• Acquired mostly in tropical regions. • Often refractory; multiple courses of treatment may be necessary.
		Alternative **Albendazole**[1]	400mg PO daily	3 days	
		or **Ivermectin**[2]	200 mcg/kg PO daily	3 days	

1. Available as 200mg tablet through TPD Special Access Program (Emergency Release). Contact pharmacy for assistance in ordering
2. Available as 3mg tablet through TPD Special Access Program (Emergency Release). Veterinary parenteral and enema formulations of ivermectin have been used in severely ill patients unable to take oral medications. Contact pharmacy for assistance in ordering.

TREATMENT OF ENTERIC PARASITIC INFECTIONS

Parasite	Symptoms	Recommended Drug	Recommended Dose[A]	Recommended Duration	Comments
HELMINTHS					
Nematodes (cont'd) **Strongyloides stercoralis**	• usually asymptomatic • may cause diarrhea +/- eosinophilia **Hyperinfection syndrome**** • ileus • bacterial sepsis • ARDS	**Ivermectin**[2] Alternative **Albendazole**[1]* Hyperinfection syndrome** **Ivermectin**[2]	200mcg/kg PO daily 400mg PO bid 200mcg/kg PO daily	2 days 7 days 7 days or until symptoms resolve	• Acquired mostly in tropical and sub-tropical regions. • Serology may be more sensitive than stool for O & P testing. • Important to eradicate in patients where immune suppression is anticipated. * Lower efficacy than ivermectin. **Immunocompromised patients may develop hyperinfection syndrome with very high mortality. Infectious Diseases consult recommended. • If initially positive, repeat stool cultures for 2 weeks after treatment to verify eradication.

1. Available as 200mg tablet through TPD Special Access Program (Emergency Release). Contact pharmacy for assistance in ordering.
2. Available as 3mg tablet through TPD Special Access Program (Emergency Release). Veterinary parenteral and enema formulations of ivermectin have been used in severely ill patients unable to take oral medications. Contact pharmacy for assistance in ordering.

TREATMENT OF ENTERIC PARASITIC INFECTIONS

Parasite	Symptoms	Recommended Drug	Recommended Dose[A]	Recommended Duration	Comments
HELMINTHS					
Nematodes (cont'd) **Ancylostoma duodenale, Necator americanus (hookworms)**	• usually asmptomatic • may cause diarrhea and eosinophilia • iron deficiency anemia	**Mebendazole** <u>Alternative</u> **Albendazole**[1]* or **Pyrantel pamoate**	100mg PO bid **or** 500mg PO 400mg PO 11mg/kg PO daily (max 1 g)	3 days 1 dose 1 dose 3 days	• Acquired mostly in tropical and subtropical regions. • Intestinal blood loss may occur with heavy infections. * Ivermectin NOT effective. * More effective than mebendazole but available only through Special Access Program.

1. Available as 200mg tablet through TPD Special Access Program (Emergency Release). Contact pharmacy for assistance in ordering.

TREATMENT OF ENTERIC PARASITIC INFECTIONS

Parasite	Symptoms	Recommended Drug	Recommended Dose[A]	Recommended Duration	Comments
HELMINTHS					
Cestodes (Tapeworms)					
Diphyllobothrium latum (fish)	• usually asymptomatic	Praziquantel	5-10mg/kg PO	1 dose	• Acquired from undercooked fresh water fish, including salmon (North Canada).
Taenia saginata (beef) Taenia asiatica (pork)	• usually asymptomatic	Praziquantel	5-10mg/kg PO	1 dose	
Taenia solium (pork)	• usually asymptomatic	Praziquantel	5-10mg/kg PO	1 dose	• May be transmitted (fecal-oral) to others resulting in tissue infection with larval forms leading to cysticercosis (most commonly manifested as neurocysticercosis [central nervous system invasion→brain cysts, acquired epilepsy]). Consultation with Infectious Diseases recommended.
Dipylidium caninum (dog)	• usually asymptomatic	Praziquantel	5-10mg/kg PO	1 dose	
Hymenolepis nana (dwarf tapeworm), Hymenolepis diminuta (rats)		Praziquantel	25mg/kg PO	1 dose	• Treatment of household contacts is recommended.

Parasite	Symptoms	Recommended Drug	Recommended Dose[A]	Recommended Duration	Comments
PROTOZOA					
Blastocystis hominis	• diarrhea • abdominal pain and cramping • nausea	<u>Asymptomatic</u> None <u>Symptomatic</u> **Metronidazole***			• Pathogenic role controversial. • Treatment recommended if symptomatic and other causes (infectious/non-infectious) of diarrhea have been excluded. • Little data available on optimal therapy. * Metronidazole resistance reported.
			<u>Adult</u> 750mg PO tid <u>Paediatric</u> 35-50mg/kg/d PO div tid	10 days 10 days	
		or **Iodoquinol**[3]	<u>Adult</u> 650mg PO tid <u>Paediatric</u> 40mg/kg/d PO div tid[3] (max 650mg/dose)	20 days 20 days	
		or **TMP/SMX**	<u>Adult</u> 1DS tab PO bid <u>Paediatric</u> 6mg/kg/d TMP PO div bid	7 days 7 days	
		or **Nitazoxanide**[4]	<u>Adult</u> 500mg PO bid <u>Paediatric</u> 1-3 y.o. 100mg PO bid <u>4-11 y.o.</u> 200mg PO bid	3 days 3 days 3 days	
Chilomastix mesnili	Non-pathogenic	None			• Found in persons exposed to poor sanitary conditions.

3. Available as 210 and 650mg tablets
4. Available as 500mg tablet or 100mg/5mL oral suspension through TPD Special Access Program (Emergency Release). Contact pharmacy for assistance in ordering.

TREATMENT OF ENTERIC PARASITIC INFECTIONS

Parasite	Symptoms	Recommended Drug	Recommended Dose[A]	Recommended Duration	Comments
PROTOZOA					
Cryptosporidium parvum & hominis	• nausea • anorexia • weight loss • watery diarrhea • abdominal cramping	Immunocompetent[*] with severe & prolonged symptoms **Nitazoxanide**[4]	<u>Adult</u> 500mg PO bid <u>Paediatric</u> 1-3 y.o. 100mg PO bid 4-11 y.o. 200mg PO bid	3 days 3 days 3 days	* Self-limiting (+/- 2 weeks) diarrhea in immuno-competent patient. **Can cause chronic diarrhea in immuno-compromised patient. No drug has proven efficacy in advanced AIDS. HAART is mainstay of therapy. Consult Infectious Diseases regarding need for therapy (nitazoxanide, paromomycin, or paromomycin + azithromycin) for immunocompromised patients.
		Immunocompromised/HIV[**] Consult Infectious Diseases[**]			
Cyclospora cayetanensis	• nausea • anorexia • weight loss • watery diarrhea • abdominal cramping	**TMP/SMX**	<u>Adult</u> 1 DS tab PO bid <u>Paediatric</u> 10mg/kg/d TMP PO div bid	7 -10 days 7-10 days	• Symptoms last an average of 7 weeks (longer in immuno-compromised patient). • Outbreaks linked to ingestion of berries imported from the tropics or subtropics.
		HIV patients **TMP/SMX**	1 DS tab PO qid then 1 DS tab PO 3x/week	10 days 2 weeks	
		Sulfa allergy **Ciprofloxacin**	500mg PO bid then 500mg PO 3x/week	7 days 2 weeks	

4. Available as 500mg tablet or 100mg/5mL oral suspension through TPD Special Access Program (Emergency Release). Contact pharmacy for assistance in ordering.

TREATMENT OF ENTERIC PARASITIC INFECTIONS

Parasite	Symptoms	Recommended Drug	Recommended Dose[A]	Recommended Duration	Comments
PROTOZOA					
Dientamoeba fragilis	• diarrhea (intermittent) • abdominal pain and bloating • nausea • anorexia • fatigue	Asymptomatic None Symptomatic **Iodoquinol**[3] or **Paromomycin**[5] Alternative **Metronidazole***	Adult 650mg PO tid Paediatric 30-40mg/kg/d PO div tid[3] (max 650mg/dose) Adult & Paediatric 25-35mg/kg/d PO div tid Adult 500-750mg PO tid Paediatric 35-50mg/kg/d PO div tid	 20 days 20 days 7 days 10 days 10 days	• Potential pathogen. • Increased incidence of coinfection with pinworm. * High failure rate.
Endolimax nana	Non-pathogenic*	None			* If symptomatic, most likely due to other cause. • Found in persons exposed to poor sanitary conditions.
Entamoeba coli, Entamoeba hartmanni	Non-pathogenic	None			• Found in persons exposed to poor sanitary conditions.

3. Available as 210 and 650mg tablets.
5. Available as 250mg capsules.

TREATMENT OF ENTERIC PARASITIC INFECTIONS

Parasite	Symptoms	Recommended Drug	Recommended Dose[A]	Recommended Duration	Comments
PROTOZOA					
Entamoeba dispar	Non-pathogenic*	None			* If symptomatic, most likely due to other cause. • Microscopically indistinguishable from E. histolytica. Consult microbiologist to discuss specialized testing if clinically indicated.
Entamoeba histolytica (Amebiasis)	• diarrhea • dysentery • liver abscess*	Asymptomatic* **Iodoquinol**[3] or **Paromomycin**[5] Symptomatic **Metronidazole** followed by **Iodoquinol**[3] or **Paromomycin**[5] (to eradicate luminal cysts)	Adult 650mg PO tid Paediatric 30-40mg/kg/d PO div tid[3] (max 2g/day) Adult & Paediatric 25-35mg/kg/d PO div tid[5] Adult 500-750mg PO tid Paediatric 35-50mg/kg/d PO div tid Dosages as above	20 days 20 days 7 days 7-10 days 7-10 days 20 days 7 days	• May be asymptomatic cyst passer. • At least three stool specimens should be examined before excluding amebiasis. * Serology is the most useful test for diagnosis of amebic liver abscess.

3. Available as 210 and 650mg tablets.
5. Available as 250mg capsules

- 469 -

TREATMENT OF ENTERIC PARASITIC INFECTIONS

Parasite	Symptoms	Recommended Drug	Recommended Dose[A]	Recommended Duration	Comments
PROTOZOA					
Giardia lamblia/ duodenalis/ intestinalis (Giardiasis)	• nausea • anorexia • watery, foul smelling diarrhea • abdominal pain and distention	**Metronidazole*** _Alternative_ Paromomycin[5]*** or Nitazoxanide[4] or Quinacrine[6]	<u>Adult</u> 250mg** PO tid <u>Paediatric</u> 15mg/kg/d PO div tid Adult & Paediatric 25-35mg/kg/d PO div tid[5] <u>Adult</u> 500mg PO bid <u>Paediatric</u> 1-3 y.o. 100mg PO bid 4-11 y.o. 200mg PO bid <u>Adult</u> 100mg PO tid <u>Paediatric</u> 6mg/kg/d PO div tid (max 300mg/day)	5-7 days 5-7 days 5-10 days 3 days 3 days 3 days 5 days 5 days	• May cause chronic diarrhea and mal-absorption. • May be asymptomatic. Treatment not routinely necessary if asymptomatic and little chance of transmission (e.g. non-institutionalized adult) * Can be used in pregnancy. **Some experts recommend higher dose (500-750mg) but not as well tolerated. ***Poorly absorbed; may be useful for treatment in pregnancy. • Refractory disease: combination therapy with metronidazole and quinacrine x 3 weeks may be effective.
Iodamoeba butschlii		None			• Non-pathogenic. • Found in patients exposed to poor sanitary conditions.

Footnotes:
4. Available as 500mg tablet or 100mg/5mL oral suspension through TPD Special Access Program (Emergency Release). Contact pharmacy for assistance in ordering.
5. Available as 250mg capsules
6. Available as 100mg tablet through TPD Special Access Program (Emergency Release). Contact pharmacy for assistance in ordering.
A. Dosage is for adult and paediatric patients **unless otherwise specified**. mg/kg/d = milligrams per kilogram per day.
Abbreviations: y.o. = years old; HAART = highly active antiretroviral therapy

ANTIMICROBIAL PROPHYLAXIS FOR THE PREVENTION OF INFECTIVE ENDOCARDITIS (IE)

ENDOCARDITIS PROPHYLAXIS RECOMMENDED
Endocarditis prophylaxis is recommended/may be considered if individual: 1. has one or more of the high risk cardiac conditions listed below under A,   **AND**   2. is undergoing one of the dental/surgical procedures listed below under B or C.
A. Cardiac Conditions Associated with Highest Risk of Adverse Outcome from Endocarditis
<ul><li>Prosthetic cardiac valves (mechanical and bioprosthetic)</li><li>Previous infective endocarditis</li><li>Congenital heart disease (CHD):<ul><li>unrepaired cyanotic CHD, including palliative shunts & conduits</li><li>completely repaired CHD with prosthetic material or device, **during the first 6 months after procedure**</li><li>repaired CHD with residual defects at or around site of prosthetic material (which inhibit endothelialization)</li></ul>NB: Except for the specific conditions listed above, prophylaxis is no longer recommended for any other form of CHD.</li><li>Cardiac transplant recipients with cardiac valvulopathy</li></ul>
B. Dental/oral procedures for which IE Prophylaxis is _Recommended in Patients with Cardiac Conditions listed in A_
<ul><li>Procedures that involve manipulation of gingival tissue or periapical region of teeth, or perforation of oral mucosa.</li></ul>
C. Respiratory tract procedures for which IE Prophylaxis _May Be Considered in Patients with Cardiac Conditions listed in A_
<ul><li>Surgical procedures that involve incision or biopsy of respiratory mucosa, e.g.<ul><li>Tonsillectomy and/or adenoidectomy</li><li>Bronchoscopy with incision of respiratory tract mucosa</li></ul></li></ul>

ANTIMICROBIAL PROPHYLAXIS FOR THE PREVENTION OF INFECTIVE ENDOCARDITIS (IE)

ENDOCARDITIS PROPHYLAXIS NOT RECOMMENDED

Dental or Surgical Procedures for which IE Prophylaxis is NOT Recommended:

Dental/oral: Routine anesthetic injections through noninfected tissue, taking of dental x-rays, placement of removable prosthodontic or orthodontic appliances, adjustment of orthodontic appliances, placement of orthodontic brackets, shedding of primary teeth, bleeding from trauma to lips or oral mucosa

Respiratory tract: Tympanostomy tube insertion. Endotracheal intubation. Surgical procedures that do not involve incision or biopsy of respiratory mucosa. Bronchoscopy without incision of respiratory tract mucosa.

GI & GU: Administration of antibiotics **solely to prevent endocarditis** is no longer recommended for patients undergoing a GU (including vaginal delivery and hysterectomy) or GI tract procedure. For select procedures (e.g. hepatobiliary, complicated urinary tract procedures), standard surgical prophylaxis may need to be modified to include enterococcal coverage.

Other: Cardiac catheterization. Implantation of cardiac pacemakers, defibrillators, stents. Incision/biopsy of surgically scrubbed skin. Circumcision. Ear/body piercing or tattooing.

ANTIMICROBIAL PROPHYLAXIS FOR THE PREVENTION OF INFECTIVE ENDOCARDITIS (IE)

SITUATION	DRUG[1]	ADULT DOSE given 30-60 minutes before the procedure[2] / ROUTE	PEDIATRIC DOSE given 30-60 minutes before the procedure[2] / ROUTE
		Dental, Oral, Respiratory Tract Procedures	
Standard	Amoxicillin	2g PO	50mg/kg PO
No oral intake	Ampicillin	2g IV/IM	50mg/kg IV/IM
Pen-allergic[4]	Clindamycin or Azithromycin[6] or Clarithromycin[6]	300-450mg[5] PO 500mg PO 500mg PO	20mg/kg PO 15mg/kg PO 15mg/kg PO
Pen-allergic, no oral intake	Clindamycin or Ceftriaxone[7] or Cefazolin[7]	600mg IV/IM 1g IV/IM 1g IV/IM	20mg/kg IV/IM 50mg/kg IV/IM 50mg/kg IV/IM

1. If patient is already receiving an antibiotic which is recommended for endocarditis prophylaxis:
   - select an antibiotic from a different class than the one the patient is already receiving (e.g. use clindamycin or a macrolide if patient receiving a β-lactam)
   - if possible, delay procedure until at least 10 days after completion of antibiotic therapy.

2. Prophylaxis should be administered as a single dose 30-60 minutes before the procedure. If the antibiotic is inadvertently not given before the procedure, it may be given up to 2 hours after the procedure.

3. Total paediatric dose should not exceed adult dose.

4. Although cephalexin is still recommended in the 2007 AHA guidelines, it is not a good option as the majority of Viridans Group Streptococci are resistant to cephalexin.

5. Although 600mg is recommended in the AHA guidelines, oral clindamycin doses > 300mg are poorly tolerated. An oral dose of 300-450mg achieves adequate serum levels and is better tolerated.

6. Azithromycin and clarithromycin offer no microbiological advantage over erythromycin but are better tolerated. Activity of all macrolides against Viridans Group Streptococci may not be optimal.

7. Cephalosporins should not be used in patients with severe/immediate-type (e.g. urticaria/angioedema, anaphylaxis) penicillin allergy.

Adapted from Wilson W, Taubert KA, Gewitz M, et al. Prevention of infective endocarditis: guidelines from the American Heart Association (AHA). Circulation 2007;116:1736-54.

BLOOD/BODY FLUID EXPOSURE

<u>Exposure</u> - percutaneous, mucosal (eyes, nose, mouth, vagina, rectum), or non-intact skin exposure to:
- blood
- body fluids (vaginal secretions, semen, CSF, synovial/pleural/peritoneal/pericardial/amniotic fluids)
- other fluids containing visible blood

NB:
- **Urine, feces, vomitus, tears and respiratory secretions are not considered infectious for bloodborne pathogens (HBV, HIV and HCV) unless contaminated with blood.**
- **Saliva** – a potential risk for HBV transmission <u>only</u>, and not a risk for HIV or HCV <u>unless</u> contaminated with blood

<u>Recipient</u> - the person who was **exposed** to the blood or body fluid of another individual

<u>Source</u> - the individual whose blood or body fluid contacted a recipient

<u>Immediate Management</u> -
1. **Cleanse with soap and water ASAP. Allow the injury to bleed freely,** but do not squeeze to promote bleeding, or apply caustic agents such as bleach. Anti-septic use is not contraindicated, but data are lacking.
2. Splashes to mucous membranes (eyes, nose, mouth) should be flushed with water ASAP for 10 minutes.
3. Remove contaminated clothing.
4. Report accident as soon as possible to Occupational Health in hospital setting or Public Health in community setting.

NB: Counseling is an essential component of blood/body fluid exposure management.

BLOOD/BODY FLUID EXPOSURE

Risk of Infection

	Transmission risk	Comments

HIV	percutaneous exposure (e.g. needlestick) 0.3%
	
	mucous membrane exposure 0.1%
	
	non-intact skin <0.1%
	
	intact skin ~ 0%
		High risk percutaneous injuries:
		• deep injury
		• visible blood in device
		• source with high viral load, e.g.,
		  ⇒ acute HIV infection
		  ⇒ end stage AIDS
		• large volume (needle removed from artery or vein of source; hollow-bore higher risk than solid needle)

Hepatitis B	percutaneous exposure (e.g. needlestick): Source HBsAg + and: • HBeAg +: 37-62% • HBeAg -: 23-37%	All health care workers should be vaccinated against Hepatitis B and response to vaccine confirmed with serology (antibodies to hepatitis B surface antigen, i.e. HBsAb or Anti-HBs)
Hepatitis C	1.8% (0-7%)	Most common blood-borne virus

BLOOD/BODY FLUID EXPOSURE

HIV Follow-up Protocol*
In all cases of exposure:
- source should have HIV serology (antibodies to HIV) done ASAP (rapid HIV test where available)
- recipient should have baseline HIV serology done ASAP

SOURCE	RECIPIENT
If source test is **negative for HIV antibodies** and there are no risk factors for acute HIV identified	Consider HIV serology in 6 months
If source test is **negative for HIV antibodies** BUT **acute HIV seroconversion illness** ("window period") is strongly suspected	HIV serology at baseline, 1, 3, and 6 months*** URGENT SPECIALIST CONSULTATION regarding *consideration* for HIV post-exposure prophylaxis (PEP)*
If source **HIV status unknown** and **low risk**	Repeat HIV serology in 1, 3, and 6 months Generally, no HIV PEP warranted
If source **HIV status unknown** and **high risk****	Repeat HIV serology in 1, 3, and 6 months*** URGENT SPECIALIST CONSULTATION regarding *consideration* for HIV PEP with significant exposures*
If source **HIV positive**	Repeat HIV serology in 1, 3, and 6 months*** URGENT SPECIALIST CONSULTATION regarding HIV PEP*

*   FOLLOW LOCAL PROTOCOL. This may include contacting Occupational Health, the Infectious Diseases specialist on call, or for non-occupational exposures, the Medical Officer of Health on call, etc..
Prophylaxis should be started as soon as possible (within 1-2 hours) after exposure (to a maximum of 72 hours).

**   High risk: high risk sexual behaviour (known HIV + partner, men who have sex with men, sexual partner who is an injection drug user [IDU] or sex trade worker, or multiple sexual partners); history of incarceration; shared needles or other drug paraphernalia; other STIs; injection drug use; tattoos/body piercing; sexual or blood contact with a known case of HIV; presence of symptoms consistent with an acute seroconversion illness with HIV; or the exposure occurred in a high risk clinic (e.g. HIV clinic).

*** Because of rare late seroconversions (especially in individuals receiving HIV PEP), some experts recommend repeating serology at 12 months, especially if source co-infected with HCV/HIV.

BLOOD/BODY FLUID EXPOSURE

Hepatitis C Follow-up Protocol*

In all cases of exposure:

- source should have hepatitis C serology (antibodies to HCV) done
- recipient should have baseline hepatitis C serology done

SOURCE	RECIPIENT
If source hepatitis C negative	Consider HCV serology in 3 and 6 months
If source hepatitis C status unknown	Repeat hepatitis C serology +/- ALT in 3 and 6 months
If source hepatitis C positive or hepatitis C status unknown and high risk**	Consider HCV qualitative RNA testing + ALT at 4-6 weeks by providing exposure history on the requisition, and repeat hepatitis C serology in 3 and 6 months*** URGENT REFERRAL to Infectious Disease/GI specialist for further management of acute HCV if lab test result is positive**** Offer counselling.

*   FOLLOW LOCAL PROTOCOL. This may include contacting Occupational Health, the Infectious Diseases specialist on call, or for non-occupational exposures, the Medical Officer of Health on call, etc..
**   High risk : injection drug user [IDU], receipt of blood or blood products before 1990 or blood-derived coagulation products after 1985, dialysis, tattoos/body piercing, sexual or blood contact with a known case of HCV, high risk sexual behavior (e.g. unprotected anal intercourse), sexual partner who is an injection drug user
***   Because of rare late seroconversions, some experts recommend repeating serology at 12 months, especially if source co-infected with HCV/HIV.
**** Currently, prophylaxis for HCV is neither available nor recommended. In the event that acute hepatitis C is diagnosed following exposure, semi-urgent (within 1 to 2 months) referral to an infectious diseases or gastroenterology/hepatology specialist for consideration of treatment should be arranged.

BLOOD/BODY FLUID EXPOSURE

Hepatitis B Follow-up Protocol*
In all cases of exposure:
- source should have Hepatitis B surface antigen (HBsAg) done
- recipient should have baseline testing done

		RECIPIENT**		
		Anti-HBs positive	Anti-HBs negative (not immunized)	Anti-HBs negative, immunized (non-responder[‡])
S O U R C E	**HBsAg positive**	No intervention	• HBIG*** & Hepatitis B vaccination series • Anti-HBs titre 1 month after vaccination series (to allow waning of HBIG antibodies) • Follow-up HBsAg at 3 and 6 months	• HBIG*** x 1 or 2[†] and vaccine booster • Anti-HBs titre at 6 months; if < 10 IU/L complete 2nd course of Hepatitis B vaccine • Follow-up HBsAg at 3 and 6 months (recent HBV vaccination can give false positive HBsAg test)
	HBsAg negative	No intervention	• Hepatitis B vaccination series • Anti-HBs titre 1 month after vaccination series	No intervention
	HBsAg status unknown/low risk	No intervention	• Hepatitis B vaccination series • Anti-HBs titre 1 month after vaccination series • Follow-up HBsAg at 3 and 6 months	• No intervention • Follow-up HBsAg at 3 and 6 months
	HBsAg status unknown/ high risk**	No intervention	• HBIG*** & Hepatitis B vaccination series • Anti-HBs titre 1 month after vaccination series (to allow waning of HBIG antibodies) • Follow-up HBsAg at 3 and 6 months	If known high risk source****: • HBIG*** x 1 or 2[†] and vaccine booster • Anti-HBs titre at 6 months; if < 10 IU/L complete 2nd course of Hepatitis B vaccine • Follow-up HBsAg at 3 and 6 months (recent HBV vaccination can give false positive HBsAg test)

* FOLLOW LOCAL PROTOCOL. This may include contacting Occupational Health, the Infectious Diseases specialist on call, or for non-occupational exposures, the Medical Officer of Health on call, etc..

BLOOD/BODY FLUID EXPOSURE

**   *If recipient has completed a hepatitis B immunization series and had an adequate response to vaccination in the past (anti-HBsAg > 10 IU/L) - no need to retest or treat. (Some provide a booster dose of vaccine following confirmed Hepatitis B exposure.)*

‡   *A non-responder is a person with inadequate response to vaccination (i.e. anti-HBsAg <10 IU/L)*

***   *Hepatitis B immune globulin - obtain from Canadian Blood Services (0.06mL/kg).* **Dose should be administered as soon as possible** *after exposure and* **within 7 days of exposure**.

****   *High risk: high risk sexual behaviour (men who have sex with men, sexual partner who is an injection drug user [IDU], multiple sexual partners), other STIs, sexual or blood contact with a known case of HBV, IDU, tattoos/body piercing, persons from endemic areas (e.g. SE Asia, Subsaharan Africa)*

†   *The option of giving one dose of HBIG and reinitiating the vaccine series is recommended for non-responders who have not completed a second 3-dose vaccine series. For persons who previously completed a second vaccine series but failed to respond, two doses of HBIG, administered 1 month apart, are recommended.*

SEXUAL ASSAULT – Adults (females & males ≥ 14 years of age)

Tests recommended in sexual assault:

- Gonorrhea: culture all penetrated orifices for N. gonorrhoeae. A nucleic acid amplification test (NAAT) should also be performed on specimens collected from the urethra (males), endocervix/urethra (females), urine (males and females) and from extragenital sites, as appropriate. This test is generally more sensitive than genital culture and may be acceptable for medico-legal purposes if confirmed by a second set of primers or, in some cases, a second test sent to another laboratory.
- Chlamydia: A nucleic acid amplification test (NAAT) should be performed on specimens collected from the urethra (males), endocervix/urethra (females), urine (males and females and from extragenital sites, as appropriate. Although culture for C. trachomatis has traditionally been used for medico-legal purposes, it is insensitive and not widely available. If available both culture and NAAT should be collected.

- Serology (baseline and follow up):

Infection	Baseline	Follow up (weeks)
Syphilis	EIA	4
HIV	Anti-HIV	4, 24
Hepatitis B	HBsAg, HBsAb	12*
Hepatitis C	Anti-HCV	12, 24

* Hepatitis B – repeat HBsAg and HBsAb if baseline was negative and patient declined HBIG.

- Pregnancy test – baseline and at 3 weeks following emergency contraception if no menses

Prophylaxis of sexually transmitted infections:

Organism/Infection	Prophylaxis	Recommended Dose & Duration
Neisseria gonorrhoeae[1]	**Cefixime** or **Ceftriaxone** Cephalosporin/severe penicillin allergy **Azithromycin**	800mg PO x 1 dose 250mg IM x 1 dose 2g PO x 1 dose
Chlamydia trachomatis	**Azithromycin** or **Doxycycline** Pregnancy/Lactation **Amoxicillin** or **Azithromycin**	1g PO x 1 dose 100mg PO bid x 7 days 500mg PO tid x 7 days 1g PO x 1 dose
Hepatitis B virus (HBV)	Prophylaxis indicated if: ○ Assailant infected with HBV ○ Requested by victim ○ Victim unlikely to return for follow up ○ Hepatitis B immunization < 3 doses **Hepatitis B immunoglobulin (HBIG)** + **Hepatitis B vaccine**	 0.06mL/kg IM once Doses at 0, 1, 6 mos.
HIV	If assailant known to be HIV positive or at high risk for HIV, e.g. known injection drug use or MSM, offer HIV post exposure prophylaxis in consultation with Regional Public Health and Infectious Diseases.	

SEXUAL ASSAULT – Adults (females & males ≥ 14 years of age)

<u>Footnotes:</u>
1. If there is suspected pharyngeal infection or oral penetration or if the source has elevated risk factors for antibiotic resistance (e.g. is an MSM or is from a region with reduced levels of cefixime susceptibility), ceftriaxone is the treatment of choice.

Emergency Contraception (EC):
<u>Preferred</u>: Levonorgestrel (Plan B®) 1.5 mg PO as a single dose
<u>Alternative</u>: Levonorgestrel 0.75 mg PO bid x 2 doses if a single 1.5 mg dose is not likely to be tolerated.   Dimenhydrinate 50 mg PO given 30 minutes before the second dose of levonorgestrel may prevent vomiting.

Notes:
- EC should be taken as soon as possible within 72 hours after exposure (efficacy declines after this, but some benefit may be achieved up to 120 hours after exposure).
- EC is contraindicated if there is evidence of an established pregnancy as confirmed by a positive pregnancy test.

Referrals:
- For sexual assault assessment and management refer to:
  - Local Sexual Assault Centre
  - Victims Services through local police service
  - Review mental state and arrange appropriate referral to mental health services if necessary

Follow up:
- If no prophylaxis was taken, follow-up should be arranged for 7–14 days after the original visit to review available laboratory test results and to repeat an STI screen to detect infections acquired at the time of the assault that were not detected at the initial examination.
- Test of cure for specific infections should follow recommendations outlined under the relevant infections. If culture used, this can be repeated at 5-7 days and if NAAT used, repeat no sooner than 4 weeks after completion of treatment.
- If empiric prophylactic therapy was given, follow-up should be arranged at 3–4 weeks.
- Arrange follow-up serologic testing as required (see table).

PROPHYLAXIS FOR CONTACTS OF COMMUNICABLE DISEASES

INVASIVE DISEASE

Neisseria meningiditis*

- Prophylaxis recommended for:
  - household contacts, including those living in the same household and individuals who share sleeping arrangements
  - close contacts:
    - child care facility or nursery school contacts
    - individuals in contact with index case's nasopharyngeal secretions (i.e. kissing on the mouth; sharing cigarettes, drinking bottles, or musical instruments) within 7 days prior to the onset of symptoms and up to 24 hours after index case starts appropriate antibiotic treatment.
  - medical personnel who have had contact with nasopharyngeal secretions (without barrier protection such as a mask) of the case such as during mouth-to-mouth resuscitation, intubation, or nasotracheal suctioning before antibiotics begun
  - index case if not treated with cefotaxime/ceftriaxone.
  - airline contacts:
    - those individuals sitting on either side of the index case (but not across the aisle) or other passengers or flight staff who have had direct contact with the respiratory secretions of the index case, and
    - the diagnosis of invasive disease occurred no more than 48 hours after air travel, and
    - the flight occurred within the previous 10 days, and
    - the total time spent aboard the aircraft was at least eight hours, including ground time.

  NB: Prophylaxis should be offered to persons who had contact with the case in the 7 days preceding the onset of illness or hospitalization of the index case. Prophylaxis can be considered for up to 10 days after last contact with an untreated case regardless of immunization status.
  Prophylaxis started > 10 days after the most recent exposure to a case is of limited or no benefit.
  Eligible contacts should also be offered meningococcal vaccine (vaccine chosen is dependent on serogroup causing disease in index case, and age of recipient).

  #### Recommended Prophylaxis

	Children	Adults
First line **Rifampin** or	< 1 month 5mg/kg PO bid x 2 days ≥ 1 month (< 60 kg) 10mg/kg PO bid x 2 days (max 600mg)	(and children > 60 kg) 600mg PO bid x 2 days
Alternative **Ceftriaxone** or	< 12 years 125mg IM single dose ≥ 12 years 250mg IM single dose	250mg IM single dose
Ciprofloxacin	≥ 9 years 500 mg PO single dose	500mg PO single dose

* Reportable to the Medical Officer of Health. Public Health will do contact investigation, follow-up, and prophylaxis.

INVASIVE DISEASE (cont'd)

Haemophilus influenzae

Type b*:
- Prophylaxis recommended for:
- Household and non-household contacts:
  - all contacts regardless of age or immunization status who have had contact or reside with at least one unimmunized or incompletely immunized contact younger than 48 months of age
  - all contacts of a fully immunized but immunocompromised child, regardless of age
  - all contacts of an unimmunized or incompletely immunized child younger than 12 months of age
    ⇒ give prophylaxis to all contacts except pregnant women
- Child care facility or nursery school contacts if ≥ 2 cases within 60 days in facility and incompletely vaccinated children attend
    ⇒ give prophylaxis to children and personnel (except if pregnant)
- Index case if any of above scenarios AND treated with ampicillin or chloramphenicol; not needed if index case treated with cefotaxime/ceftriaxone.
- Unimmunized or incompletely immunized children should also receive a dose of vaccine and be scheduled for completion of the recommended age-specific immunization schedule.

Prophylaxis should be offered to persons who had contact with the case in the 7 days preceding the onset of illness or hospitalization of the index case. Prophylaxis can be considered for up to 10 days after last contact with an untreated case.

Non type b:
NB: The need for prophylaxis of index cases of **invasive non type b** Haemophilus disease and their contacts has not been established but may be prudent. It is the opinion of the authors that at least the index case should receive rifampin prophylaxis.

Recommended Prophylaxis

	Children < 12 years	Children ≥ 12 years & Adults
Rifampin	< 1 month 10mg/kg PO daily x 4 days ≥ 1 month and < 12 years 20mg/kg PO daily x 4 days (max 600mg)	600mg PO daily x 4 days

* Reportable to the Medical Officer of Health. Public Health will do contact investigation, follow-up, and prophylaxis.

PROPHYLAXIS FOR CONTACTS OF COMMUNICABLE DISEASES

INVASIVE DISEASE (cont'd)

Group A Streptococcal (GAS) Disease*

Chemoprophylaxis recommended for household/close contacts** of a confirmed severe case of:

- Streptococcal Toxic Shock Syndrome
- soft tissue necrosis (including necrotizing fasciitis, myositis, gangrene)
- meningitis
- GAS pneumonia
- other life threatening conditions (e.g. bacteremia)
- a confirmed case of invasive GAS resulting in death

Chemoprophylaxis should be given as soon as possible and preferably within 24 hours of case identification, but is still recommended for up to 7 days after last contact with infectious case.

household contacts: All contacts living in the same household as the index case who have spent at least 4 hours/day on average or 20 hours/week with the case within 7 days of index case becoming ill and up to 24 hours after start of treatment of the index case

close contacts:
- Non-household persons who share the same bed with the case or had sexual relations with the case
- Persons who have had direct mucous membrane contact with the oral or nasal secretions of a case (e.g. mouth-to-mouth resuscitation, open mouth kissing) or direct contact with an open skin lesion of the case
- Injection drug users who have shared needles with the case
- Selected long-term care facility contacts
- Selected child care contacts
- Selected hospital contacts

who have been exposed to the case within 7 days of index case becoming ill and up to 24 hours after start of treatment of the index case.

Recommended Prophylaxis

	Children	Adults
First Line **Cephalexin**	25-50mg/kg/day div bid-qid x 10 days (max 1g/day)	250mg PO qid x 10 days **or** 500mg PO bid x 10 days
Second Line **Erythromycin** or	20-30mg/kg/day div bid-qid x 10 days (base) (max 500mg/dose)	500mg PO bid x 10 days (base)
Clarithromycin or	15rng/kg/day PO div bid (max 500mg/day) x 10 days	250mg PO bid x 10 days
Clindamycin	8-16mg/kg/day div tid-qid x 10 days	150mg PO qid x 10 days

* Reportable to the Medical Officer of Health. Public Health will do contact investigation and follow-up.

PROPHYLAXIS FOR CONTACTS OF COMMUNICABLE DISEASES

INFLUENZA

NB: It is essential to check resistance patterns of the current season's influenza strains.

- Amantadine is active against susceptible Influenza A (**not active against Influenza B**).
- Oseltamivir and zanamivir are active against susceptible Influenza A <u>and</u> B.

- Antiviral prophylaxis indicated:
    - ⇒ for control of Influenza outbreaks among high risk residents of institutions
    - ⇒ as an adjunct to late vaccination of people at high risk
    - ⇒ as sole agent for prophylaxis during an influenza outbreak in high risk individuals where vaccination cannot be given
    - ⇒ as a supplement to vaccination in high risk individuals with impaired immune response to the vaccine
    - ⇒ for unvaccinated persons who provide hands on patient care for high risk individuals during an outbreak.
- Duration of antiviral prophylaxis is 10 days, or duration of outbreak, whichever is longer.

> **NB: Antiviral prophylaxis should NOT replace annual influenza vaccination.**

Recommended Oseltamivir[†] Dosage

Age		Dosage
1-12 years	≤ 15kg	30mg PO daily
	> 15-23kg	45 mg PO daily
	> 23-40kg	60mg PO daily
	> 40kg	75mg PO daily
≥ 13 years	Clcr > 60 mL/min	75mg PO daily
	Clcr > 30-60mL/min	30mg PO daily
	Clcr 10-30 mL/min	30mg PO q2days

[†] Prophylaxis should be started within 48h of exposure.
Clcr=creatinine clearance

Recommended Zanamivir[†] Dosage

Age	Dosage
≥ 7 years	10mg inhaled by mouth daily

[†] Prophylaxis should be started within 48h of exposure.

INFLUENZA (cont'd)

Recommended Amantadine Dosage by Age and Renal Status

Age	Dosage
No renal impairment	
1-9 years[A]	5mg/kg divided once or twice daily (max daily dose 150mg)
10-64 years	200mg divided once or twice daily[B]
≥ 65 years	100mg once daily[C]

Creatinine clearance (mL/min/1.73m^2)	Dosage with capsules		Daily dosage with solution (10mg/mL)
	10-64 years old	**> 65 years old**	**> 65 years old***
≥ 80	100mg twice daily	100mg once daily	100mg (10mL)
60-79	Alternating daily doses of 200mg and 100mg	Alternating daily doses of 100mg and 50mg	75mg (7.5mL)
40-59	100mg once daily	100mg every 2 days	50mg (5mL)
30-39	200mg twice weekly	100mg twice weekly	25mg (2.5mL)
20-29	100mg three times/week	50mg three times/week	25mg (2.5mL)
10-19	Alternating weekly doses of 200mg and 100mg	Alternating weekly doses of 100mg and 50mg	No daily dose**

A. Use in children < 1 year of age has not been evaluated adequately.
B. Dosage reduction to 100mg/day is recommended for people with a seizure disorder as they may be at risk for more frequent seizures with the higher dosage.
C. The reduced dosage is recommended to minimize the risk of toxic effects, as renal function generally declines with age and side effects have been reported more frequently in the elderly.

Calculation of estimated creatinine clearance:

Females	Clcr (mL/min) =	$\dfrac{(140 - age) \times IBW^* (kg)}{Scr\ (\mu mol/L)}$	* If ABW < IBW, use ABW.
Males	Clcr (mL/min) =	Clcr (female) x 1.2	

* Give 100mg (10mL) on day 1, then follow dosing in chart, according to creatinine clearance, on subsequent days.
** If outbreak continues, repeat 100mg dose every 7 days during the outbreak.

PROPHYLAXIS FOR CONTACTS OF COMMUNICABLE DISEASES

PERTUSSIS (Whooping Cough)*

- Adults are important reservoirs of B. pertussis (by 12 years post-immunization there is no demonstrable protection against pertussis).
  - All adolescents in Canada are given a booster of dTap (diphtheria-tetanus-acellular pertussis vaccine).

- Prophylaxis should be given to the following significant contacts (immunized or un-immunized):
  - Individuals who are *vulnerable persons** AND are residing in the same household as the case
  - Individuals who are *vulnerable persons** AND have had face to face exposure and/or have shared confined air with the confirmed case for > 1 hour and/or other significant exposure decided upon on a case by case basis (e.g. being coughed on by a confirmed case)
  - Individuals who are residing in households (or working in or attending day care centres and family day homes) in which a *vulnerable person** also lives (or attends on a regular basis)
    * *Vulnerable persons:*
      - *Infants < 1 year of age (because of increased rate of mortality)*
      - *Pregnant women in the third trimester (because of risk of disease transmission to neonate)*
- Antibiotic post exposure prophylaxis should be offered to all eligible contacts (regardless of immunization status) as soon as possible after first contact with index case and within 21 days of onset of cough in the index case.

Recommended Prophylaxis

	Children	Adults
Azithromycin	10mg/kg PO first day (max 500mg) then 5mg/kg PO daily (max 250mg) x 4 days	500mg PO first day then 250mg PO daily x 4 days
Clarithromycin	15mg/kg/d PO div bid (max 1g/day) x 7 days	250-500mg PO bid x 7 days
Erythromycin	40mg/kg/d PO div tid x 7 days (estolate) (max 1g/day)	250-500mg PO qid x 7 days (base)
<u>Alternative</u> **TMP/SMX** (> 2 months of age)	≤ 40 kg: 4-6mg TMP/kg/d PO div bid x 10 days > 40 kg: 8mg TMP (max 320mg)/kg/d PO div bid x 10 days	1 DS tab PO bid x 10 days

* Reportable to the Medical Officer of Health. Public Health will do contact investigation, follow-up, and prophylaxis.

PROPHYLAXIS FOR CONTACTS OF COMMUNICABLE DISEASES

VARICELLA ZOSTER

Varicella zoster immune globulin (VZIG) provides passive immunization against Varicella Zoster virus

Indication for VZIG:

In the following high risk non-immune individuals within 96 hours of significant exposure to an active case of chickenpox :

- immunocompromised individuals with congenital, acquired immunodeficiency disease, or immunosuppression due to disease or therapy, e.g. > 20mg/day prednisone or equivalent for > 2 weeks
- susceptible pregnant women who have never had chickenpox or shingles (Varicella IgG negative)
- newborns whose mothers develop chickenpox within 5 days before delivery or within 48 hours after delivery
- hospitalized premature infants exposed during the first 4 weeks of life (If < 28 weeks gestation or ≤ 1000 grams, give VZIG regardless of maternal status.)
- exposed infants 29-37 weeks gestation if mother not immune at the time of birth.

- If VZIG is indicated, it should be given ASAP (maximum 96 hours after exposure). Canadian Blood Services should be contacted to arrange for release and delivery of VZIG.

- Susceptible health care workers should contact Occupational Health if exposed to chickenpox.
- Healthy susceptible individuals should contact physician if exposed.
  ⇒ Acyclovir can reduce severity of symptoms if started promptly (within 24h of rash).
  ⇒ Varicella vaccine has been shown to be effective in preventing or reducing the severity of disease if given to susceptible individuals within 72 hours and no longer than 5 days after exposure. Consider for post-exposure management in:
    - Susceptible non-pregnant healthcare workers and hospitalized patients in consultation with Infectious Diseases physician
    - Susceptible household or close contacts of high risk individuals (immunocompromised, chronic health problem)
    - Unique cases in special circumstances on a case by case basis with Medical Officer of Health

* Varicella is reportable to Public Health.

INFECTION PREVENTION AND CONTROL

USE ROUTINE PRACTICES* AND PRECAUTIONS FOR EVERY CONTACT AND ALL INDIVIDUALS RECEIVING CARE.

*Routine Practices = Hand Hygiene; Risk Assessment with use of appropriate barriers; Equipment Cleaning and Disinfection; etc.

NB: Infection Control in the OFFICE SETTING should focus on ROUTINE PRACTICES, including hand hygiene, personal protective equipment, handling of sharps, syringe and multi-dose vial safety (New Needle. New Syringe. Every Time) and Reprocessing of Medical Equipment (cleaning, disinfection, sterilization) – Who is responsible for reprocessing? Is their training adequate? Has the office sterilizer been approved for the tasks expected? How are sterilization parameters monitored? Do Not Re-use Single-Use Medical Devices.

HAND HYGIENE IS THE SINGLE MOST IMPORTANT STEP IN PREVENTING THE TRANSMISSION OF INFECTION.

Perform Hand Hygiene: (the Canadian Patient Safety Institute "4 Moments of Hand Hygiene")
- Before contact with patients or their environment (including before putting on gloves)
- Before an aseptic procedure (e.g. placement or handling of intravascular lines or urinary catheters)
- After contact with body fluids/blood/mucous membranes/non-intact skin
- After contact with patients or their environment (including after removing gloves)

Hand Hygiene Products:
The type of hand hygiene product selected depends on the clinical setting.
Recommendations:
Waterless Antiseptic Hand Agents (alcohol-based hand sanitizers/rubs – ABHR)
- Preferred product in most situations, e.g. before/after care of all patients including individuals with antibiotic resistant organisms, immunosuppression, or those at higher risk of infection (e.g. neonatal/pediatric/adult intensive care, burn units, dialysis units, transplant units) and where invasive procedures are performed (e.g. operating rooms, delivery rooms, treatment rooms).

Plain Soap and Water is preferred in 3 situations:
- When hands are visibly dirty or contaminated with blood or body fluids.
- During food handling
- When caring for patients with vomiting or diarrhea (soap & water may be more effective than ABHR for Noroviruses and C. difficile)

Antiseptic Agents may be an option but should be restricted to the following higher risk clinical areas or situations:
- where there are patients who are immunosuppressed or at high risk of infection (e.g. neonatal/pediatric/adult intensive care, burn units, dialysis units, transplant units)
- where invasive procedures are performed (e.g. operating rooms, delivery rooms, treatment rooms)
NB: Antibacterial soaps may promote antimicrobial resistance and are NOT effective against viruses or fungi.

INFECTION PREVENTION AND CONTROL

APPROPRIATE PERSONAL PROTECTIVE EQUIPMENT/BARRIERS (GLOVES, GOWNS, MASKS, AND EYE PROTECTION) MUST BE WORN TO PREVENT EXPOSURE TO BLOOD OR BODY FLUIDS.

Gloves

NB: Gloves do not replace hand hygiene.
- Perform hand hygiene before and after using gloves
- Are worn to prevent gross soiling of hands with blood and body fluids and excretions
- Must always be changed between each patient contact
- Should be used only once and thrown out

Gowns

- Are worn to protect clothing and exposed skin from soiling and/or contamination
- Should be fluid-resistant if exposure to significant amounts of blood or body fluids is anticipated
- Should be used only once and then placed in the appropriate receptacle

Masks

- A surgical/procedure mask should be worn:
  - if splashing or aerosolization of blood and/or body fluids is anticipated
  - when performing invasive procedures on the respiratory tract (e.g. suctioning, intubating)
  - when caring for individuals with cough and fever of unknown etiology
- A fit-tested N95 respirator/mask should be worn for infections spread by the airborne route, whether suspected or confirmed (e.g. tuberculosis, chicken pox, measles)
- Masks should be removed (by handling ties or elastics), and discarded following use (followed by hand hygiene)

Eye Goggles/Face Shield

- Should be worn to protect eyes from splashes or aerosols of blood or body fluids
- Should protect from the sides as well as the front
- **NB**: Prescription eye glasses do not provide adequate eye protection.

INFECTION PREVENTION AND CONTROL PRECAUTIONS[*]

Organism	Infective Material	Mode of Transmission	Precautions[**]					Duration of Precautions
			Single Room	Gloves	Gowns	Mask		
Colonization and/ or infection with: **Methicillin - resistant Staphylococcus aureus (MRSA)** **Vancomycin – intermediate or resistant Staphylococcus aureus (VISA/VRSA)**	Body fluids or secretions containing organism	Direct contact or droplet Inanimate objects from patient room often harbor organisms	Acute care: Yes **NB:**Cohorting may be an option for MRSA if insufficient single rooms. Long term care: Assess each situation individually.	Acute Care: Worn upon entry into care room and removed prior to exit Long Term Care: If in direct contact with colonized or infected body fluids/secretions Perform hand hygiene at all times when entering or leaving patient room, including before and after glove use.	Acute Care: Worn upon entry into care room and removed prior to exit Long Term Care: If in direct contact with colonized or infected body fluids/ secretions	Acute Care: If nasal carrier or if in contact with respiratory secretions Long Term Care: If in contact with respiratory secretions from individual with pneumonia or tracheostomy		• Consult Infection Prevention and Control (IP&C) regarding precautions and screening. • Always consult IP&C prior to discontinuation of precautions.

NB: Other multiresistant organisms may be transmitted nosocomially. Consultation with Infection Prevention and Control is recommended.

* Consult with IP&C as local guidelines may vary.

**Use of disposable dishes is not recommended to prevent transmission of antibiotic-resistant organisms.

INFECTION PREVENTION AND CONTROL PRECAUTIONS*

Organism	Infective Material	Mode of Transmission	Precautions**					Duration of Precautions
			Single Room	Gloves	Gowns	Mask		
Colonization and/or infection with:								
Vancomycin - resistant Enterococci (VRE)	Body fluids or secretions containing organism	Direct contact / Inanimate objects from patient room often harbor organisms	Acute Care: Yes NB:Cohorting may be an option for VRE if insufficient single rooms. / Long term care: Assess each situation individually	Acute Care: Worn upon entry into care room and removed prior to exit / Long Term Care: If in direct contact with colonized or infected body fluids/secretions / Perform hand hygiene at all times when entering or leaving patient room	Acute Care: Worn upon entry into care room and removed prior to exit / Long Term Care: If direct contact with colonized or infected body fluids/ secretions	No	No	• Consult Infection Prevention and Control (IP&C) regarding precautions and screening. • Always consult with IP&C prior to discontinuation of precautions.

NB: Other multiresistant organisms may be transmitted nosocomially. Consultation with Infection Prevention and Control is recommended.

* Consult with IP&C as local guidelines may vary.

**Use of disposable dishes is not recommended to prevent transmission of antibiotic-resistant organisms.

INFECTION PREVENTION AND CONTROL PRECAUTIONS*

Organism	Infective Material	Mode of Transmission	Precautions**					Duration of Precautions
			Single Room	Gloves	Gowns	Mask		
Colonization and/ or infection with:								
Extended-spectrum ß-lactamases (ESBL) (most commonly seen in E. coli and Klebsiella spp)	Body fluids or secretions containing organism	Direct contact	Acute Care: Contact site Infection Prevention and Control personnel for specific instructions	Acute Care: Contact site Infection Prevention and Control personnel for specific instructions	Acute Care: Contact site Infection Prevention and Control personnel for specific instructions	No		• Consult Infection Prevention and Control (IP&C) regarding precautions.
AmpC cephalosporinase-producing Klebsiella spp, Salmonella spp, & Proteus mirabilis			Long term Care: Assess each situation individually	Long Term Care: If in direct contact with colonized or infected body fluids/secretions	Long Term Care: If direct contact with colonized or infected body fluids or secretions	No		
Carbapenemase-producing Enterobacteriaceae (including NDM-1 and KPC)				Hand hygiene at all times when entering or leaving patient room				

NB: Other multiresistant organisms may be transmitted nosocomially. Consultation with Infection Prevention and Control is recommended.
* Consult with IP&C as local guidelines may vary.
**Use of disposable dishes is not recommended to prevent transmission of antibiotic-resistant organisms.

INFECTION PREVENTION AND CONTROL PRECAUTIONS*

Organism	Infective Material	Mode of Transmission	Precautions**					Duration of Precautions
			Single Room	Gloves	Gowns	Mask		
Infection with:								
Clostridium difficile	Body fluids or secretions containing organism; usually feces	Direct contact Inanimate objects from patient room often harbor organisms	Acute Care: Yes Long term Care: Assess each situation individually	Acute Care: Worn upon entry into care room and removed prior to exit Long Term Care: If in direct contact with colonized or infected body fluids/secretions Perform hand hygiene at all times when leaving patient room	Acute Care: Worn upon entry into care room and removed prior to exit Long Term Care: If direct contact with colonized or infected body fluids/secretions	No	No	• Consult Infectious Diseases regarding clinical management of **non-resolving cases.** • Contact site Infection Prevention and Control for issues regarding precautions, including when precautions may be discontinued. Typically, precautions may be discontinued when the patient is both asymptomatic and able to resume good bowel routine for 48 – 72 hours though some favour prolonged isolation. • Routine repeat laboratory testing of stool is NOT necessary.

NB: Other multiresistant organisms may be transmitted nosocomially. Consultation with Infection Prevention and Control is recommended.
* Consult with IP&C as local guidelines may vary.
**Use of disposable dishes is not recommended to prevent transmission of antibiotic-resistant organisms.

ANTIMICROBIAL PROPHYLAXIS IN DENTISTRY

The following categories of patients require antimicrobial prophylaxis for dental procedures/surgery:

I. Patients at risk of bacterial endocarditis (see Endocarditis Prophylaxis section)

II. Patients with orthopedic joint prostheses (see Table 2)

III. High risk dental surgical procedures (see Table 3)

IV. Immunocompromised patients (see Table 1)

- The risk of sepsis following dental procedures in immunocompromised patients should not be much higher than the general population.
- Certain conditions that may be associated with increased risk of infection include but are not limited to: neutropenia and neutrophil dysfunction, severe malnourishment, poorly controlled diabetes, and certain haematologic malignancies/disorders.

For these conditions recommend:

Table 1. PROPHYLAXIS OF DENTAL PROCEDURES IN IMMUNOCOMPROMISED PATIENTS

Antibiotic	Adult Dose	Paediatric Dose
amoxicillin	2g PO x 1 dose 1h before	50mg/kg (max 2g) PO x 1 dose 1h before
β-lactam allergy		
clindamycin	300-450mg[1] PO x 1 dose 1h before	20mg/kg (max 300mg) PO x 1 dose 1h before

1. Although clindamycin 600mg is recommended in some guidelines, oral clindamycin doses > 300mg are poorly tolerated. A dose of 300-450mg achieves adequate serum levels and is better tolerated.

ANTIMICROBIAL PROPHYLAXIS IN DENTISTRY

Table 2. PROPHYLAXIS OF DENTAL PROCEDURES IN PATIENTS WITH PROSTHETIC JOINTS

- **Long term antibiotic prophylaxis in patients with prosthetic joints is NOT recommended.**

- **Routine prophylaxis of dental procedures in patients with prosthetic joints is NOT recommended as:**
  - there are inadequate data to support its use
  - dental procedure-induced bacteremias are a very rare ($\leq 0.05\%$) cause of prosthetic joint infections
  - major professional associations (CDA, ADA, AAOM, BSAC) do not recommend routine prophylaxis. NB: Although the AAOS recently recommended prophylaxis for all patients with prosthetic joints undergoing dental procedures, this is not supported by scientific data and represents expert opinion only.
  - risks (adverse/allergic reactions, C. difficile infection, antimicrobial resistance) and costs of antibiotic prophylaxis are greater than any benefit.

Prophylaxis may be considered for the following high risk cases:
  - Joint replacement procedure < 2 years previous
  - Previous joint infection
  - Patients with inflammatory arthropathies (rheumatoid arthritis, systemic lupus erythematosus)

NOTE: **Prophylaxis is NOT required for fixation devices, such as screws, plates, pins, and nails.**

Table 2a.   RECOMMENDED ANTIBIOTIC REGIMEN

Antibiotic	Adult Dose	Paediatric Dose
amoxicillin	2g PO x 1 dose 1h before	50mg/kg (max 2g) PO x 1 dose 1h before
β-lactam allergy		
clindamycin	300-450mg PO x 1 dose 1h before	20mg/kg (max 300mg) PO x 1 dose 1h before

For above high risk patients with poor oral hygiene, consider rinsing with chlorhexidine mouthwash for 1 minute immediately **prior** to dental procedure. **NB: Prolonged use of chlorhexidine prior to, or following, the dental procedure is NOT recommended as it may result in selection of antimicrobial resistant oral bacteria.**

ANTIMICROBIAL PROPHYLAXIS IN DENTISTRY

Table 3. RECOMMENDED DRUG REGIMENS FOR SURGICAL PROPHYLAXIS IN DENTISTRY

SURGERY/PROCEDURE	ADULT DOSE/ ROUTE/DURATION	PAEDIATRIC DOSE[1]/ ROUTE/DURATION	COMMENTS
NB: **For high risk groups** (patients at risk of bacterial endocarditis, immunosuppressed patients or patients at risk of prosthetic joint infection), refer to Tables 1-3 for prophylaxis recommendations.			
- The following recommendations for prophylaxis are for patients not belonging to high risk groups.			
- **Antibiotic prophylaxis should always be given pre-operatively.**			
- The value of post-operative antibiotic doses has not been well validated in dental surgery but may be of benefit in certain invasive/complicated procedures.			
- **Established infections require treatment NOT prophylaxis.** Refer to Recommended Empiric Therapy of Selected Dental Infections.			
DENTOALVEOLAR SURGERY (tooth extraction, cystectomies, alveoplasty, apical surgery)			
Simple/minimally invasive oral surgical procedures	NO surgical prophylaxis indicated	NO surgical prophylaxis indicated	
Alveolar (Dry socket) osteitis	NO surgical prophylaxis indicated	NO surgical prophylaxis indicated	
Complicated oral surgical procedures (e.g. difficult third molar extraction)	• amoxicillin 2g PO x 1 dose 1h pre-op or • penicillin G 2MU IV ≤ 30 min pre-op β-lactam allergy: • clindamycin 300mg PO x 1 dose 1h pre-op or • clindamycin 300-600mg IV ≤ 30 min pre-op	• amoxicillin 50mg/kg PO x 1 dose 1h pre-op or • penicillin G 50,000U/kg IV ≤ 30 min pre-op β-lactam allergy: • clindamycin 20mg/kg PO x 1 dose 1h pre-op or • clindamycin 20mg/kg IV ≤ 30 min pre-op	

1. Total paediatric dose should not exceed adult dose.

ANTIMICROBIAL PROPHYLAXIS IN DENTISTRY

Table 3. RECOMMENDED DRUG REGIMENS FOR SURGICAL PROPHYLAXIS IN DENTISTRY

SURGERY/PROCEDURE	ADULT DOSE/ ROUTE/DURATION	PAEDIATRIC DOSE[1]/ ROUTE/DURATION	COMMENTS
ENDOSSEOUS IMPLANTS			
Endosseous implants	• amoxicillin 2g PO 1h pre-op ± amoxicillin 500mg PO q8h x 24h post-op* • chlorhexidine mouthwash[†] β-lactam allergy: • clindamycin 300mg PO 1h pre-op ± clindamycin 300mg PO q6h x 24h post-op* • chlorhexidine mouthwash[†] [†] rinse with chlorhexidine mouthwash for 1 minute immediately **prior** to dental procedure**	• amoxicillin 50mg/kg 1h pre-op ± amoxicillin 25mg/kg PO q8h x 24h post-op* • chlorhexidine mouthwash[†] β-lactam allergy: • clindamycin 20mg/kg PO 1h pre-op ± clindamycin 20mg/kg/d PO div qid x 24h post-op* • chlorhexidine mouthwash[†] [†] rinse with chlorhexidine mouthwash for 1 minute immediately **prior** to dental procedure**	* The value of postoperative antibiotic use has not been proven [Cochrane Review 2010]. **Prolonged use of chlorhexidine prior to, or following, the dental procedure is NOT recommended as it may result in selection of antimicrobial resistant oral bacteria.

1. Total paediatric dose should not exceed adult dose. mg/kg/d = milligrams per kilogram per day

ANTIMICROBIAL PROPHYLAXIS IN DENTISTRY

Table 3. RECOMMENDED DRUG REGIMENS FOR SURGICAL PROPHYLAXIS IN DENTISTRY

SURGERY/PROCEDURE	ADULT DOSE/ ROUTE/DURATION	PAEDIATRIC DOSE[1]/ ROUTE/DURATION	COMMENTS
PERIODONTAL SURGERY			
Gingivectomy	NO surgical prophylaxis indicated	NO surgical prophylaxis indicated	* Use of antimicrobial prophylaxis in these procedures is controversial. A single pre-operative dose of antibiotic may be indicated in some cases depending on extent of surgery, anatomical location, and oral hygiene of patient.
Replaced flaps Apically positioned flaps Osseous surgery (no implants)	Surgical prophylaxis not routinely indicated*	Surgical prophylaxis not routinely indicated*	
Regenerative techniques	• amoxicillin 2g PO x 1 dose 1h pre-op + • chlorhexidine mouthwash[†] β-lactam allergy: • clindamycin 300mg PO x 1 dose 1h pre-op + • chlorhexidine mouthwash[†] [†]rinse with chlorhexidine mouthwash for 1 minute immediately **prior** to dental procedure*	• amoxicillin 50mg/kg PO x 1 dose 1h pre-op + • chlorhexidine mouthwash[†] β-lactam allergy: • clindamycin 20mg/kg PO x 1 dose 1h pre-op + • chlorhexidine mouthwash[†] [†]rinse with chlorhexidine mouthwash for 1 minute immediately **prior** to dental procedure*	- A short course of chlorhexidine post-op is recommended. * Prolonged use of chlorhexidine prior to, or following, the dental procedure is NOT recommended as it may result in selection of antimicrobial resistant oral bacteria. - Some experts advocate tetracycline antibiotic use for their anti-inflammatory properties.
ENDODONTICS			
Conservative endodontic procedures e.g. root canal therapy	NO surgical prophylaxis indicated	NO surgical prophylaxis indicated	

1. Total paediatric dose should not exceed adult dose.

ANTIMICROBIAL PROPHYLAXIS IN DENTISTRY

Table 3. RECOMMENDED DRUG REGIMENS FOR SURGICAL PROPHYLAXIS IN DENTISTRY

SURGERY/PROCEDURE	ADULT DOSE/ROUTE/DURATION	PAEDIATRIC DOSE/ROUTE/DURATION	COMMENTS
MAXILLOFACIAL SURGERY			
Orthognathic surgery	**Mandibular*** • penicillin G 2MU IV ≤ 30 min pre-op + penicillin VK 300-600mg PO qid x 7 days post-op **Maxillary*** • ampicillin 2g IV < 30 min pre-op + amoxicillin 500mg PO tid x 7 days post-op β-lactam allergy: • clindamycin 300-600mg IV ≤ 30 min pre-op + clindamycin 300mg PO qid x 7 days post-op	**Mandibular*** • penicillin G 50,000U/kg IV ≤ 30 min pre-op + penicillin VK 40mg/kg/d PO div qid or penicillin G 100,000U/kg/d IV div q6h x 7 days post-op **Maxillary*** • ampicillin 50mg/kg IV < 30 min pre-op + amoxicillin 25mg/kg PO tid x 7 days post-op β-lactam allergy: • clindamycin 20mg/kg IV ≤ 30 min pre-op + clindamycin 20mg/kg/d PO div qid x 7 days post-op	* If extraoral incisions, use clindamycin (added S. aureus coverage). - Consider chlorhexidine mouthwash x 7 days.

ANTIMICROBIAL PROPHYLAXIS IN DENTISTRY

Table 3. RECOMMENDED DRUG REGIMENS FOR SURGICAL PROPHYLAXIS IN DENTISTRY

SURGERY/PROCEDURE	ADULT DOSE/ ROUTE/DURATION	PAEDIATRIC DOSE[1]/ ROUTE/DURATION	COMMENTS
MAXILLOFACIAL SURGERY			
Major bone grafting • intraoral	• penicillin G 2MU IV ≤ 30 min pre-op + penicillin VK 300-600mg PO qid x 3-7 days post-op <u>Alternative:</u> • clindamycin 300-600mg ≤ 30 min IV pre-op + clindamycin 300mg PO qid x 3-7 days	• penicillin G 50,000U/kg IV ≤ 30 min pre-op + penicillin VK 40mg/kg/d PO div qid x 3-7 days post-op <u>Alternative:</u> • clindamycin 20mg/kg IV ≤ 30 min pre-op + clindamycin 20mg/kg/d PO div qid x 3-7 days post-op	
• extraoral	• clindamycin 300-600mg IV ≤ 30 min pre-op + clindamycin 300-600mg IV x 1 dose post-op <u>Alternative:</u> • cefazolin 1g IV ≤ 30 min pre-op + cefazolin 1g IV x 1 dose post-op	• clindamycin 20mg/kg IV ≤ 30 min pre-op + clindamycin 20mg/kg IV x 1 dose post-op <u>Alternative:</u> • cefazolin 25mg/kg IV ≤ 30 min pre-op + cefazolin 25mg/kg IV x 1 dose post-op	
Temporomandibular joint surgery	• cefazolin 1g IV ≤ 30 min pre-op <u>Alternative:</u> • clindamycin 300-600mg IV ≤ 30 min pre-op	• cefazolin 25mg/kg IV ≤ 30 min pre-op <u>Alternative:</u> • clindamycin 20mg/kg IV ≤ 30 min pre-op	

1. Total paediatric dose should not exceed adult dose. mg/kg/d = milligrams per kilogram per day

ANTIMICROBIAL PROPHYLAXIS IN DENTISTRY

Table 3. RECOMMENDED DRUG REGIMENS FOR SURGICAL PROPHYLAXIS IN DENTISTRY

SURGERY/PROCEDURE	ADULT DOSE/ ROUTE/DURATION	PAEDIATRIC DOSE/ ROUTE/DURATION	COMMENTS
FACIAL TRAUMA			
Facial trauma			
• open reduction*	• ampicillin 2g IV < 30 min pre-op + amoxicillin 500mg PO tid x 7 days post-op if prosthetic material placed β-lactam allergy: • clindamycin 300-600mg IV ≤ 30 min pre-op + clindamycin 300mg PO qid x 7 days post-op if prosthetic material placed	• ampicillin 50mg/kg IV < 30 min pre-op + amoxicillin 25mg/kg PO tid x 7 days post-op if prosthetic material placed β-lactam allergy: • clindamycin 20mg/kg IV ≤ 30 min pre-op + clindamycin 20mg/kg/d PO div qid x 7 days post-op if prosthetic material placed	* If extraoral incisions, use clindamycin (added S. aureus coverage). - Consider chlorhexidine mouthwash x 7 days.
• closed reduction	• ampicillin 2g IV ≤ 30 min pre-op β-lactam allergy: • clindamycin 300-600mg IV ≤ 30 min pre-op	• ampicillin 50mg/kg IV ≤ 30 min pre-op β-lactam allergy: • clindamycin 20mg/kg IV ≤ 30 min pre-op	
ORTHODONTICS			
Orthodontic adjustments	NO surgical prophylaxis indicated	NO surgical prophylaxis indicated	
Subgingival band placement	NO surgical prophylaxis indicated	NO surgical prophylaxis indicated	

1. Total paediatric dose should not exceed adult dose. mg/kg/d = milligrams per kilogram per day

RECOMMENDED EMPIRIC THERAPY OF SELECTED DENTAL INFECTIONS[A]

Table 1. SPECTRUM OF ACTIVITY OF ANTIMICROBIAL AGENTS AGAINST SELECTED ORAL MICROORGANISMS

	Viridans Group Streptococci*	Anaerobic Gram negative bacilli	Aggregati-bacter spp	Capnocyto-phaga spp	Eikenella corrodens	Actinomyces spp	Comments
Penicillin	+/-	+/-	+/-	+	+	+	- Use penicillin V as it results in higher plasma levels than penicillin G.
Amoxicillin	+/-	+/-	+/-	+	+	+	- Achieves higher serum concentrations than oral penicillin; recommended in prophylaxis of dental infections.
Amoxicillin-clavulanate	+/-	+	+/-	+	+	+	- BID dosing now recommended. - Alternative in dental infections.
Oral Cephalosporins**	-	-	+/-	-	-	-	- Not recommended in prophylaxis/ treatment of dental infections. - >90% of Viridans Group Streptococci are resistant to cephalexin.
Erythromycin	+/-	-	-	-	-	+	- Poor activity against most dental pathogens.
Azithromycin/ Clarithromycin	+/-	-	-	-	-	+	- Offer no microbiological advantage over erythromycin in the treatment of dental infections.
Ciprofloxacin/ Levofloxacin	+/-	-	+	+	+	-	- Not recommended in prophylaxis/ treatment of dental infections (no anaerobic coverage).
Clindamycin	+/-	+/-	-	+	-	+	- Alternative in the prophylaxis/ treatment of dental infections.
Metronidazole	-	+	-	-	-	-	- No aerobic coverage; use in combination with penicillin.
Doxycycline/ Tetracycline	+/-	-	+	+	+	+	- Anti-inflammatory properties may have role in periodontal infections.

* Includes S. anginosus, S. mitis, S. mutans, S. salivarius, and S. sanguinis groups.
**Includes agents such as cephalexin, cefixime, cefuroxime axetil, cefprozil.

RECOMMENDED EMPIRIC THERAPY OF SELECTED DENTAL INFECTIONS[A]

Table 2. MICROORGANISMS ASSOCIATED WITH DENTAL INFECTIONS*

Aerobic Gram Positive Cocci	• Viridans Group Streptococci
	    ▪ Streptococcus anginosus
	    ▪ Streptococcus mitis
	    ▪ Streptococcus mutans
	    ▪ Streptococcus salivarius
	    ▪ Streptococcus sanguinis

Aerobic Gram Positive Bacilli	• Rothia dentocariosa
Aerobic Gram Negative Coccobacilli	• Aggregatibacter spp • Campylobacter spp • Capnocytophaga spp • Eikenella spp • Haemophilus spp
Anaerobic Gram Positive	• Actinomyces spp • Anaerobic Gram positive cocci • Anaerobic Gram positive bacilli
Anaerobic Gram Negative Bacilli	• Porphyromonas spp • Fusobacterium spp • Prevotella spp • Bacteroides spp
Spirochetes	• Treponema spp

* Aerobic Gram negative bacilli and Staphylococcus aureus rarely cause dental infections. They may be the causative agents in patients with serious underlying disease.

RECOMMENDED EMPIRIC THERAPY OF SELECTED DENTAL INFECTIONS[A]

Infection	Recommended Empiric Therapy	Recommended Dose[B]/Duration	Comments
- Most dental infections are polymicrobial (aerobic & anaerobic bacteria). Normal oral flora consists of >500 bacterial species. - The etiology of dental infections is multifactorial. Organisms that are part of the normal flora of the mouth (see Table 2) may be associated with dental infections. - Local antibiotic therapy (+/- local delivery systems) is not routinely recommended as it offers no advantage over conventional mechanical debridement. - The routine use of mouthwashes/rinses for infection control/occupational risk exposure is not recommended. - **NB: Prolonged use of chlorhexidine is NOT recommended as it may result in selection of antimicrobial resistant oral bacteria.** - For treatment of fungal/yeast infections of the oral cavity, see Recommended Empiric Therapy of Fungal Infections.			
Odontogenic			
Root caries	1. **Repair all carious lesions.** 2. **Patient education and oral hygiene instruction.** 3. **Optimize the use of fluorides.** 4. **Institute dietary changes.**		

High Risk Patients*	<u>Unresponsive to above</u>
	Chlorhexidine gluconate 0.12% mouthwash**
		Rinse with 15 mL PO for 30 seconds bid (after tooth-brushing) x 3 weeks then reevaluate	* High risk:
			  • ≥ 3 root caries in last 3 years
			  • recent full mouth reconstruction
			  • severe periodontal disease
			  • extensive gingival recession
			  • xerostomia
			
			**There is some evidence of benefit in root caries, but not in enamel caries.

RECOMMENDED EMPIRIC THERAPY OF SELECTED DENTAL INFECTIONS[A]

Infection	Recommended Empiric Therapy	Recommended Dose[B]/Duration	Comments
Odontogenic			
Endodontic Abscesses (dentoalveolar, periapical)	First line therapy **Surgical drainage & debridement** If unable to achieve optimal drainage **Penicillin VK** +/- **Metronidazole*** β-lactam allergy **Clindamycin**	300-600mg PO qid x 7 days 500mg PO bid x 7 days 150-300mg PO qid x 7 days	- **Antibiotics are NOT recommended without drainage and debridement.** * Addition of metronidazole recommended if signs of fascial space infection or systemic symptoms develop.
Dry socket (fibrinolytic alveolitis)	The benefit of antimicrobial therapy has not been established and is **not recommended.**		- Pain management essential. - Post extraction complication (usually of mandibular 3rd molar). - An infectious etiology has been proposed but not substantiated.
Periodontal			
Gingivitis	- Inflammation of the soft tissues around teeth without loss of periodontal support.		
Acute Herpes simplex I	Immunocompetent Primary **Acyclovir** or **Famciclovir** or **Valacyclovir** Recurrent **No therapy indicated** Immunocompromised* **Acyclovir** or **Famciclovir** or **Valacyclovir**	Adult 400mg PO tid x 7 days Paediatric 40-60mg/kg/d PO div 4-5x/d 500mg PO bid x 7 days 500mg-1g PO bid x 7 days 400mg PO 5x/day x 7-10 days 500mg PO bid x 7-10 days 500mg-1g PO bid x 7-10 days	* If immunocompromised, medical consultation advised. Adult HIV patients and transplant recipients may benefit from suppressive acyclovir therapy 200-400mg PO bid-tid. If paediatric patient, consider admission to hospital.

RECOMMENDED EMPIRIC THERAPY OF SELECTED DENTAL INFECTIONS[A]

Infection	Recommended Empiric Therapy	Recommended Dose[B]/Duration	Comments
Periodontal			
Gingivitis (cont'd) **Chronic**	First line therapy **Personal plaque/calculus control and professional debridement essential** **Patient education and oral hygiene instruction** **Correction of plaque retentive factors*** Unresponsive to above, add **Chlorhexidine gluconate 0.12% mouthwash** **Antibiotics not recommended**	Rinse with 15 mL PO for 30 seconds bid (after tooth-brushing) x 3 weeks then reevaluate	- In refractory cases, evaluation of systemic factors recommended: • diabetes • pregnancy • viral infection • endocrine dysfunction • vitamin deficiency/malnutrition • reduced host defences (eg. HIV, blood dyscrasias, medication +/or radiation therapy induced) • xerostomia • smoking. - In refractory cases, desquamative gingivitis should be differentially diagnosed from mucocutaneous disorders such as: • lichen planus • pemphigus • cicatricial pemphigoid • squamous cell carcinoma. * e.g. overcontoured crowns, open margins, caries, etc.

RECOMMENDED EMPIRIC THERAPY OF SELECTED DENTAL INFECTIONS[A]

Infection	Recommended Empiric Therapy	Recommended Dose[B]/Duration	Comments
Periodontal			
Acute necrotizing ulcerative gingivitis (ANUG or "trench mouth")	First line therapy **Personal plaque/calculus control and professional debridement essential**		- Frequently seen in HIV patients. - Oxygenating agents such as hydrogen peroxide or sodium perborate (Amosan®) may be used as adjunctive therapy.
	Systemic symptoms* +/- unresponsive to above **Penicillin VK**	300-600mg PO qid x 7 days	* **NB: Antibiotic use should be reserved for patients showing systemic signs and symptoms.**
	β-lactam allergy **Clindamycin**	150-300mg PO qid x 7 days	
Pericoronitis	- Painful infection developing around impacted/partially erupted teeth.		
	Systemic symptoms **Penicillin VK** +/- **Metronidazole**	300-600mg PO qid x 7days 500mg PO bid x 7 days	- Pain management essential. - Consider removal of the offending tooth.
	β-lactam allergy **Clindamycin**	150-300mg PO qid x 7 days	

RECOMMENDED EMPIRIC THERAPY OF SELECTED DENTAL INFECTIONS[A]

Infection	Recommended Empiric Therapy	Recommended Dose[B]/Duration	Comments
Periodontal			
Periodontitis	- Inflammation of the gingiva & adjacent attachment apparatus associated with loss of attachment due to destruction of the periodontal ligament & loss of adjacent supporting bone.		
Early onset (< 35 years): • prepubertal • juvenile • rapidly progressive	<u>First line therapy</u> **Personal plaque/calculus control and professional debridement essential** **Consider referral to a periodontal specialist**		- May involve host defense abnormalities. - Associated with severe & rapid periodontal destruction. - Aggregatibacter *actinomycetemcomitans* plays a prominent role. <u>Prepubertal</u> - Rare condition that usually affects deciduous teeth. - Neutropenia observed. <u>Juvenile</u> - Age of onset between 10-20 years. <u>Rapidly Progressive</u> - Age of onset between 20-30 years.

RECOMMENDED EMPIRIC THERAPY OF SELECTED DENTAL INFECTIONS[A]

Infection	Recommended Empiric Therapy	Recommended Dose[B]/ Duration	Comments
Periodontal			
Periodontitis (cont'd)			
Adult			

Chronic	<u>First line therapy</u>
	Personal plaque/calculus control and professional debridement essential
	
	Antibiotics not recommended
			- Therapeutic response may be adversely affected by:
			  1. Underlying systemic conditions (e.g. diabetes melitus, Crohn's disease etc.)
			  2. Reduced host defenses (eg. HIV, blood dyscrasias, medication +/or radiation therapy induced, etc.)
			  3. Smoking (increases the risk of poor response to treatment **5 fold**).

Refractory	<u>First line therapy</u> **Personal plaque/calculus control and professional debridement essential** <u>Unresponsive to above</u> **Tetracycline*** or **Doxycycline*** or **Doxycycline (Periostat®)**** <u>Alternative</u> **Penicillin VK** +/- **Metronidazole**	250mg PO qid x 7 days 100mg PO bid x 7 days 20mg PO bid x 3-12 months 300-600mg PO qid x 7 days 500mg PO bid x 7 days	- Progressive destruction of periodontal attachment despite diligent mechanical treatment. - If not responding, consider referral. * Some experts advocate tetracycline antibiotics for their anti-inflammatory properties. ** Collagenase inhibitor approved for use as an adjunct to scaling and root planing. Duration of therapy depends on severity of gum disease. - Since Aggregatibacter may be found in up to 1/3 of cases, clindamycin not optimal.

RECOMMENDED EMPIRIC THERAPY OF SELECTED DENTAL INFECTIONS[A]

Infection	Recommended Empiric Therapy	Recommended Dose[B]/Duration	Comments
Periodontal			
Periodontal abscess	First line therapy **Personal plaque/calculus control and professional debridement essential** Systemic symptoms +/- unresponsive to above* Paediatric **Penicillin VK** +/- **Metronidazole** β-lactam allergy **Clindamycin** Adult **Penicillin VK** +/- **Metronidazole** β-lactam allergy **Clindamycin** or **Tetracycline**** or **Doxycycline****	Paediatric 40mg/kg/d PO div tid or qid x 7 days 15-30mg/kg/d PO div bid x 7 days 30mg/kg/d PO div qid x 7 days Adult 300-600mg PO qid x 7 days 500mg PO bid x 7 days 150-300mg PO qid x 7 days 250mg PO qid x 7 days 100mg PO bid x 7 days	- If recurrent, consider referral or extraction. - Surgical drainage of both the pocket and the pulp chamber must be considered when there is a combined periodontal-endodontic lesion. * The role of antibiotics in the treatment of periodontal abscess is not established. ** Some experts advocate tetracycline antibiotics for their anti-inflammatory properties (controversial).

- 511 -

RECOMMENDED EMPIRIC THERAPY OF SELECTED DENTAL INFECTIONS[A]

Infection	Recommended Empiric Therapy	Recommended Dose[B]/Duration	Comments
Periodontal			
Post-operative peri-implantitis	First line therapy **Personal plaque/calculus control and professional debridement essential**		* If implant mechanically unstable, or extensive abscess develops, removal of implant recommended.
	Moderate - severe/Abscess* **First line therapy** + **Penicillin VK** +/- **Metronidazole**	300-600mg PO qid x 7 days 500mg PO bid x 7 days	
	β-lactam allergy **Clindamycin**	150-300mg PO qid x 7 days	
	Adjunctive Therapy **Chlorhexidine gluconate 0.12% mouthwash**	Rinse with 15 mL PO for 30 seconds bid (after tooth-brushing) x 3 weeks	

RECOMMENDED EMPIRIC THERAPY OF SELECTED DENTAL INFECTIONS[A]

Infection	Recommended Empiric Therapy	Recommended Dose[B]/Duration	Comments
Oral			
Fascial space infections	*First line therapy* **Surgical drainage essential**		- May require immediate hospitalization and maintenance of the airway.
	Paediatric **Penicillin** + **Metronidazole**	150,000-250,000u/kg/d IV q6h x 10 days 30mg/kg/d IV div q12h x 10 days	
	β-lactam allergy **Clindamycin**	40mg/kg/d IV div q8h x 10 days	
	Unresponsive/Severe **Piperacillin-tazobactam**	240-300mg piperacillin/kg/d IV div q6-8h x 10 days	
	Adult **Penicillin** + **Metronidazole**	2 MU IV q4-6h x 10 days 500 mg IV q12h x 10 days	
	β-lactam allergy **Clindamycin**	600 mg IV q8h x 10 days	
	Unresponsive/Severe **Piperacillin-tazobactam**	3.375g q6h x 10 days	

A. These are empiric antibiotic recommendations based on local susceptibility patterns, and need to restrict and rationalize antibiotic use. Antibiotics listed for each condition are not all inclusive, nor are they all approved by TPD for the listed indication. Choice of empiric antibiotic therapy should be based on the patient's age, allergies, co-morbidities, and clinical condition, as well as cost and convenience of the dosage regimen. Empiric antibiotic therapy should be modified to narrower spectrum antibiotic(s) according to culture and susceptibility (C&S) results.

B. Usual **adult** dose in patients with normal renal and hepatic function, unless otherwise specified. Pediatric doses are reported as mg/kg/d = milligrams per kilogram per day. Total paediatric dose should not exceed adult dose.

ANTIMICROBIALS IN PREGNANCY

* Legend:
FDA risk categories:

A. Controlled studies in women fail to demonstrate a risk to the fetus.

B. Animal studies have not revealed toxicity but there are no adequate human studies, or animal studies have shown toxicity that was not confirmed in human studies.

C. Animal studies have revealed toxicity and there are no adequate human studies, or studies in humans and animals are not available. Drug should only be given if potential benefit justifies the potential risk to the fetus.

D. Positive evidence of human fetal risk, but the benefits from use in pregnant women may be acceptable despite the risk.

X. Human and/or animal studies have shown a risk to the fetus, and risks outweigh benefits. Contraindicated in pregnancy.

** For information on antiretroviral agents see:

- U.S. Department of Health & Human Services Guidelines - Treatment/Prevention - Perinatal Guidelines - Supplement: Safety and Toxicity of Individual Antiretrovirals in Pregnancy (www.aidsinfo.nih.gov/)
- Antiretroviral Pregnancy Registry (www.apregistry.com/).

Abbreviations:
BLI = β-lactamase inhibitor, G6PD = glucose-6-phosphate dehydrogenase, TMP/SMX – trimethoprim/sulfamethoxazole, WHO = World Health Organization

***Adapted from: *Briggs GG, et al. Drugs in pregnancy and lactation. 9th ed. 2011.*

ANTIMICROBIALS IN PREGNANCY

DRUG	FDA RISK CATEGORY*	RECOMMENDATION***	COMMENTS
ANTIBACTERIAL AGENTS			
β-Lactams			
Penicillins	B	Compatible with pregnancy	
Penicillins & BLI	B		No human data suggesting toxic effects.
Cephalosporins	B	Compatible with pregnancy	
Doripenem	B	No human data - probably compatible	Probably compatible with pregnancy based on the safety of other β-lactams.
Ertapenem	B	No human data - probably compatible	Probably compatible with pregnancy based on the safety of other β-lactams.
Imipenem	C	Limited human data - animal data suggest low risk	Animal studies have not shown teratogenic effects or fetal malformations but have shown an increase in embryonic loss. No human data on use in the 1st trimester, however 3 references consider it to be safe during the perinatal period.
Meropenem	B	Limited human data - animal data suggest low risk	Probably compatible with pregnancy based on the safety of other carbapenems in the perinatal period.
Aztreonam	B	No human data - animal data suggest low risk	If the drug is indicated, it should not be withheld because of pregnancy.
Aminoglycosides			
Amikacin	C	Human data suggest low risk	Fetal cranial nerve VIII toxicity resulting in hearing loss has occurred with some aminoglycosides (e.g. streptomycin). Ototoxicity due to in utero exposure, however, has not been reported with these agents. Dose-related nephrotoxicity has been observed in fetal rats.
Gentamicin	C		
Tobramycin	C		
Streptomycin	D	Human data suggest risk	See Antimycobacterials.

DRUG	FDA RISK CATEGORY*	RECOMMENDATION***	COMMENTS
ANTIBACTERIAL AGENTS (cont'd)			
Macrolides			
Azithromycin	B	Limited human data - animal data suggest low risk	
Clarithromycin	C	Limited human data – animal data suggest high risk (including increase in embryonic loss)	
Erythromycin	B (excluding estolate)	Compatible with pregnancy	Estolate salt associated with maternal hepatotoxicity.
Quinolones			Interpretation of animal data controversial as variable rates and types of fetal effects have been observed in animals. Human data for ciprofloxacin, norfloxacin, and ofloxacin have not revealed a predictable pattern of anomalies but a causal relationship cannot be excluded. Because of this and the available animal data, quinolones should be used with caution, especially in the first trimester. Other authors conclude that quinolones should be contraindicated in pregnancy as safer alternatives usually exist.
Ciprofloxacin	C	Human data suggest low risk	
Norfloxacin	C		
Ofloxacin	C		
Levofloxacin	C	No human data – risk extrapolated from data for other quinolones.	
Moxifloxacin	C		
Others			
Chloramphenicol	C	Compatible with pregnancy BUT use with caution in final stage of pregnancy	May be associated with gray baby syndrome (characterized by abdominal distention, vomiting, flaccidity, cyanosis, circulatory collapse, and death).

ANTIMICROBIALS IN PREGNANCY

DRUG	FDA RISK CATEGORY*	RECOMMENDATION***	COMMENTS
ANTIBACTERIAL AGENTS (cont'd)			
Others (cont'd)			
Clindamycin	B	Compatible with pregnancy	
Daptomycin	B	Limited human data – animal data suggest low risk	Animal studies do not show a risk to the fetus, however there have been no controlled human studies. There are three case reports describing the use of daptomycin in the 2nd and 3rd trimesters. High molecular weight should limit exposure of the fetus. If the antibiotic is required, it should not be withheld because of pregnancy.
Fosfomycin	B	Compatible with pregnancy	Fosfomycin does cross the placenta but the lack of teratogenicity in animals and the apparently safe use of fosfomycin during human pregnancy indicate that the drug presents a low risk, if any, to the fetus.
Linezolid	C	Compatible – maternal benefit > fetal risk	Animal studies have shown no teratogenicity but embryo, fetal and maternal toxicity were observed. Safer alternatives should be used if possible. If not, and linezolid must be used, maternal benefit appears to outweigh unknown fetal risk.

ANTIMICROBIALS IN PREGNANCY

DRUG	FDA RISK CATEGORY*	RECOMMENDATION***	COMMENTS
ANTIBACTERIAL AGENTS (cont'd)			
Others (cont'd)			
Metronidazole	B	Human data suggest low risk	The latest studies, which examined thousands of women exposed to metronidazole during pregnancy, including a Medicaid cohort study, a large case-control study, and two meta-analyses, have concluded that there is no evidence that using metronidazole during pregnancy increases the rate of major birth defects above the baseline rate or that there are any detectable adverse effects on fetuses.
Nitrofurantoin	B	Human data suggest risk in 3rd trimester	Nitrofurantoin should be avoided at term (38-42 weeks), during labor and delivery, or when the onset of labor is imminent, due to potential for hemolytic anemia in the newborn. Otherwise, considered safe.
Sulfonamides *(For TMP/SMX, see also Trimethoprim)*	C (D if near term)	Human data suggest risk in 3rd trimester	Jaundice, hemolytic anemia, and kernicterus may occur in the newborn if given at term therefore avoid maternal use at term. Otherwise, sulfonamides are a low teratogenic risk.
Tetracyclines	D	Contraindicated in 2nd and 3rd trimesters of pregnancy	Associated with abnormal development of fetal teeth and bone, congenital defects, and maternal liver toxicity.
Tigecycline	D	Human data suggest risk in 2nd and 3rd trimesters	Tigecycline can permanently discolor the teeth if used in the second half of pregnancy. Use in the 1st trimester probably does not represent a major risk to the fetus, but use in later trimesters should be avoided.

ANTIMICROBIALS IN PREGNANCY

DRUG	FDA RISK CATEGORY*	RECOMMENDATION***	COMMENTS
ANTIBACTERIAL AGENTS (cont'd)			
Others (cont'd) Trimethoprim (For TMP/SMX, see also Sulfonamides)	C	Human and animal data suggest risk	Although case reports and controlled trials have not demonstrated an increase in fetal abnormalities, other data are suggestive that structural defects may occur when trimethoprim is used in the 1st trimester or up to 12 weeks prior to conception (perhaps because it is a folate antagonist).
Vancomycin	B	Compatible with pregnancy	No reports of congenital defects in humans.

ANTIMICROBIALS IN PREGNANCY

DRUG	FDA RISK CATEGORY*	RECOMMENDATION***	COMMENTS
ANTIFUNGAL AGENTS			
Amphotericin B	B	Compatible with pregnancy	No reports linking use during various stages of pregnancy with congenital defects. Preferred therapy for susceptible fungal infections during pregnancy.
Anidulafungin	C	No human data – animal data suggest low risk	There are no reports of anidulafungin (or caspofungin or micafungin) use in human pregnancy. Animal reproduction data show skeletal teratogenic effects. Best course is to avoid anidulafungin in pregnancy; however, if the woman's condition requires it, the benefit probably outweighs the unknown risk. The lowest possible dose should be used.
Caspofungin	C	No human data – animal data suggest risk	There are no reports of caspofungin (or anidulafungin or micafungin) use in human pregnancy. Animal data are suggestive of risk, especially if exposure occurs in the 1st trimester. Therefore, if indicated, avoid maternal treatment in the 1st trimester, if possible.
Fluconazole	C (single dose for vaginal candidiasis) D (all other indications/doses)	Human data suggest low risk at low doses Human data suggest risk at doses > 400mg/day	Short course, low dose (≤ 150 mg/day) fluconazole therapy, such as that prescribed for vaginal fungal infections, has not been associated with an increased incidence of congenital defects. Congenital anomalies reported in infants with maternal dose of 400-800 mg/day during the first trimester. High doses in rats produced teratogenic and embryotoxic effects.

ANTIMICROBIALS IN PREGNANCY

DRUG	FDA RISK CATEGORY*	RECOMMENDATION***	COMMENTS
ANTIFUNGAL AGENTS (cont'd)			
Flucytosine	C	Contraindicated in 1st trimester	Teratogenic in some animal species. Use of flucytosine in 2nd and 3rd trimesters resulted in no defects in the newborns (n=3 cases).
Itraconazole	C	Human data suggest low risk	Human data suggest risk of anomalies is low. Cases of malformations in human infants have been reported (n=14), however 2 prospective cohort studies (n=198 and n=206) showed no significant risk. Avoid use in 1st trimester if possible.
Ketoconazole	C	**Oral:** Limited human data - animal data suggest risk **Topical:** No human data – probably compatible.	Embryotoxic and teratogenic in rats in high doses. A population-based, case-control study failed to demonstrate a higher incidence of congenital malformations in infants of mothers exposed to ketoconazole versus controls.
Micafungin	C	No human data – animal data suggest moderate risk	There are no reports of micafungin (or anidulafungin or caspofungin) use in human pregnancy. Animal data are suggestive of moderate risk, especially if exposure occurs in the 1st trimester. Therefore, if indicated, avoid maternal treatment in the 1st trimester, if possible.

ANTIMICROBIALS IN PREGNANCY

DRUG	FDA RISK CATEGORY*	RECOMMENDATION***	COMMENTS
ANTIFUNGAL AGENTS (cont'd)			
Posaconazole	C	No human data. Animal data suggest risk.	Teratogenic in high doses in animal studies. Best to avoid posaconazole during pregnancy, especially in the 1st trimester. However, if the woman's condition requires posaconazole, the benefit probably outweighs the unknown risk. The lowest possible dose should be used.
Terbinafine	B	No human data. Animal data suggest low risk (no harmful effects seen).	Due to the lack of human pregnancy data however, therapy should be delayed, if possible, until after delivery.
Voriconazole	D	No human data. Animal data suggest risk.	Teratogenic and embryotoxic in animal studies.
Vaginal Products			
Clotrimazole	B	Compatible with pregnancy	Systemic absorption from the skin and vagina is minimal. Three large surveillance studies found no association between clotrimazole and birth defects.
Miconazole	C	Compatible with pregnancy (topical)	Small amounts are absorbed from the vagina. Use in pregnant patients with vulvovaginal candidiasis has not been associated with an increase in congenital malformations.
Nystatin	C	Compatible with pregnancy	Poor systemic absorption after oral administration and topical or mucosal application.
Terconazole	C	Human data suggest low risk.	

ANTIMICROBIALS IN PREGNANCY

DRUG	FDA RISK CATEGORY*	RECOMMENDATION***	COMMENTS
ANTIPARASITIC AGENTS			
Atovaquone +/- proguanil	C	Compatible with pregnancy; maternal benefit outweighs embryo/fetal risk.	Limited human pregnancy experience., including lack of 1st trimester exposure prevents risk assessment however a 2004 review concluded that while not recommended, it can be used if no alternatives exist. Maternal benefit outweighs the fetal risk so the drug should not be withheld in pregnancy.
Chloroquine	C	Compatible with pregnancy; maternal benefit outweighs embryo/fetal risk	Drug of choice in pregnancy for prophylaxis and treatment of susceptible malaria strains.
Ivermectin	C	Human data suggest low risk	Ivermectin was teratogenic in three animal species, but only at doses at or near those producing maternal toxicity. No teratogenicity or toxicity attributable to ivermectin has been observed in limited human pregnancy experience. WHO states that use after the 1st trimester is probably acceptable
Mebendazole	C	Human data suggest low risk	Embryotoxic and teratogenic in rats but not in other animal species.
Mefloquine	C	Compatible with pregnancy	If indicated, mefloquine should not be withheld in pregnancy because the maternal and fetal risk from malaria far outweighs the unknown potential of developmental toxicity.
Pentamidine	C	Compatible with pregnancy; maternal benefit outweighs embryo/fetal risk	Safety in human pregnancy not established however if pentamidine must be used during pregnancy, aerosolized administration may be preferred over IV administration as it results in lower systemic concentrations.

ANTIMICROBIALS IN PREGNANCY

DRUG	FDA RISK CATEGORY*	RECOMMENDATION***	COMMENTS
ANTIPARASITIC AGENTS (cont'd)			
Praziquantel	B	Limited human data; animal data suggest moderate risk	Not teratogenic in animals however human pregnancy experience limited to one case. May be mutagenic/carcinogenic in humans therefore use only if parasite causing maternal clinical illness or public health problems.
Primaquine	C	Limited human data; probably compatible with pregnancy	May cause hemolytic anemia in a fetus with G6PD deficiency. If possible, withhold drug until after delivery.
Pyrimethamine	C	Compatible with pregnancy; maternal benefit outweighs embryo/fetal risk	Folic acid (5 mg/day) supplementation recommended, especially during first trimester, to prevent folate deficiency.
Quinine	D	Human data suggest risk	Human case reports of teratogenicity, usually associated with use of quinine in toxic doses as an abortifacient. Although no increased teratogenic risk has been documented with therapeutic doses, quinine use during pregnancy should be avoided.

ANTIMICROBIALS IN PREGNANCY

DRUG	FDA RISK CATEGORY*	RECOMMENDATION***	COMMENTS
ANTIMYCOBACTERIAL AGENTS			
Dapsone	C	Compatible with pregnancy; maternal benefit outweighs embryo/fetal risk	Has been used extensively without producing major fetotoxicity or birth defects. If used in combination with pyrimethamine for malaria prophylaxis, folic acid (5 mg/day) supplementation recommended.
Ethambutol	B	Compatible with pregnancy	No reports of congenital defects. Part of the regimen of choice for tuberculosis treatment in pregnancy: ethambutol, isoniazid, and rifampin plus pyridoxine.
Isoniazid	C	Compatible with pregnancy; maternal benefit outweighs embryo/fetal risk	Does not appear to be teratogenic. Part of the regimen of choice for tuberculosis treatment in pregnancy: ethambutol, isoniazid, and rifampin plus pyridoxine.
Pyrazinamide	C	Compatible with pregnancy; maternal benefit outweighs embryo/fetal risk	No relevant animal data, but there are a small number of human pregnancy exposures reported with no fetal harm. Therefore, if indicated, pyrazinamide should not be withheld in pregnancy.
Rifampin	C	Compatible with pregnancy	Although animal studies have revealed teratogenic and embryotoxic effects, it is not a proven teratogen in humans and is used with isoniazid, pyridoxine, and ethambutol as part of the regimen for tuberculosis treatment in pregnancy. If used, prophylactic vitamin K is recommended to prevent hemorrhagic disease of the newborn.
Streptomycin	D	Human data suggest risk	Streptomycin may cause fetal ototoxicity resulting in deafness in newborns. However, the risk of this toxicity is low if there is appropriate dose monitoring and the duration of fetal exposure is limited.

ANTIMICROBIALS IN PREGNANCY

DRUG	FDA RISK CATEGORY*	RECOMMENDATION***	COMMENTS
ANTIVIRAL AGENTS**			
Acyclovir	B	Compatible with pregnancy	No adverse effects to the fetus or newborn have proved attributable to the drug. Acyclovir is also used in neonates.
Amantadine	C	Limited human data- animal data suggest risk.	A higher number of birth defects (n=5) than expected (n=2) was observed in a small number of 1st trimester exposures (n=51). The drug is best avoided in the first trimester.
Famciclovir	B	Limited human data. Animal data suggest low risk.	
Foscarnet	C	Compatible with pregnancy; maternal benefit outweighs embryo/fetal risk	Very limited human data (2 case reports) showed no defects. Animal studies have resulted in skeletal anomalies. If foscarnet must be used (i.e. sight-threatening CMV retinitis), monitor both mother and fetus for renal toxicity.
Ganciclovir	C	Compatible with pregnancy; maternal benefit outweighs embryo/fetal risk.	Animal studies have demonstrated mutagenicity/carcinogenicity/teratogenicity/embryotoxicity. Six human case reports of ganciclovir use in human pregnancy showed no fetal defects. Because of the potential for fetal toxicity and the known toxic effects in animals, some experts recommend that ganciclovir should only be used during pregnancy for life-threatening disease or in immunocompromised patients with major CMV infections, such as retinitis. Avoid use in first trimester if possible.

ANTIMICROBIALS IN PREGNANCY

DRUG	FDA RISK CATEGORY*	RECOMMENDATION***	COMMENTS
ANTIVIRAL AGENTS** (cont'd)			
Oseltamivir	C	Compatible with pregnancy; maternal benefit outweighs embryo/fetal risk.	Available human data suggest that oseltamivir is unlikely to cause adverse pregnancy or fetal outcomes.
Valacyclovir	B	Compatible with pregnancy	
Valganciclovir	C	Compatible with pregnancy; maternal benefit outweighs embryo/fetal risk.	No data available on use of valganciclovir in human pregnancy. See ganciclovir.
Zanamivir	C	Compatible with pregnancy; maternal benefit outweighs embryo/fetal risk.	Low systemic bioavailability after oral inhalation limits the amount of drug available for crossing the placenta, however lack of human data prevents full assessment of risk.

ANTIMICROBIALS IN LACTATION

In the vast majority of cases, lactating women on antibiotic therapy do NOT need to interrupt breastfeeding. In almost all cases where antibiotics are clinically indicated, the benefits of breastfeeding outweigh the risks, where present, of antibiotic exposure. In general, drugs taken by the nursing mother reach the infant in much smaller amounts than that for a fetus when the mother takes the drug during pregnancy.

Legend:

1. Risk categories (from *Hale TW. Medications and mothers' milk. Accessed on-line August 2011-12*)
   - **L1 = SAFEST**: Drug used in a large number of breastfeeding women without affecting infant, or studies indicate that the possibility of harm to infant is remote, or the drug is not orally bioavailable in infants.
   - **L2 = SAFER**: Drug used in a limited number of breastfeeding women without affecting infant, and/or risk to infant by using drug is remote.
   - **L3 = MODERATELY SAFE**: There are no controlled studies. The risk of adverse effects in the infant is possible, or studies show only minimal non-threatening adverse reactions. Benefit versus risk to the infant must be considered.
   - **L4 = POSSIBLY HAZARDOUS**: There is evidence of risk to the breastfed infant or breast milk production, but the benefits to the mother may outweigh the risk to the infant (e.g. in life-threatening situations or when safer drugs cannot be used).
   - **L5 = CONTRAINDICATED**: Studies show a significant and documented risk to infants, or it is a drug that has a high risk of causing significant harm. The drug is contraindicated in breastfeeding, as the possible harm to the infant outweighs any potential benefits from breastfeeding.

2. **AAP ratings:** Recommendations from American Academy of Pediatrics (AAP), published in *Pediatrics 2001;108:776-89.*
   ✓ = approved - drug is usually compatible with breastfeeding.

3. **Relative infant dose (RID):** An estimate of the theoretical infant's dose in milk divided by the mother's dose (in mg/kg/day). An infant dose < 10% of the maternal dose is usually considered safe, but some with RID > 10% are also safe (e.g. fluconazole metronidazole). [Ito S. NEJM 2000;343:118-26.]

Abbreviations: AAP = American Academy of Pediatrics; G6PD = Glucose-6-phosphate dehydrogenase; GI = gastrointestinal; TMP/SMX – trimethoprim/sulfamethoxazole, WHO = World Health Organization

ANTIMICROBIALS IN LACTATION

DRUG	RISK CATEGORY[1]	AAP RATING[2]	RELATIVE INFANT DOSE[3]	COMMENTS
ANTIBACTERIAL AGENTS				
β-Lactams				
Penicillins				Small amount of penicillins excreted in human milk. Possible allergic sensitization or disruption of GI flora. Observe infant for rash or diarrhea.
Amoxicillin	L1	✓	1%	
Ampicillin	L1		0.2-0.5%	
Cloxacillin	L2		0.4-0.8%	
Penicillin G	L1	✓		
Piperacillin	L2			Concentrations in milk expected to be very low due to extremely low concentrations secreted into milk and poor oral absorption.
Ticarcillin	L1	✓	0.2%	Less than 1% of maternal dose transferred into milk; poor oral absorption.
Aztreonam	L2	✓	0.2-1%	
Penicillins + β-lactamase Inhibitors				Small amount of penicillins excreted in human milk. Possible allergic sensitization or disruption of GI flora. Observe infant for rash or diarrhea.
Amoxicillin/ clavulanate	L1		0.9%	Clavulanate: Excretion into breast milk likely occurs due to low molecular weight, but effect in infants unknown – probably compatible with breastfeeding.
Piperacillin/ tazobactam	L2			Tazobactam is excreted into breast milk in low concentrations – probably compatible with breastfeeding.
Ticarcillin/ clavulanate	L1	✓	0.2%	Clavulanate: Excretion into breast milk likely occurs due to low molecular weight, but effect in infants unknown – probably compatible with breastfeeding.

ANTIMICROBIALS IN LACTATION

DRUG	RISK CATEGORY[1]	AAP RATING[2]	RELATIVE INFANT DOSE[3]	COMMENTS
Cephalosporins				Excreted in human milk in small concentrations. Possible allergic sensitization or disruption of GI flora. Observe infant for rash or diarrhea.
Cefaclor	L1		0.4-0.8%	
Cefazolin	L1	✓	0.8%	Excreted in human milk in insignificant amounts, and oral absorption by the infant would be poor.
Cefepime	L2		0.3%	Excreted in human milk in small amounts. May disrupt GI flora – observe infant for diarrhea or thrush.
Cefixime	L2			Excreted in human milk in limited amounts, but oral absorption by the infant would be poor (bioavailability 30-50%).
Cefotaxime	L2	✓	0.3%	Excreted in human milk, but oral absorption by the infant would be poor.
Cefoxitin	L1	✓	0.1-0.3%	Excreted in human milk in very low amounts.
Cefprozil	L1	✓	3.7%	
Ceftaroline	L3			No data in human milk but unlikely to cause adverse effects. May disrupt GI flora, observe infant for diarrhea or thrush.
Ceftazidime	L1	✓	0.9%	No progressive ceftazidime accumulation in human milk.
Ceftriaxone	L1	✓	4.1-4.2%	Excreted in human milk in small amounts and oral absorption by the infant would be poor.
Cefuroxime	L2		0.6-2%	Excreted in human milk in small amounts and oral absorption by the infant would be poor.
Cephalexin	L1		0.5-1.5%	Excreted in human milk in small amounts.

ANTIMICROBIALS IN LACTATION

DRUG	RISK CATEGORY[1]	AAP RATING[2]	RELATIVE INFANT DOSE[3]	COMMENTS
Carbapenems				
Doripenem	L3			Observe infant for diarrhea. No human data but levels in milk will likely be low. Low oral bioavailability. Observe infant for diarrhea and changes in gut flora.
Ertapenem	L2		0.1-0.4%	Excreted in human milk in small amounts.
Imipenem	L2			Transfer into breast milk probably minimal.
Meropenem	L3			Transfer into breast milk probably minimal.
Aminoglycosides				Small amount excreted in human milk; poor systemic absorption by infant, resulting in subtherapeutic, clinically irrelevant serum levels in nursing infants. Nephrotoxicity and ototoxicity in the infant would not be expected; could produce minor changes in gut flora. No data on infant exposure with extended interval aminoglycoside dosing.
Amikacin	L2			
Gentamicin	L2	✓	2.1%	
Tobramycin	L3		2.6%	
Macrolides				
Azithromycin	L2		5.9%	Excreted in human milk. Predicted infant dose 0.4 mg/kg/day (vs. 5-10mg/kg/day pediatric dose).
Clarithromycin	L1		2.1%	Observe infant for diarrhea or thrush.
Erythromycin	L3 – early postnatally	✓	1.4-1.7%	Excreted in human milk. L3 rating early postnatally is due to documented risk of hypertrophic pyloric stenosis in the newborn. Azithromycin or clarithromycin may be better choices.

ANTIMICROBIALS IN LACTATION

DRUG	RISK CATEGORY[1]	AAP RATING[2]	RELATIVE INFANT DOSE[3]	COMMENTS
Quinolones				Based on their low molecular weight, high lipid solubility and low protein binding, these drugs are expected to be found in breast milk. Ofloxacin, levofloxacin, and norfloxacin are probably the better choices for breastfeeding women due to lower milk levels. Observe infant for diarrhea.
Ciprofloxacin	L3	✓	2.1-6.3%	Excreted in human milk. Observe infant for diarrhea. Tooth discoloration possible.
Levofloxacin	L3		10.5-17.2%	Milk levels similar to maternal plasma levels. Observe infant for diarrhea and changes in gut flora.
Moxifloxacin	L2 – ophth L3 – PO, IV			No human data. Excretion into the milk of lactating animals and its molecular weight suggest that moxifloxacin would be excreted into breast milk. Consider using ofloxacin or levofloxacin for which published data in lactation are available.
Norfloxacin	L3			Not detected in human milk following maternal administration of a single 200 mg dose.
Ofloxacin	L2	✓	3.1%	Breast milk concentrations equal to maternal plasma levels. Ofloxacin levels in breast milk lower than with ciprofloxacin or levofloxacin.
Others				
Chloramphenicol	L4	Effect on nursing infant unknown but may be of concern.	3.2%-8.5%	Excreted in human milk. Possible bone marrow suppression and allergic sensitization.

ANTIMICROBIALS IN LACTATION

DRUG	RISK CATEGORY[1]	AAP RATING[2]	RELATIVE INFANT DOSE[3]	COMMENTS
Others (cont'd) Clindamycin	L2	✓	1.6%	Small amount excreted in human milk. Observe infant for diarrhea, including pseudomembranous colitis (rare).
Daptomycin	L1		0.1%	Limited human data - probably compatible. Low levels in milk, poor oral absorption; would not be expected to cause any adverse effects in breastfed infants but observe infant for changes in gut flora, diarrhea, or GI complaints.
Fosfomycin	L3			Limited human data - probably compatible. Levels in milk are ~10% of maternal plasma level and not likely to produce untoward effects in infant.
Linezolid	L3			Excreted in the milk of lactating rats at concentrations similar to those in plasma. Low molecular weight suggests linezolid would be excreted into breast milk. If linezolid is used during lactation, monitor infant for toxicity (e.g. myelosuppression, thrombocytopenia), and changes in GI flora or diarrhea. Infant would ingest approximately 1.7 mg/kg/day with a maternal dose of 1200 mg/day.
Metronidazole	L2	Effect on nursing infant unknown but may be of concern.	12.6%-13.5%	No adverse effects in the infant have been reported in numerous studies. Observe infant for diarrhea. Commonly used in neonates.

ANTIMICROBIALS IN LACTATION

DRUG	RISK CATEGORY[1]	AAP RATING[2]	RELATIVE INFANT DOSE[3]	COMMENTS
Others (cont'd) Nitrofurantoin	L2	✓	6.8%	Small amount excreted in human milk. Use with caution in infants at risk for G6PD deficiency and newborns at risk for hyperbilirubinemia.
Sulfonamides				Low breast milk levels as most sulfonamides bind extensively to plasma proteins, are water soluble and acidic.
Sulfamethoxazole (For TMP/SMX, see also Trimethoprin)	L3			Use with caution in premature/weakened infants, infants at risk for G6PD deficiency and newborns at risk for hyperbilirubinemia.
Tetracyclines	L4 risk category with chronic maternal use			Excreted in human milk; poor systemic absorption by nursing infant. Short term (< 3 weeks) use is acceptable. Could alter GI flora. L4 risk category with chronic maternal use: Although no harmful effects have been reported in breastfed infants, tetracyclines may theoretically cause dental staining and inhibition of bone growth. Avoid chronic use.
Doxycycline	L3 – acute L4 – chronic		4.2 – 13.3%	More lipophilic and lower binding to milk calcium than tetracycline thus may distribute more readily into breast milk.
Minocycline	L2 – acute L4 – chronic		0.2 – 1.4%	More lipophilic lower binding to milk calcium than tetracycline thus may distribute more readily into breast milk.
Tetracycline	L2 – acute L4 – chronic	✓	0.6%	

ANTIMICROBIALS IN LACTATION

DRUG	RISK CATEGORY[1]	AAP RATING[2]	RELATIVE INFANT DOSE[3]	COMMENTS
Others (cont'd)				
Tigecycline	L3			Limited oral bioavailability; unlikely that the infant would absorb clinically relevant levels over a brief time. Prolonged use (> 3 weeks) not recommended; can cause tooth discoloration.
Trimethoprim	L2	✓	9%	Small amount excreted in human milk. As it interferes with folate metabolism, long term use should be avoided or infant should be supplemented with folic acid.
(For TMP/SMX, see also Sulfonamides)				
Vancomycin	L1		6.7%	Low levels excreted in human milk; poor systemic absorption by nursing infant. Could potentially alter GI flora.
ANTIFUNGAL AGENTS				
Amphotericin B	L3			No human data on excretion in milk, although unlikely the amount excreted in milk would be clinically significant as virtually unabsorbed orally (<9%), high protein binding, and large molecular weight. Used clinically in neonates.
Anidulafungin	L3			No human data, although highly unlikely that it will transfer into breast milk due to its large molecular weight, high protein binding, large volume of distribution, and lack of oral bioavailability in the infant. Observe infant for signs and symptoms of histamine release (e.g., rash, facial swelling, pruritus) and GI complaints.

ANTIMICROBIALS IN LACTATION

DRUG	RISK CATEGORY[1]	AAP RATING[2]	RELATIVE INFANT DOSE[3]	COMMENTS
ANTIFUNGAL AGENTS (cont'd)				
Caspofungin	L3			No human data; probably compatible. Excreted in the milk of lactating rodents. Oral bioavailability poor, so unlikely that the amount excreted in human milk would be clinically significant. Observe infant for signs and symptoms of histamine release (e.g., rash, facial swelling, pruritus) and GI complaints.
Clotrimazole	L1			Little or no absorption after topical/intravaginal/oral administration and limited oral absorption by the breastfed infant.
Fluconazole	L2	✓	16.4-21.5%	No complications from exposure to breast milk have been found. Commonly used in neonates.
Flucytosine	L4			No human data on excretion in milk, although has been used in neonates. Based on potential toxicity to the infant, breastfeeding is not recommended.
Itraconazole	L2		0.2%	Excreted in human milk. Potential effects to the nursing infant are not known, but oral absorption by the infant unlikely. However, itraconazole, when administered to newborn rats, can produce significant bone toxicity. Fluconazole, if clinically appropriate, would be the preferred choice.
Ketoconazole	L2	✓	0.3%	< 1% of maternal dose is excreted in human milk.

ANTIMICROBIALS IN LACTATION

DRUG	RISK CATEGORY[1]	AAP RATING[2]	RELATIVE INFANT DOSE[3]	COMMENTS
ANTIFUNGAL AGENTS (cont'd)				
Micafungin	L3			No human data; probably compatible. High molecular weight, low lipid solubility, and high protein binding suggest excretion into breast milk would be low. Excreted in rat milk. Observe infant for signs and symptoms of histamine release (e.g. rash, facial swelling, pruritus) and GI complaints.
Miconazole	L2			Little or no absorption after topical/intravaginal administration. Used in pediatric patients less than 1 year of age.
Nystatin	L1			Extremely poor oral absorption, undetectable in maternal plasma; not likely to be found in breast milk. Commonly used in neonates for oral candidiasis (thrush).
Posaconazole	L3			No human data on excretion in milk; potential toxicity. Excreted in rat milk. Posaconazole should not be used in nursing mothers unless the potential benefit to the mother clearly outweighs the potential risk to the infant.

ANTIMICROBIALS IN LACTATION

DRUG	RISK CATEGORY[1]	AAP RATING[2]	RELATIVE INFANT DOSE[3]	COMMENTS
ANTIFUNGAL AGENTS (cont'd)				
Terbinafine	L2			Topical cream and spray: the small amount absorbed through the skin is unlikely to affect the nursing infant. Oral formulation is excreted in human milk. Potential effects to the nursing infant are not known. Excretion in breast milk after 500 mg oral dose in 2 volunteers was 0.03 – 0.13% of the total maternal dose. Because the duration of therapy is usually prolonged (6 or 12 weeks for onychomycosis), the potential for serious toxicity in a nursing infant may be increased and women taking terbinafine probably should not breastfeed.
Voriconazole	L4			No human data. It may be excreted in breast milk due to its relatively low molecular weight. Based on potential toxicity to the infant, breastfeeding is not recommended.

ANTIMICROBIALS IN LACTATION

DRUG	RISK CATEGORY[1]	AAP RATING[2]	RELATIVE INFANT DOSE[3]	COMMENTS
ANTIPARASITIC AGENTS				
Atovaquone	L3			No human data. Based on potential toxicity to the infant, breastfeeding is not recommended.
Chloroquine	L2	✓	0.6-1.1%	Although the amount excreted in human milk is not considered to be harmful to the nursing infant, it is insufficient to provide adequate protection against malaria. Monitor infant for adverse effects (diarrhea, GI distress, hypotension).
Hydroxychloroquine	L2	✓	2.9%	Mostly metabolized to chloroquine. No adverse effects reported but should monitor infant for blood dyscrasias or retinal damage. See also chloroquine.
Ivermectin	L3	✓	1.3%	Excreted in human milk. No adverse effects reported.
Mebendazole	L3			Unlikely that the negligible amount excreted in human milk would be clinically significant due to poor oral absorption (2-10%) and high protein binding.
Mefloquine	L2		0.1-0.2%	Only 3 - 4% of maternal dose is excreted in human milk. No adverse effects have been reported in nursing infants, however with continued maternal use drug accumulation may occur (plasma half-life = 10 – 21 days).

ANTIMICROBIALS IN LACTATION

DRUG	RISK CATEGORY[1]	AAP RATING[2]	RELATIVE INFANT DOSE[3]	COMMENTS
ANTIPARASITIC AGENTS (cont'd)				
Pentamidine	NA			No data in lactating women using inhaled/IM/IV formulations, however systemic concentrations achieved via aerosol are low thus milk levels are probably nil, and poor oral absorption thus IM/IV therapy probably safe. WHO Rating: Compatible with breastfeeding.
Praziquantel	L2		0.05%	Excreted in human milk, but concentrations likely too low to harm infant.
Primaquine	L3			No human data on excretion in milk. Maternal plasma levels are low, suggesting milk levels might be low. Contraindicated in babies with G6PD deficiency.
Pyrimethamine	L3	✓	45.8%	Excreted in human milk. Possible carcinogenesis may preclude use in infants. May cause bone marrow suppression but this has not been reported in breast fed infants.
Quinine	L2	✓	0.7-1.3%	Excreted in human milk. Babies at risk for G6PD should not be breastfed until diagnosis ruled out.
ANTIMYCOBACTERIAL AGENTS				
Dapsone	L4	✓	6.3-22.5%	Significant amount excreted in human milk; nursing infant may be at risk of developing hemolytic anemia. Should be used very cautiously, if at all, even though it received AAP rating as compatible with lactation.
Ethambutol	L2	✓	1.5%	Small amount excreted in human milk.

ANTIMICROBIALS IN LACTATION

DRUG	RISK CATEGORY[1]	AAP RATING[2]	RELATIVE INFANT DOSE[3]	COMMENTS
ANTIMYCOBACTERIAL AGENTS (cont'd)				
Isoniazid	L3	✓	1.2-18%	Excreted in human milk. Observe infant for liver toxicity and neuritis: fatigue, weakness, malaise, anorexia, nausea, vomiting; and vision changes. Recommend mother breast feed prior to taking medication to avoid the peak drug level that occurs at 1-2 hours post dose.
Pyrazinamide	L3		1.5	Excreted in human milk. Observe infant for liver toxicity: fatigue, weakness, malaise, anorexia, nausea, vomiting; and thrombocytopenia, rash, and arthralgia.
Rifampin	L2	✓	5.3-11.5%	Small amount excreted in human milk.
Streptomycin	L3	✓	0.3-0.6%	Excreted in human milk; poor systemic absorption by infant.
ANTIVIRAL AGENTS				
Acyclovir	L2	✓	1.1 -1.5%	Excreted in human milk; poor systemic absorption by infant. Commonly used in neonates.
Amantadine	L3			Small amount excreted in human milk. No adverse effects reported in nursing infants but can cause a major reduction in maternal prolactin levels so should be avoided in breastfeeding mothers or at least used with caution observing milk production.

ANTIMICROBIALS IN LACTATION

DRUG	RISK CATEGORY[1]	AAP RATING[2]	RELATIVE INFANT DOSE[3]	COMMENTS
ANTIVIRAL AGENTS (cont'd)				
Antiretrovirals				Centers for Disease Control and Prevention recommend that HIV-infected women in developed countries NOT breastfeed in order to avoid postnatal transmission of HIV to the infant.
Famciclovir	L2			No human data on excretion in milk. Significant amount excreted in rat milk. Since there is a potential for toxicity, acyclovir would be the preferred choice.
Foscarnet	L4			No human data on excretion in milk. Significant amount excreted in rat milk. Based on potential toxicity to the infant, breastfeeding is not recommended.
Ganciclovir	L3			No human data on excretion in milk. Based on potential toxicity to the infant, breastfeeding is not recommended (although the drug has been used in neonates for congenital CMV infections).
Oseltamivir	L2		0.5%	Small amounts of oseltamivir and its metabolite have been detected in breast milk. The CDC recommends that women taking oseltamivir continue breast feeding.
Valacyclovir	L1		4.7%	No human data on excretion in milk, however it is rapidly and almost completely converted to acyclovir, which is considered to be safe in breastfeeding.

ANTIMICROBIALS IN LACTATION

DRUG	RISK CATEGORY[1]	AAP RATING[2]	RELATIVE INFANT DOSE[3]	COMMENTS
ANTIVIRAL AGENTS (cont'd)				
Valganciclovir	L3			Metabolized to ganciclovir. Very water soluble and lipophobic which suggests milk levels would be low. Oral absorption in infant likely low. Based on potential toxicity to the infant, breastfeeding is not recommended (although ganciclovir has been used in neonates for congenital CMV infections).
Zanamivir	L3			No human data on excretion in milk, however due to its poor systemic absorption and extremely low maternal plasma levels, it is unlikely that there would be adverse effects in breastfed infants.

EXPOSURE TO SELECTED* COMMUNICABLE DISEASES DURING PREGNANCY

Infectious Agent	Potential Effect on Fetus	Rate of Perinatal Transmission	Maternal Screening	Prevention
The best way to prevent many of these infections is to maintain careful handwashing practices and keep all adult immunizations up to date.				
Cytomegalovirus (CMV) Primary or Reactivated	• Congenital Syndrome[†] especially: ⇒ hearing loss ⇒ hepatosplenomegaly ⇒ jaundice ⇒ microcephaly ⇒ developmental delay ⇒ visual impairment	Maternal infection: • primary – 30-70% (primary infection associated with more severe fetal infection) • reactivated – 30-40% • 0.2-2.4% of all live births are affected by intra-uterine CMV infections.	- Routine screening not currently recommended.	- Handwashing (especially when changing diapers).
Hepatitis B	• Hepatitis • Cirrhosis and/or liver cancer (as an adult)	Untreated: • 5-20% if HBeAg negative mother • 70-90% if HBeAg positive mother • Transmission usually at time of delivery Treated: • If HBIG and HBV vaccine given 24h after birth – 5-15%	- Routine HbsAg (performed in 1st trimester).	- HBIG (Hepatitis B immune globulin) and HBV vaccine should be given to baby within 12h of birth. - If non-immune mother exposed in pregnancy give HBIG and HBV vaccine. - If high risk non-immune mother, vaccinate in pregnancy.

EXPOSURE TO SELECTED* COMMUNICABLE DISEASES DURING PREGNANCY

Infectious Agent	Potential Effect on Fetus	Rate of Perinatal Transmission	Maternal Screening	Prevention
Hepatitis C	• Hepatitis • Cirrhosis and/or liver cancer (later in life)	• High maternal viral load is predictive of vertical transmission (up to 5%). • Potential increased risk of transmission if mother co-infected with HIV (5.4%).	- Screening HCV-Ab recommended in high risk pregnant patients: ⇒injection drug users and their partners ⇒ blood transfusion before 1992 ⇒ undiagnosed hepatitis. - Viral load testing may be considered. ⇒ consult Infectious Diseases or Hepatologist and Maternal/Fetal specialist.	- Avoid high risk behavior (e.g. IVDU) - Currently no post exposure prophylaxis available.
Herpes Simplex Primary or Recurrent	In Utero: Primary • Congenital Syndrome[†] (rare) Neonatal: Primary and Recurrent • Mucocutaneous lesions • Disseminated disease • Encephalitis	• Transmission occurs at time of delivery in up to 90% of cases. Vaginal delivery: • primary – 30-50% • recurrent – 2-5% • Neonatal HSV infection affects 1/17,000 births (half of these related to primary infection). • 59% of neonatal disease is skin/eye/mouth • 23% encephalitis • 18% disseminated disease	- Consult Virology lab in event of suspected primary infection in pregnancy. - Inspect for lesions at time of delivery (maternal shedding can occur in the absence of lesions).	Primary infection: - Consult Infectious Diseases for treatment. - If it occurs in 3rd trimester, consider pre-labour booked caesarean section. Recurrent infection: - In women with known recurrent disease, recommend prophylaxis at 36 weeks to delivery with acyclovir 400mg PO tid. - If lesions present at time of delivery, recommend caesarean section.

EXPOSURE TO SELECTED* COMMUNICABLE DISEASES DURING PREGNANCY

Infectious Agent	Potential Effect on Fetus	Rate of Perinatal Transmission	Maternal Screening	Prevention
Human Immunodeficiency Virus (HIV)	• Neonatal/childhood HIV infection	- 25% (rate reduced to less than 1% with suppressive triple antiretroviral therapy) - majority of infants infected in 3rd trimester or at time of delivery. - transmission may also occur with breastfeeding (5-20%).	- Routine HIV antibody (performed in 1st trimester). - Repeat in 3rd trimester if high risk for HIV.	- Avoid high risk behavior. - For documented HIV exposure in pregnancy, consult Infectious Diseases. - If HIV positive, consult Infectious Diseases and Maternal/Fetal specialist or experts in perinatal HIV disease. - Avoid breastfeeding.
Parvovirus B$_{19}$ (Fifth disease)	• Fetal loss • Hydrops • Anemia • Congestive heart failure	Risk of infection: 17-33%	- Routine screening not recommended. - If maternal exposure or suspect infection, contact Virology lab re: Parvovirus IgG and IgM and/or PCR. Note: PCR can be performed on blood or amniotic fluid.	- Droplet precautions. - If mother seroconverts in pregnancy, consult Maternal/Fetal specialist for in utero assessment of fetal anemia and if intrauterine blood transfusions are required.
Rubella	• Fetal loss • Congenital Syndrome† especially: ⇒ hearing loss ⇒ congenital heart failure ⇒ cataracts ⇒ thrombocytopenia/purpura	• 1st trimester – 67-85% (infection in 1st trimester associated with more severe fetal infection) • 11-16 weeks – 55% • > 16 weeks – 45%	- Routine Rubella IgG performed in 1st trimester. - If maternal rubella suspected, perform Rubella IgM.	- Vaccination before or after pregnancy (not during). - In acute infection – droplet precautions. - In neonatal infection acquired congenitally, use contact precautions for at least 1 year unless nasopharyngeal and urine cultures repeatedly negative after 3 months.

EXPOSURE TO SELECTED* COMMUNICABLE DISEASES DURING PREGNANCY

Infectious Agent	Potential Effect on Fetus	Rate of Perinatal Transmission	Maternal Screening	Prevention
Toxoplasma gondii	• Fetal loss • Congenital Syndrome[†] especially: ⇒ chorioretinitis ⇒ hydrocephalus ⇒ intracerebral calcification	• 1st trimester – 10-25% (increased risk for severe perinatal infection) • 2nd trimester – 30-54% • 3rd trimester – 60-65%	- Routine screening not recommended. - If maternal exposure or suspect infection, contact lab re: Toxoplasma IgG/IgM/IgA.	- Wash hands: • before eating • after handling raw meat • after contact with soil/cat feces. - Pregnant woman should avoid: • eating raw or rare beef, pork, or lamb • contact with cats of unknown feeding history • cleaning litter boxes. - If mother has suspected acute toxoplasma infection in pregnancy, consult Infectious Diseases and Maternal/Fetal specialist re: antimicrobial therapy, amniocentesis, and need for further therapy to decrease fetal effects.

EXPOSURE TO SELECTED* COMMUNICABLE DISEASES DURING PREGNANCY

Infectious Agent	Potential Effect on Fetus	Rate of Perinatal Transmission	Maternal Screening	Prevention
Varicella Zoster (VZV) Primary infection or Perinatal period	Primary • Congenital Syndrome† especially: ⇒ limb hypoplasia ⇒ ocular abnormalities ⇒ CNS abnormalities • Dermatomal scarring Perinatal period • Chicken pox +/- • Encephalitis	• Congenital VZV syndrome: ⇒ < 13 weeks – 1% risk ⇒ 13-20 weeks – 2% risk NB: Neonatal VZV – if mother develops varicella < 5 days before to 2 days after delivery – 30% risk of neonatal fatality.	- Routine screening recommended if no history of chicken pox. - If pregnant woman (with no history of previous chicken pox) is exposed, perform STAT Varicella IgG/IgM. - If suspect primary infection, contact Virology lab re: VZV testing: • DFA of lesions - best test or • serology (IgG and IgM).	- Non-immune women should be vaccinated before or after pregnancy (not during). - Non-immune women exposed during pregnancy should receive VZIG (within 96 hours of exposure). - If pregnant woman or neonate develops varicella, consult Infectious Diseases/Infection Control. - Exposed neonate should receive VZIG prophylaxis. (See Prophylaxis for Contacts of Communicable Diseases for VZIG indications.) If mother develops varicella < 5 days before to 2 days after delivery – give prophylactic acyclovir to baby. - If severe neonatal VZV infection develops despite VZIG, start high dose acyclovir.

Note: If siblings at home have chicken pox and mother has positive chicken pox history, can send baby home. If negative maternal history, delay sending baby home until 7 days after onset of infection in siblings.

* NB: This list is not all inclusive. There are other infections, including syphilis, lymphocytic choriomeningitis virus, Coxiella burnetii, and tuberculosis, which may be associated with congenital infection. Consult with Infectious Diseases recommended.

† Congenital Syndrome – One or more of the following: jaundice, hepatosplenomegaly, microcephaly, CNS abnormalities, ocular abnormalities, thrombocytopenia/purpura, hemolytic anemia, intracerebral calcifications, hearing loss, intrauterine growth retardation, prematurity.

PREVENTION OF PERINATAL INFECTION

Intrapartum Antimicrobial Prophylaxis of Group B Streptococcus (GBS)

- At 35-37 weeks, obtain single swab from lower vagina and anorectum (Indicate on requisition if patient β-lactam allergic as lab will perform susceptibility testing for clindamycin and vancomycin)
- Give intrapartum prophylactic antibiotics[†] upon commencement of labour[‡] if:
  ⇒ culture positive for GBS or
  ⇒ GBS bacteriuria during present pregnancy or
  ⇒ previous baby with invasive GBS disease or
  ⇒ unknown GBS status and patient has one or more of the following risk factors:
    • pre-term labour (< 37 weeks gestation)
    • prolonged rupture of membranes ($\geq$ 18h) and/or labour expected to last $\geq$ 18h at term ($\geq$ 37 weeks)
    • maternal fever ($\geq$ 38°C)

  [†] If patient receiving treatment for amnionitis with antibiotics reliably active against GBS (ampicillin, penicillin, vancomycin), additional prophylactic antibiotics are not needed.
  [‡] NB: For elective Caesarean delivery before onset of labor and with intact membranes, the risk of early-onset GBS disease in the infant is extremely low and intrapartum antimicrobial prophylaxis is not recommended regardless of GBS colonization status of the mother.

Antimicrobial Regimen	Dose & Duration	Comments
Penicillin*	5MU IV given ideally at least 4h prior to delivery then 2.5MU IV q4h until delivery or labour stops	* Penicillin preferred because: • narrow spectrum • less likely to select resistant organisms.
Alternative **Ampicillin**	2g IV given ideally at least 4h prior to delivery then 1g IV q4h until delivery or labour stops	- Ampicillin + gentamicin recommended if chorioamnionitis suspected.
Nonsevere β-lactam allergy **Cefazolin**	2g IV given ideally at least 4h prior to delivery then 1g IV q8h until delivery or labour stops	
Severe β-lactam allergy/ anaphylaxis **Clindamycin****	900mg IV q8h until delivery or labour stops	**Significant clindamycin resistance – check susceptibility.
Alternative if clindamycin resistance or unknown susceptibility to clindamycin **Vancomycin**	15mg/kg (max 2g) IV q12h until delivery or labour stops	

1. Centers for Disease Control and Prevention. Prevention of perinatal Group B streptococcal disease. Revised guidelines from CDC, 2010. MMWR 2010;59(No. RR-10):1-31.
2. Committee on Infectious Diseases and Committee on Fetus and Newborn, American Acadamy of Pediatrics. Policy statement – Recommendations for the prevention of perinatal Group B streptococcal (GBS) disease. Pediatrics 2011;128:611-6.

PREVENTION OF PERINATAL INFECTION

Antimicrobial Prophylaxis for Preterm (< 37 weeks gestation) Rupture of Membranes	
• In the asymptomatic stable patient with preterm rupture of membranes, prophylaxis with one of the following regimens is recommended:	
Antimicrobial Regimen	**Dose & Duration**
Oral **[Erythromycin**	250mg PO qid x 10 days
+	
Amoxicillin]	250mg PO tid x 10 days
or Parenteral **[Erythromycin**	250mg IV q6h x 48 hours
+	
Ampicillin]	2g IV q6h x 48 hours
followed by **[Erythromycin**	250mg PO qid x 5 days
+	
Amoxicillin]	250mg PO tid x 5 days

1. Yudin MH, van Schalkwyk J, Van Eyk N, et al. Antibiotic therapy in preterm premature rupture of the membranes. JOGC 2009;Sep:863-7.

PERINATAL HIV PROTOCOL

For the current version of the Alberta Health Services Edmonton Zone protocol for Reducing the Rate of Perinatal HIV Transmission for Mothers and Babies, see www.bugsanddrugs.ca

GUIDE TO GRAM STAIN INTERPRETATION

This is meant to be a general guide only.
- The organism list for each bacterial morphology type is not all inclusive.
- Bacterial morphology may be altered by antibiotic therapy, and some transport/culture media.
- Clinical correlation is essential when choosing empiric therapy.

Bacterial Morphology	Probable Organisms
GRAM POSITIVE	
• Cocci in clusters/clumps	Staphylococcus spp Micrococcus/Macrococcus spp Pediococcus spp Aerococcus spp
• Cocci in pair/chains	Streptococcus spp Gemella spp Enterococcus spp Anaerobic cocci
• Bacilli (small) non spore forming	Listeria spp Corynebacterium spp Erysipelothrix spp Propionibacterium spp Actinomyces spp Other anaerobic bacilli
• Bacilli (large) +/- spores	Clostridium spp Bacillus spp Lactobacillus spp
• Bacilli branching/beaded/ filamentous	Nocardia spp Actinomyces spp Streptomyces spp
GRAM NEGATIVE	
• Bacilli	Enterobacteriaceae P. aeruginosa Stenotrophomonas maltophilia Other nonfermentative bacilli
• Coccobacilli/pleomorphic bacilli	Aggregibacter spp Cardiobacterium hominis Eikenella corrodens Haemophilus influenzae/parainfluenzae Kingella spp Bacteroides spp Brucella spp Pasteurella spp Other anaerobic bacilli
• Fusiform bacilli	Fusobacterium spp Capnocytophaga spp
• Curved bacilli	Campylobacter spp Vibrio spp
• Diplococci	Neisseria spp Moraxella catarrhalis Acinetobacter spp

COMMENSAL AND PATHOGENIC ORGANISMS FOR SPECIFIC BODY SITES

RESPIRATORY TRACT

Normal Oropharyngeal Flora*	May be part of normal flora but may be potential pathogens in lower respiratory tract**
Viridans group Streptococci	Streptococcus pneumoniae
Non haemolytic Streptococci	Haemophilus influenzae/parainfluenzae
Coagulase negative Staphylococci	Moraxella catarrhalis
Anaerobes (Prevotella spp, Porphyromonas spp, Fusobacterium spp)	Staphylococcus aureus
	β-haemolytic Streptococci
Neisseria spp (except N. gonorrhoeae)	Enterobacteriaceae
Corynebacterium spp	Pseudomonas aeruginosa
Micrococcus/Macrococcus spp	Other non-fermentative bacilli
Rothia spp	Neisseria meningitidis
Lactobacillus spp	Candida spp
Enterococcus spp	Corynebacterium pseudodiphtheriticum
Bacillus spp	Pasteurella spp

* Some of these organisms may be involved in polymicrobial infections (aspiration pneumonia, bronchiectasis)
** Quality of sputum is assessed microscopically. Only adequate specimens are cultured.
Potential pathogens are reported when ≥ normal flora or if predominant organism seen on Gram stain.

COMMENSAL AND PATHOGENIC ORGANISMS FOR SPECIFIC BODY SITES

EYES

Normal Flora	Potential Pathogens
Coagulase negative Staphylococci	Haemophilus influenzae
Viridans group Streptococci	Streptococcus pneumoniae
Non-haemolytic Streptococci	Staphylococcus aureus
Corynebacterium spp	Moraxella spp
Neisseria spp (except N. gonorrhoeae)	β-haemolytic Streptococci
Acinetobacter spp	Neisseria gonorrhoeae
Anaerobic Gram cocci (multiple species)	Pseudomonas aeruginosa*
Propionibacterium spp	Enterobacteriaceae*

* These organisms may cause keratitis (trauma or contact lens related), rather than conjunctivitis.

EARS

Normal Flora	Potential Pathogens
Coagulase negative Staphylococci	Streptococcus pneumoniae
Viridans group Streptococci	Moraxella catarrhalis
Non-haemolytic Streptococci	Haemophilus influenzae
Corynebacterium spp	Staphylococcus aureus
Neisseria spp	β-haemolytic Streptococci
Acinetobacter spp	Pseudomonas aeruginosa*
Bacillus spp	Enterobacteriaceae*
Anaerobic cocci (multiple species)	Other Gram negative bacilli*
Propionibacterium spp	Anaerobes**

* These organisms may be colonizers of external canal. Correlation with Gram stain and clinical presentation recommended.
**May be involved in chronic otitis media but not acute otitis media.

COMMENSAL AND PATHOGENIC ORGANISMS FOR SPECIFIC BODY SITES

URINARY TRACT*

Common Contaminants	Potential Pathogens
Lactobacillus spp	Enterobacteriaceae
Viridans group Streptococci	Staphylococcus saprophyticus
Non-haemolytic Streptococci	Enterococcus spp
Aerococcus viridans	β-haemolytic Streptococci (group A&B)
Neisseria spp	Pseudomonas aeruginosa
Corynebacterium spp (other than C. urealyticum)	Other non-fermentative bacilli
Coagulase negative Staph (other than S.	Streptococcus bovis
Gardnerella vaginalis**	Staphylococcus aureus
Anaerobes	Candida spp
Oligella spp**	Haemophilus influenzae/parainfluenzae
Actinomyces spp**	Corynebacterium urealyticum
	Aerococcus urinae
	Streptococcus pneumoniae
	Actinobaculum spp

* Work-up/reporting of urine samples based on colony count/clinical information/number and type of organisms:
10^8 cfu/L - significant indication of urinary tract infection
10^7 cfu/L - significant with signs/symptoms. Lab will work up 1 or 2 organisms at this colony count if relevant diagnosis.
10^6 cfu/L - low colony count - may be significant in females with pyuria/dysuria syndrome. Lab will work up if pure
uropathogen and history provided.
≥ 3 organisms - mixed-probable contamination. Lab will work up a uropathogen > 80% predominant.
** Occasionally may cause urinary tract infections.

COMMENSAL AND PATHOGENIC ORGANISMS FOR SPECIFIC BODY SITES

GENITAL TRACT

Normal Flora	Potential Pathogens
Lactobacillus spp	*Pathogens:*
Viridans group Streptococci	Neisseria gonorrhoeae - cervicitis
Non-haemolytic Streptococci	Chlamydia trachomatis - cervicitis
Enterococcus spp	Herpes simplex
Coagulase negative Staphylococci	Trichomonas vaginalis - vaginitis
Gardnerella vaginalis	*Potential Pathogens:**
Corynebacterium spp	Candida spp
β-haemolytic Streptococci (group B,C,G)	β-haemolytic Streptococci (group A)
Enterobacteriaceae	Staphylococcus aureus
Anaerobes	Actinomyces spp (IUCD-related)
Cancida spp	Neisseria meningitidis
	Pasteurella spp
	Pseudomonas aeruginosa
	*Pregnancy:***
	β-haemolytic Streptococci (group B)
	Listeria monocytogenes
	Haemophilus influenzae
	Streptococcus pneumoniae

* Other organisms may be involved post surgical/post abortion/post partum.
** Potential for disease in fetus/newborn.

COMMENSAL AND PATHOGENIC ORGANISMS FOR SPECIFIC BODY SITES

SKIN/SOFT TISSUE

Normal Skin Flora	Superficial/ Skin[1]	Potential Pathogens Superficial Wounds (< 2 cm)[2]	Deep Wounds(> 2cm)[3]
Coagulase negative Staph	Staphylococcus aureus	Staphylococcus aureus	Staphylococcus aureus
Viridans group Streptococci	β-haemolytic Streptococci (group A,B,C,G)	β-haemolytic Streptococci (group A,B,C,G)	β-haemolytic Streptococci (group A,B,C,G)
Non-haemolytic Streptococci	Pseudomonas aeruginosa	Enterobacteriaceae	Enterobacteriaceae
Corynebacterium spp	Candida spp	Pasteurella multocida	Pseudomonas aeruginosa
Bacillus spp	Dermatophytes	Pseudomonas aeruginosa	Other non- fermentative bacilli
Acinetobacter spp		Other non-fermentative bacilli	Pasteurella multocida
Moraxella spp		Mycobacterium spp	Enterococcus spp
Peptostreptococcus spp		Haemophilus spp	Candida spp
Propionibacterium spp		Nocardia spp	Streptococcus anginosus group
Candida spp		Bacillus anthracis	Eikenella corrodens
		Erysipelothrix rhusiopathiae	Anaerobes
		Vibrio spp	Bacillus cereus
			Corynebacterium spp
			S. lugdunensis/S. schleiferi
			Other coagulase negative Staph
			Erysipelothrix rhusiopathiae
			Capnocytophaga spp
			Vibrio spp
			Actinomyces spp
			Nocardia spp
			Fungal pathogens
			Mycobacterium spp
			Bacillus anthracis

1. Superficial/skin: rash/abrasion/impetigo/folliculitis/balanitis/boils/acne
2. Superficial wounds (< 2 cm in depth): wounds/incisions/ulcers/sebaceous cysts/catheter site/cellulitis/abscesses
3. Deep wounds (> 2 cm in depth): wounds/incisions/ulcers/abscesses

INDEX

Bold numbers indicate empiric therapy recommendations for **ADULT** patients.

INDEX

Bold numbers indicate empiric therapy recommendations for **ADULT** patients.

INDEX

Bold numbers indicate empiric therapy recommendations for **ADULT** patients.

INDEX

Bold numbers indicate empiric therapy recommendations for **ADULT** patients.

INDEX

Bold numbers indicate empiric therapy recommendations for **ADULT** patients.

INDEX

Bold numbers indicate empiric therapy recommendations for **ADULT** patients.

INDEX

Bold numbers indicate empiric therapy recommendations for **ADULT** patients.

AFTERWORD

The effort to produce Bugs & Drugs 2012 includes two significant milestones.

First, updating the content since the last version (2006) represents an incredible undertaking. The volume of relevant literature has increased greatly over the last 6 years, and without the dedication, perseverance and patience demonstrated by Edith Blondel-Hill & Susan Fryters over the last year and a half, this revision would not have been possible.

Second, Bugs & Drugs 2012 is the first version to have a smartphone application. The people from Saint Street and Myrna Pickering have transformed the hardcopy content into an easy-to-navigate mobile tool that continues the Bugs & Drugs function of helping clinicians make informed decisions.

Two years in the making, projects of this magnitude require support and dedication to succeed. Many people have contributed their time and effort at various stages of this project and for that I am very grateful. In addition to those already acknowledged in the Foreword, the following people have also made key contributions at various times throughout this project: Kim Dreher, Mary Carson, Dr. Martin Lavoie, Dean Blue, Sandy Saiko, Karen Horon, Anoop Johal, Patty Oliver, Jacqueline Beaucage, Robert Warnock, Jeff Whissell, and Andrew Goddard. Finally, this project continues to be possible with the extensive support and encouragement of Gail Hufty.

Rob Vretenar, BSc Pharm
Director, Program Performance & Quality
Pharmacy Services, AHS